Emerging Trends in Indigenous Language Media, Communication, Gender, and Health

Kehinde Opeyemi Oyesomi
Covenant University, Nigeria

Abiodun Salawu
North-West University, South Africa

A volume in the Advances in Human Services and Public Health (AHSPH) Book Series

IGI Global
DISSEMINATOR OF KNOWLEDGE

Published in the United States of America by
IGI Global
Medical Information Science Reference (an imprint of IGI Global)
701 E. Chocolate Avenue
Hershey PA, USA 17033
Tel: 717-533-8845
Fax: 717-533-8661
E-mail: cust@igi-global.com
Web site: http://www.igi-global.com

Library of Congress Cataloging-in-Publication Data

Names: Oyesomi, Kehinde Opeyemi, 1978- editor. | Salawu, 'Biodun, editor.
Title: Emerging trends in indigenous language media, communication, gender, and health / Kehinde Opeyemi Oyesomi, Abiodun Salawu, editors.
Description: Hershey, PA : Medical Information Science Reference, [2020] | Includes bibliographical references and index. | Summary: "This book explores trends in the areas of indigenous language media, communication, gender, and health" -- Provided by publisher.
Identifiers: LCCN 2019036390 (print) | LCCN 2019036391 (ebook) | ISBN 9781799820918 (h/c) | ISBN 9781799820925 (eISBN)
Subjects: MESH: Health Communication | Ethnic Groups | Communications Media | Information Dissemination
Classification: LCC RA423.2 (print) | LCC RA423.2 (ebook) | NLM WA 590 | DDC 362.101/4--dc23
LC record available at https://lccn.loc.gov/2019036390
LC ebook record available at https://lccn.loc.gov/2019036391

This book is published in the IGI Global book series Advances in Human Services and Public Health (AHSPH) (ISSN: 2475-6571; eISSN: 2475-658X)

British Cataloguing in Publication Data
A Cataloguing in Publication record for this book is available from the British Library.

Advances in Human Services and Public Health (AHSPH) Book Series

ISSN:2475-6571
EISSN:2475-658X

Editor-in-Chief: Jennifer Martin, RMIT University, Australia

MISSION

The well-being of the general public should be a primary concern for any modern civilization. Ongoing research in the field of human services and public healthcare is necessary to evaluate, manage, and respond to the health and social needs of the global population.

The **Advances in Human Services and Public Health (AHSPH)** book series aims to publish high-quality reference publications focused on the latest methodologies, tools, issues, and strategies for managing the health and social welfare of the public. The AHSPH book series will be especially relevant for healthcare professionals, policy makers, government officials, and students seeking the latest research in this field.

COVERAGE

- Poverty
- Healthcare Reform
- Public Welfare
- Access to Healthcare Services
- Medicare and Medicaid
- Social Work
- Domestic Violence
- Youth Development
- Assistance Programs
- Public Funding

IGI Global is currently accepting manuscripts for publication within this series. To submit a proposal for a volume in this series, please contact our Acquisition Editors at Acquisitions@igi-global.com or visit: http://www.igi-global.com/publish/.

The Advances in Human Services and Public Health (AHSPH) Book Series (ISSN 2475-6571) is published by IGI Global, 701 E. Chocolate Avenue, Hershey, PA 17033-1240, USA, www.igi-global.com. This series is composed of titles available for purchase individually; each title is edited to be contextually exclusive from any other title within the series. For pricing and ordering information please visit http://www.igi-global.com/book-series/advances-human-services-public-health/102256. Postmaster: Send all address changes to above address.

Titles in this Series

For a list of additional titles in this series, please visit:
https://www.igi-global.com/book-series/advances-human-services-public-health/102256

Impact of Textile Dyes on Public Health and the Environment
Khursheed Ahmad Wani (Government Degree College, Bijbehara, India) Nirmala Kumari Jangid (Banasthali Vidyapith, India) and Ajmal Rashid Bhat (Government Degree College, Bijbehara, ndia)
Information Science Reference • © 2020 • 335pp • H/C (ISBN: 9781799803119) • US $245.00

Handbook of Research on Health Systems and Organizations for an Aging Society
César Fonseca (Universidade de Évora, Portugal) Manuel José Lopes (Universidade de Évora, Portugal) David Mendes (Universidade de Évora, Portugal) Felismina Mendes (Universidade de Évora, Portugal) and José García-Alonso (University of Coimbra, pain)
Medical Information Science Reference • © 2020 • 323pp • H/C (ISBN: 9781522598183) • US $365.00

Cases on Cross-Cultural Counseling Strategies
Bonnie C. King (Midwestern State University, USA) and Tiffany A. Stewart (Midwestern State University, USA)
Medical Information Science Reference • © 2020 • 380pp • H/C (ISBN: 9781799800224) • US $245.00

Environmental Exposures and Human Health Challenges
Paraskevi Papadopoulou (Deree – The American College of Greece, Greece) Christina Marouli (Deree – The American College of Greece, Greece) and Anastasia Misseyanni (Deree – The American College of Greece, Greece)
Medical Information Science Reference • © 2019 • 449pp • H/C (ISBN: 9781522576358) • US $255.00

Forecasting and Managing Risk in the Health and Safety Sectors
Luisa Dall'Acqua (Scientific Lyceum TCO, Italy & University of Bologna, Italy)
Medical Information Science Reference • © 2019 • 304pp • H/C (ISBN: 9781522579038) • US $245.00

For an entire list of titles in this series, please visit:
https://www.igi-global.com/book-series/advances-human-services-public-health/102256

IGI Global
DISSEMINATOR OF KNOWLEDGE

701 East Chocolate Avenue, Hershey, PA 17033, USA
Tel: 717-533-8845 x100 • Fax: 717-533-8661
E-Mail: cust@igi-global.com • www.igi-global.com

Editorial Advisory Board

Table of Contents

Detailed Table of Contents

Indigenous communication is an indispensable medium of communication in the socio-cultural tradition of Africans. These systems have been used to promote co-operation, mobilization, and participation among African people. This chapter takes into account indigenous communication roles of traditional birth attendants in maternal wellbeing and maternal health practices during pregnancy and childbirth in both Nigerian and South African communities. The significant motivation behind the examination is to assess the indigenous communication role of traditional birth attendants in maternal health practices in the two nations through empirical studies. After careful review of the studies, it is shown and discovered that TBAs in both Nigeria and South Africa assist pregnant women based on their religious or traditional beliefs. The researchers therefore recommend that health professionals should train TBAs in modern maternal health practices. This will go a long way to help them know their restrictions and possibly refer mothers and their children for emergency services and attention as needed.

This chapter examines the use of indigenous languages during antenatal care (ANC) sessions among mothers in Lagos state. Authors investigate factors that influence the use of indigenous languages, the most preferred mode of presentation, and how the languages affect reception, participation, and knowledge of mothers on safe motherhood practices. Using in-depth interviews with nurses and observations during the ANC sessions, the study found that indigenous languages engender participation and are effective in building self-esteem, trust, and confidence of mothers. Songs in the indigenous language, particularly Yoruba language, help mothers retain and recall safe motherhood messages easily. Mothers generally demonstrate their understanding during the question and answer sessions, while also serving as agents of information reinforcement among themselves using indigenous languages. In view of the occasional need for interpreters, the study recommends that health workers should be encouraged to take courses in indigenous languages within their region as a second language.

Communication is a vital aspect of human existence. It pervades man's existence and society, forming an integral part of human life. Communication is the means through which human beings express their feelings. Indigenous communication serves as the traditional means of conveying messages, all social and value exchanges of indigenous practice like the health practices. Traditional health practices include the use of knowledge skills, practices based on indigenous belief, experiences of culture used in maintenance of health-prevention, treatment and diagnosis in traditional health practices. This chapter examines and documents traditional health practices on how Yorùbás care for pregnancy, child delivery, and their babies. Such traditional health practices have existed since before the advent of modern health practices, thereby using indigenous communication for preservation and dissemination of valuable information that is significant for Yorùbá generations.

The importance of health communication and information cannot be over emphasized especially with issues related to sickle cell disorder. Sickle cell disorder, common among Africans, has a lot of myths and misconceptions tied to it, so this chapter unearths and explores how indigenous communication can facilitate learning and understanding of the disorder majorly in rural areas and some urban areas where knowledge of the disorder is assessed low using the focus group discussion. It also reveals the importance of incorporating indigenous language and communication techniques in increasing awareness and eradicating stereotypes as regards sickle cell disorder. The findings of this chapter reflect that misinformation occurs due to lack of proper understanding of language used in sickle cell health communication-related issues. Hence, this chapter proposes that health education about the concept of SCD should be executed majorly in indigenous languages and through the indigenous media platforms.

All over the world, the issues of health and ill health have generated heightened attention among health professionals and communication experts. This is expected in view of the prevalence of increasingly life-threatening ailments. It is therefore not surprising that matters bordering on health have been elevated to the front burner of policy and decision making both at the national and multinational levels. This chapter, therefore, observes that the reason most health information doesn't get to the intended audiences and produce the desired effect is because they are not communicated in the most intelligible language to the people. Indigenous language media are potential channels through which health information could reach the grassroots where more than 70 percent of the nation's populations are resident. It also perceived that health communication could be made to produce more effect in this digital era as more citizen journalists could be raised to communicate in the indigenous language.

HIV/AIDS has become a challenge to every society all over the world. The indigenous media could serve as channels through which information dissemination about knowledge; prevention and treatment are used as weapons to curtail its devastating effect. Despite the advancement in media technologies, information about HIV/AIDS is still limited in the rural areas, as they seemed marginalized because of their socio-economic status as well as their literacy level. Therefore, this chapter examines how the grassroot media can be utilized effectively to reach the indigenous people in a way that their cultural values will reflect in all media campaign against HIV/AIDS. It was observed that health messages about HIV/AIDS could be disseminated effectively using the various indigenous media. Health message designers are therefore implored to take advantage of these indigenous media to generate local contents which could consequently be disseminated through the mediums of radio and television for wider reach.

Section 3
Indigenous Language Media/Communication and Radio/Television Programming

Sexual and reproductive health-related communication in Africa is culturally regulated. This chapter analyses the handling of sexually offensive expressions on Zimbabwe's African language radio stations. The conceptual lens for this study is grounded in the indigenous knowledge systems perspective, which underscores indigenous communication systems as indispensable assets for African cultural communities. The chapter shows that African language radio stations are expedient channels for sexual and reproductive health-related communication in the contemporary society. However, this study shows the widespread use of inconceivable sexually explicit language and ineffective euphemisms in a manner that diminishes the relevance of the radio programmes. Therefore, the chapter maintains that it is imperative to remodel African language radio's language use conventions in programmes that relate to sexual and reproductive health issues in ways that match the cultural traditions of the respective audience.

lack of practical synergy between government, policy implementation committee, and media organizations. Exploring the values of indigenous language in development media theory, this chapter sets out to demonstrate merits of media support in health policy execution via dynamics of indigenous language programmes towards achieving sustainable development goals. The chapter therefore recommends that constitutional gap in health provision should be bridged to eliminate the question of accountability at all levels and on the long run decentralize health education; and it will make it much easier for state government to embark on holistic health communication strategies that suits their geopolitical terrain.

This conceptual work examines corporate communication as a tool for coordinating universities' internal and external messages in Nigeria. It explores universities' attempts to harness, link-up, and interact with their publics. This chapter presents effective corporate communication as the unifying principle in many institutional decisions. It emphasizes that sometimes, universities' efforts to communicate effectively and profitably with their host communities end up in futility especially where indigenous language is a key environmental factor. University-neighbour relationship globally ought to be symbiotic and mutually-reinforcing. This chapter reviews scholarly commentaries on corporate communication, the relevance of indigenous language to community relations; and highlights in conclusion, the implications for universities in neglecting indigenous language during community engagements. It recommends that universities should motivate their employees to apply indigenous languages in enhancing understanding between the institutions and their host communities.

Diabetes is a major health challenge in the world, but it can be effectively managed or controlled through diabetes information and education. However, none has dwelt on the language dynamics of communication interactions despite the fact that Nigeria is a multi-lingual nation. Therefore, the study investigates the language challenges

Preface

It is no gainsaying that there is a symbiosis between communication and development. Therefore, the language and the media through which the communication is done cannot but be important. Specifically, the media that use indigenous languages are important for the purpose of information, mobilisation and continuity i.e. survival of the language and culture (Salawu 2004a, 2004b). The language in which a development message is disseminated is a very important aspect of the message treatment. It is posited that the indigenous language of any community is the best suited for the purpose of conveying any message, whatsoever, to the said community (Nwuneli, 1985: 203). There is ample literature in support of the fact that people would understand information better in their indigenous language than in a foreign language, no matter the length of time the (foreign) language has been with them (Ngugi, 1986: 116; Chieka, 1982; Eyoh, 1986: 111). So, it does not matter the level of corrosion or corruption a native language has suffered as a result of the influence of a foreign language, the (native) language still remains the language that speaks in the idiom of the people. Without using the language of the people, development will only be communicated *at* the people; not *to* the people, and not *with* the people.

My Model of Indigenous Language for Development Communication (Salawu, 2001) graphically explains this.

In the model, the Source is a change agent which could be a development agency, a non-governmental organisation, a government body or a media organisation. The Message is basically development-oriented and it is constructed in the indigenous language of the community for which the development programme is meant. The Receiver(s) are the owners of the language. They understand the development messages better in this language and they can express themselves better in it; thus, facilitating robust interaction between them and the Source.

This model actually derives its strength from the myriad of studies (McNamara, 1965; Klein, 1994; Okombo and Rubgumya, 1996; Luckett, 1994; Fafunwa et al, 1989) already carried out which, undoubtedly, confirmed the effectiveness of mother-tongue or indigenous language (L1) for instructional purposes. Similarly, in a study conducted by me (Salawu, 2001, 2004a), respondents (all of Yoruba origin)

Figure 1. Model of indigenous language for development communication
Source: Salawu, 2001

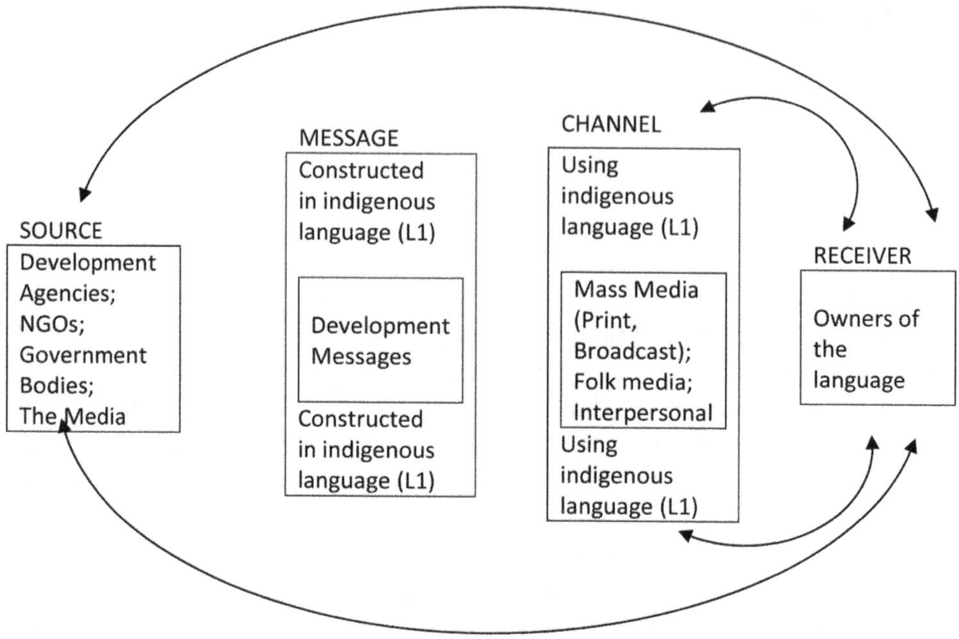

to copies of a questionnaire distributed adjudged Yoruba language newspapers more effective than the English language newspapers in the dissemination of development messages. In other words they understand development messages in Yoruba language newspapers better than in English language newspapers.

This point is what chapters in this current book also try to grapple with. Health and gender are two critical issues in development studies. Chapters in the book have focused on how communication in indigenous languages has been used to promote these causes. The fourteen-chapter book is divided into four sections. The first section entitled 'Indigenous language media/communication and safe motherhood practices' is made up of five chapters. The first chapter by Oyesomi et al examines the role of indigenous language communication in maternity health practices in South Africa and Nigeria. In the second chapter, Ogunyombo and Bello interrogate the use of indigenous language in antenatal sessions by mothers in Lagos and how it helps them retain and recall safe motherhood messages. This is followed by, in chapter 3, Taiwo's examination of traditional health practices and how Yorùbás care for pregnancy, child delivery and their babies. This is followed by, in Chapter4, Ifeanyichukwu Aloysius' exploration of indigenous language media's role in the battle against maternal mortality and the quest for safe motherhood practices. The author argues that indigenous language media are central in the fight since they have the upper hand against mainstream English language media in penetrating the rural areas. The last chapter of this section, that is chapter 5, by Funmi Falobi, looks at the role of indigenous language media in engendering safe motherhood practices in Lagos State.

The second section of the book, titled 'Indigenous language media/communication and health related issues' is made up of three chapters. The section opens with chapter 6 which examines the "Peculiarities of Indigenous language media and communication techniques in tackling myths and misconceptions as regards sickle cell disorder". The authors, Opeyemi Oredola and Kehinde Oyesomi, explore 'how indigenous (language) communication can facilitate learning and understanding of the disorder in rural areas and some urban areas...' The remaining two chapters (7 and 8) in the section by Owolabi and Ajikanle-Nurudeen, and Ogundoyin respectively interrogate the deployment of indigenous language media and digital based media for purposes of health communication.

The third section of the book entitled 'Indigenous language media/communication and radio/television programming' opens with, in chapter 9, Mpofu and Salawu's examination of the handling of sexually offensive expressions on Zimbabwe's indigenous language radio stations. They examine how these are put across in a conservative society where sexual issues are not openly discussed. They argue that the use of euphemisms and inconceivable sexually explicit language diminish the usefulness of the radio programmes. This is followed by Adeyeye et al's analysis, in Chapter 10, of the use of radio for agricultural programming purposes. They deploy diffusion of innovations theory and theory of planned behaviour and conclude 'that indigenous language use in agricultural radio programming engages agricultural programme producers and farmers through their opinion leaders'. In Chapter 11, Okorie et al examine 'the perception of young Africans of American values as portrayed in popular entertainment programs'.

The last section of the book, which is made up of three chapters, opens in chapter 12 with Olujoke and Olunike's examination of issues, trends and perspectives in health education and indigenous language media. They argue that the Nigerian government's lack of interest in policy implementation, media's hunt for profit and audience's diminishing preference for indigenous language media exacerbate the problem of poor health practices. They argue that the use of media, specifically indigenous language programmes, could be very useful in attaining sustainable development. This chapter is followed by, in chapter 13, Ekanem et al's interrogation of Nigerian Universities' corporate communication practices. They argue that the universities ignore indigenous languages media in their corporate communication endeavours thereby negatively impacting their efforts. The last chapter by Chinyere Azuka Mbaka 'investigates the language challenges faced by persons living with diabetes (PLWDs) and diabetes educators (DEs) in the course of diabetes education in the urban and semi-urban centres of Nigeria'. The author concludes by suggesting the need to produce and utilise pamphlets in indigenous languages for interactions between diabetes educators and people living with diabetes.

REFERENCES

Chieka, I. (1982). The Place of Local Languages in Nigeria today. In B. Ikara (Ed.), Nigerian Languages and Cultural Development. Lagos: The National Language Center, Federal Ministry of Education. Pp. 96 – 118.

Eyoh, H. N. (1986). Theatre of Relevance: An Interview with Ngugi Wa Thiong'o. African Theatre Review: Vol. 1. *No.2, April* (pp. 110–114). Ibadan: Heineman Educational Books.

Fafunwa, A. B., Macauley, I., & Sokoya, F. (1989). *Education in mother tongue: the Ife Primary education research project 1970 – 1978*. Ibadan: UPL.

Klein, C. (1994). The need to maintain mother tongue. *Die Suid-African* Special issue on education.

Luckett, K. (1994). National Additive bilingualism: Towards a language plan for South African education. *South African Journal of Applied Language Studies*, *2*(1), 23–39.

Macnamara. (1965). The problems of solving difficulties of bilingual children. *Bulletin of the British Psychological Society, 18:* 58-59.

Ngugi, W. T. (1986). *Decolonising the Mind: The Politics of Language in African Literature*. London, UK: James Currey.

Nwuneli, O. (1985). Communication and Social Development in Nigeria. In O. Nwuneli (Ed.), *Mass Communication in Nigeria: A Book of Reading* [sic]. (pp. 185–210). Enugu: Fourth Dimension Publishing.

Okombo, O., & Rubgumya, C. (1996). Synopsis of research findings on languages of instruction and their implication for education policies in Africa. *ADEA Newsletter*, *8*(4), 11–14.

Salawu, A. (2001). An Evaluation of Development Communication Content of Yoruba Newspapers in Nigeria. (Ph.D dissertation), University of Ibadan, Nigeria.

Salawu, A. (2004a). A readership survey of Yoruba newspapers for development messages. *Journal of Social Sciences*, *8*(3), 197–202. doi:10.1080/09718923.2004.11892414

Salawu, A. (2004b). A determination of the use of indigenous language newspapers by development agencies. *Unilag Sociological Review*, *5*, 1–19.

Section 1

Indigenous Language Media/Communication and Safe Motherhood Practices

Chapter 1
Indigenous Communication's Role in Traditional Birth Attendants in Maternal Health Practices:
A Selective Examination of Empirical Studies in Nigeria

Kehinde Opeyemi Oyesomi
https://orcid.org/0000-0002-5318-0442
Covenant University, Nigeria

Toluwanimi Onakoya
Covenant University, Nigeria

Kevin Onyenankeya
https://orcid.org/0000-0001-5814-8823
University of Fort Hare, South Africa

Ayobami Busari
Covenant University, Nigeria

DOI: 10.4018/978-1-7998-2091-8.ch001

ABSTRACT

Indigenous communication is an indispensable medium of communication in the socio-cultural tradition of Africans. These systems have been used to promote co-operation, mobilization, and participation among African people. This chapter takes into account indigenous communication roles of traditional birth attendants in maternal wellbeing and maternal health practices during pregnancy and childbirth in both Nigerian and South African communities. The significant motivation behind the examination is to assess the indigenous communication role of traditional birth attendants in maternal health practices in the two nations through empirical studies. After careful review of the studies, it is shown and discovered that TBAs in both Nigeria and South Africa assist pregnant women based on their religious or traditional beliefs. The researchers therefore recommend that health professionals should train TBAs in modern maternal health practices. This will go a long way to help them know their restrictions and possibly refer mothers and their children for emergency services and attention as needed.

INTRODUCTION

In contemporary years, there has been growing discussion over the expediency of Traditional Birth Attendants (TBAs) in maternal health practices. Critics of Traditional Birth Attendants are of the opinion that TBAs have done little to advance maternal health practices because of the orthodox way of practicing maternal health which is not safe for the mother and the child and this is believed to have frustrated the efforts made by maternal health advocates to reduce maternal mortality. Supporters of Traditional Birth Attendants on the other hand, have articulated the importance for a continuous partnership with Traditional Birth Attendants as a tactic and approach to improve access to essential maternity health care in rural areas specially to achieve momentous decrease in maternal mortality.

Maternal mortality is high in most African nations, especially in areas where access to formal human services is constrained. This builds the danger of mortality for both mother and kid with extreme maternal and neonatal wellbeing entanglements. Physical separation and monetary impediments are two noteworthy imperatives that keep network individuals from getting to, utilizing prepared health institutional and services (Mfrekemfon & Okere, 2015).

Indigenous communication assumes a gigantic part in maternal health practices, particularly in the rustic regions of Africa where indigenous communication methods are still to a great extent utilized. As Oyesomi, Salawu and Olorunyomi (2017) note that the traditional media system is people-oriented. Since indigenous communication are rooted in the culture of the people and traditional birth attendants are basically in such communities, the paper examined the role played by traditional birth attendants in maternal health care practices through selective examination of empirical studies in both South Africa and Nigeria.

Traditional Birth Attendants and Maternal Health Practices

There are two basic groups that help and care for women during pregnancy, childbirth and post-childbirth; Skilled Birth Attendants (SBAs) and Traditional Birth Attendants (TBAs) (Lindsey, 2016). A skilled birth attendant

...is an accredited health professional—such as a midwife, doctor, or nurse—who has been educated and trained to proficiency in the skills needed to manage normal (uncomplicated) pregnancies, childbirth and the immediate postnatal period, and in the identification, management and referral of complications in women and new norms. (WHO, 2004).

Since the reception of the Primary Health Care (PHC) approach in Nigeria in 1979, government has perceived the requirement for coordinating traditional birth specialists (TBAs) into the PHC framework and had thus started TBAs preparing programs (Ofili & Okojie, 2005). Women are bound to use SBA with the accessibility of skilled staff, reinforcing of the wellbeing framework and with affordable charges for maternal wellbeing administrations (Adewemimo, Msuya, Olaniyan & Adegoke, 2013). The lack of skilled birth workers has been recognized as a central point in charge of the rising maternal and baby death rate. There is adequate proof that traditional birth specialist gave maternal medicinal services has adverse effects maternal wellbeing (Unyime, Idongesit & Akpabio, 2016).

However, Traditional birth attendants were known to aid women in childbirth before the arrival of progressive medicine. They helped women with pregnancy care, during labour and with postnatal processes (PATH, 2010). Most traditional birth attendants are matured women who are generally accepted by the community and are known for their skills in home delivery (Makoe, 2000; Abdulhamid, Lawal, Tahir, Harande, & Usman, 2017).

Most Traditional Birth Attendants speak the same language with the women they attend to. As Omojola, Odiboh, & Amodu, 2018, Oyero, Oyesomi, Abioye, Ajiboye & Kayode Adedeji 2018, Folayan, et al. 2018, Oyesomi & Salawu, 2019, Oyesomi, Salawu, & Onyenankeya, 2019 note that the language of communication is critical in conveying messages to the people. Various research works have endeavored to determine the indigenous role of TBA's have in communities and to determine if they can reduce the mortality rate of pregnant women and mothers. 'There are several literatures expansively discussing the importance of the TBAs and their effect thereof. This empirical study examined the role played by TBAs in Maternal Health Practices in Nigeria and South Africa.

The Indigenous Communication Role of Traditional Birth Attendants in Maternal Health Practices

Since indigenous communication is rooted in the rural community, developing countries make extensive use of Traditional Birth Attendants (TBAs) in providing primary maternity care in such communities (Mfrekemfon P., 2015). TBAs are known to provide emotional support, give advice and also provide health care to pregnant women and mothers. TBAs have been the resource for women during childbirth in the rural areas even till date (Abdulhamid, et al., 2017). TBAs' profession in Nigeria has been handed over from one generation to another in all communities. TBAs may not have received any prior formal education and training in health care provision. Most often than not TBAs are self-trained or go through a form of apprenticeship.

The duties of TBAs begin immediately after a woman becomes pregnant till after delivery. They are consulted about the steps and stages during pregnancy and the appropriate procedures to follow (Abdulhamid, et al., 2017; Kayombo, 2013). They are consulted from the first to second week after delivery. The necessity of TBAs arises from the lack of adequate health care services and poor access to the minimal health care facilities that do exist (Ebuehi & Akintujoye, 2012). However, TBAs are known to have little to no formal educational training such as obstetricians and gynecologists but they come across as affordable and accessible to those in rural and urban communities.

TBAs give advice to pregnant women and nursing mothers primarily based on experience and knowledge acquired informally through the traditions and practices of the communities where they originated (Mfrekemfon P., 2015). In the Northern part of Nigeria, TBAs are known to have a considerable knowledge of herbal medicines used in the treatment of pregnant women. Most TBAs are known to be elderly, thereby declaring expertise and raising more confidence that they are aware of what they are doing. Hausa people of Northern Nigeria know Traditional birth attendants as "Unguwan zoma" or "Sarguwa", while the Fulani's know them as "Ungozomajo" considered most times to be mid-aged or elderly women who focus on child delivery and the post-partum care of the mother and child (Abdulhamid, et al., 2017). A notable inference is that most studies have shown that most TBAs are considered elderly to show they have years of knowledge in their grasps (Amutah-Onukagha, et al., 2017; Ebuehi & Akintujoye, 2012; Adewemimo, Msuya, Olaniyan, & Adegoke, 2013)

TBAs provide source of comfort, trust and counsel for mothers and pregnant women. The traditional birth attendants are known to be very close to the people and the women believe and have trust in them so much (Mfrekemfon P., 2015). They are highly respected and their advice is taken dearly and put into use. This trust and respect is brewed by the facts that TBAs speak the local language, are part of the community, live in their immediate surroundings and share mostly the same belief and culture (Mfrekemfon P., 2015; Abdulhamid, et al., 2017). This has helped cement trust in the community towards TBAs.

Nigeria is shown to be amongst the top five countries with highest rates of maternal mortality with about 40,000 pregnant women dying in the country in 2013 (Abdulhamid, et al., 2017). The presence of TBAs is becoming more and more important as it can make impact on reducing infant and maternal deaths. The roles of TBAs are essential and cannot be replaced by professional health care facilities. Instead it is important that more Traditional Birth Attendants are trained to cater for complications in pregnancies as well as other things.

Indigenous Communication, Traditional Birth Attendants and Maternal Health: Nigeria in Focus

In a study conducted by Ofili & Okojie (2005), it was pointed out that consistently, roughly 600,000 women die of pregnancy-related causes. Ninety-eight percent of these death happen in developing nations, and for each woman who dies, at any rate 30 others endure wounds and, frequently, perpetual incapacity. The Nigerian government since 1979, acknowledged the possibility of the need to coordinate TBAs into PHC framework and have therefore started TBAs preparing programs. Ofili & Okojie (2005) studies on the "Assessment of the role of traditional birth attendants in maternal health care in Oredo Local Government Area, Edo State Nigeria from January to May 2002" found out that ten TBAs were enlisted in the Primary Health Care unit of Oredo LGA; of these, three were at that point dead while seven were as yet alive. Snowball examining strategy was utilized to enroll the TBAs for the examination.

All the TBAs recognized inside the LGA agreed to take part in the investigation and were in this manner incorporated into the research. Each of the seven TBAs on the register of the LGA was followed to their homes. The help of the TBAs were requested in distinguishing different TBAs. In all, 45 TBAs were found. It was reported that of the 45 TBAs talked with, forty-four (97.8%) were female. The lion's share (62.2%) gained their aptitudes through apprenticeship with relatives, while 8.9% had no prior training.

The administrations given by the TBAs went from pre-natal consideration given by 53.3%, delivery, 97.8%, treatment of barrenness, 60.0%, handling premature birth, 13.3% and circumcision of infants, 28.9%. Arrangements utilized in the treatment of line stump included methylated soul utilized by 42.2% of the respondents, natural arrangements, 28.9%, dry warmed sand, 11.1% and motor oil, 6.7%. A portion of the drugs utilized (creature compost, flies, scarification stamps, and cow pee) to treat patients could fill in as wellsprings of disease. Techniques for hazard evaluation during pre-natal consideration, the executives of conveyance confusions, record keeping among TBAs were seen as poor. Disease avoidance strategies utilized were likewise seen as poor, with the greater part (51.1%) not utilizing any type of preventive measures during systems.

While Adewemimo et al. (2013) led their very own investigation in Funtua local government of Kastina state, to discover if the individuals disparaged Skilled Birth Attendants or favored the Traditional Birth Attendants. As indicated by the researchers, a multistage inspecting system was utilized to choose the examination populace. The multistage examining included three phases. At stage one, a provincial LGA (Funtua) was purposively chosen. At stage two, we haphazardly (balloting) chose two political wards (Tun-dunya and Goya) out of the 11 political wards in Funtua though at stage three, utilizing precise examining they chose 400 women of regenerative age from Tundunya and Goya. Test size for each ward was gotten by utilizing likelihood corresponding to measure. 190 women were selected in Tundunya and 210 women from the Goya political ward.

The study showed that rather than use the skilled birth attendance, the TBAs are most preferred due to certain reasons despite the attendant risks involved in their activities. In general, this study showed that the proportion of women in the study area utilising SBA during pregnancy, at birth and during postnatal period was very low. Mother's education, husband's occupation, knowledge of danger signs and place of last childbirth were found to be significant predictors of SBA utilisation. Enabling factors for TBA utilisation were husband's approval, availability of staff and affordability of maternal health services. However, barriers to SBA utilisation described by mothers include unavailability of staff, lack of enabling environment and poverty/

Unyime et al., (2016) carried out their findings by similar method, cross sectional study utilizing organized, approved, and pre-tried polls. The survey was structured and used to get pertinent data from the recognized women in different local government areas of Akwa Ibom state. The polls comprised of both open and shut finished inquiries. The data on the poll included socio-statistic information, for example, age, sex, religion, conjugal status, and so forth. Notwithstanding inquiries on statistic data, the survey included inquiries on contribution with the support of Traditional birth chaperons, explanations behind disparaging them, recurrence of utilization of traditional birth specialist administrations, inclination between conventional birth orderly administrations and present day medicinal services administrations among other data.

Mfrekemfon & Okere (2015I in a study, evaluate the role of TBAs in health care system, respondents accepted that TBAs could assume significant jobs in family arranging, screening for high-chance pregnant moms, ripeness/fruitlessness treatment, and maternal and youngster care administrations. Rural inhabitants like to utilize the services of TBAs as contrasted and their urban partners. Purposes behind their inclination included: the choice of home delivery, TBAs' accessibility, openness, modest work, and country occupants' confidence in the viability of their services. Having an inspirational disposition toward TBA services and fulfillment with work got from TBAs was likewise altogether connected with the individuals who had ever utilized their services.

Ugboaja, Oguejiofor, Oranu and Igwegbe (2018) studies on the use of traditional birth attendants in Sagamu, Ogun State, Nigeria. The study revealed high patronage of traditional birth homes shows that the patronage of TBA services as observed in this study is high. Factors influencing the high patronage of TBAs as found in this study are proximity to patients; ready accessibility of traditional birth attendants; friendly, loving, and caring nature of TBAs in the provision of their services; low cost of TBAs services as well as religious and traditional beliefs. The researchers suggest that in view of the substantial number of deliveries that take place with the TBAs, there is need to train and integrate of TBAs into the existing maternal health-care delivery system. This will help to reduce maternal mortality.

Indigenous Communication, Traditional Birth Attendants and Maternal Health: South Africa in Focus

Discoveries from South African among a group known as Eastern Cape uncover that indigenous health practices are an imperative health resource in the community, and many traditional healers are women. Abrahams (2002) considered indigenous health practices and self-medication among pregnant ladies in Cape Town, and found that the dominant part of Xhosa speaking women take after indigenous health practices for both themselves and their children in view of the need to "fortify" the womb against witchcraft or divination, to forestall youth diseases, and to treat indications they see that biomedical administrations would not have the capacity to treat. Self-medicine with non-recommended medications, herbs and Dutch cures was normal among Afrikaans speaking women.

In pregnancy, herbs or minerals are regularly utilized as a tonic to clean the womb, to ease delivery, to induce labour, and to shield the child from danger and have a sound kid (Henda and Peltzer, 2005; Van der Kooi and Theobald, 2006;

Varga and Veale, 1997). Nolte (1998) says that Traditional Birth Attendants (TBAs) can be portrayed in South Africa as a moderately aged or elderly woman with no formal preparing, who gained her skill through experience and takes care of women during the course of their pregnancy, labour and the postnatal period in various ways. This may incorporate exhortation or guidelines with respect to what to eat, what not to eat, provision of natural remedies for pain, disorder or distress, offering solace to moms; among others. They likewise help with the delivery of the child and provide advice to the new mother on the best way to look after the infant after it is conceived (Department of Health, 2004). Various authors have demonstrated traditional birth attendants in the delivery of health care to the mother and child in South Africa (Nolte, 1998; Jepson and MacDonald, 1988; Selepe and Thomas, 2000; Troskie, 1997).

In an interview by the researchers with an indigene of the community, it is discovered that indigenous women are by and large the key holders of traditional food and medicinal practice, yet may speak just their local dialects, and are frequently unused to speaking with individuals outside of their locale. Thus, indigenous ladies regularly encounter outrageous bias in their contact with the outside world, especially in health and social services. This pushes them to depend exclusively on indigenous health practices, of which maternal health is a major concern. Indigenous women seldom get appropriate care in a western health care system and this is especially hazardous during pregnancy. Indigenous women have higher rates of maternal mortality than non-indigenous women.

Bulterys et al (2002) note that "traditional or trained" birth attendants could assume a core role by reaching pregnant women not currently receiving formal antenatal care and by assisting with delivery of primary services designed to prevent HIV transmission. Trained birth chaperons could regulate the arrangement of nevirapine to ladies contaminated with HIV who conceives an offspring at home and to their babies. They could likewise advise women and their spouses on the best way to reduce the risk of HIV being transmitted to the child, concentrating especially on the postpartum period. An alternate view is held by Berger (2003) contending that the traditional birth attendants cannot be relied upon to do HIV/AIDS avoidance and treatment exercises (to direct HIV tests or convey antiretroviral medications to women conceiving an offspring at home) owing to their lack of skills and abilities. This argument is valid however in the developed nations of the world. In developing countries, this contention is faulty.

WHO (2004) takes note that traditional birth chaperons have the potential for enhancing maternal and infant health at community level. While administering non- prescribed medications may not cause any clinical issues, they might be risky, may meddle with suitable health-seeking behaviour and prevent consistence with breastfeeding as prescribed by the World Health Organization (Bland et al., 2004;

Mabina et al., 1997; Varga and Veale, 1997). Traditional health-care attendants are exceedingly esteemed people who are whose counsels are often sought for the "procurement of traditional preparations for infant use" (Sibeko et al, 2005; Varga and Veale, 1997).

Although some health care providers stay suspicious of traditional remedies, most concur that traditional healers can assume a vital integral part in health care provision (Bodeker et al., 2006; Baggaley et al., 1996; Burnett et al., 1999; Bulterys et al., 2002). Utilization of traditional drugs on newborn children and discussion with traditional healers appear to be normal. The significance of perceiving and directly utilizing traditional medications is emphasized in this study. Health programs that disregard this issue might miss critical chances to give instruction and limit drug interactions. Health care providers must open lines of correspondence with traditional healers and with moms to augment achievement. Given the utilization of conventional pharmaceuticals, incorporating traditional healers into wellbeing activities could be a well thought strategy for meeting specific wellbeing needs (Bodeker et al., 2006; Ndulo et al., 2001; Nations and Souza, 1997).

THEORETICAL FRAMEWORK

This study adopted the multi-step flow theory. Multi step flow theory leans on the assumption that ideas do not go to the wider population directly, but instead, they flow from the mass media to opinion leaders, after which they get disseminated to a much wider population. The multi-step flow theory was propounded 1944 by Paul Lazarsfeld. This theory holds that opinion leaders play a major role of intervention, as they 'intervene' between the media's message, and the reaction of the audience to that message. They wield considerable amount of effect on persons similar to them on the basis of personality, demography and a host of other socio-economic factors. Hence, much more than the conventional media would influence the actions of audience members, these opinion leaders would, owing to the fact that the audience identifies more with a leader than a newspaper article. Using this theory, we realize that information is largely affected by the communal norms present in the society it enters.

In relation to this study therefore, traditional birth attendants are considered the opinion leaders whom the people revere and trust the most, regardless of what the newspapers and other conventional media say. Women in the rural areas, both in Nigeria and South Africa have revealed the power of opinion leaders, as they continually turn to traditional birth attendants whenever the issue of childbirth and other surrounding concerns arise. In many of these rural societies, traditional birth attendants are mature women whose skills in home delivery are widely known and accepted by members of that community (Makoe, 2000; Abdulhamid, Lawal, Tahir, Harande, & Usman, 2017). This supports the multi-step theory which holds on to the bane of a better relationship with and identification to these opinion leaders, rather than the information being provided by the conventional media. If the opinion leaders (traditional birth attendants) buy into a piece of information being circulated by the mas media, poaching it and applying it to the members of the audience (mothers and pregnant women) would be much easier, than a direct dissemination of information from the media to members of the audience.

Comparison Between the Status of TBAs in South Africa and In Nigeria

Traditional Birth Attendants aided women in childbirth before the arrival of modern medicine. They are still present till date, helping in rural and also urban areas in developing countries. They are notably known to help women South Africa and Nigeria, there are footprints are particularly seen in rural with pregnancy care, during labor and with postnatal care using indigenous practices (Ngunyulu & Mulaudzi, 2009). TBAs, according to studies, are particularly prominent in areas. (Peltzer & Henda, 2006; Amutah-Onukagha, et al., 2017) There are similarities as well as wide differences in TBA practices in both countries.

TBAs cross countries mixed their health care practices with deep traditional and religious practices (Abdulhamid, et al., 2017; MAKOAE, 2000; Peltzer & Henda, 2006). In Gaedei & Versteegii, 2011, it was explained that TBAs in South Africa protected postnatal women from evil spirits by detaching the new mother. This was shown in the statement

Evil things can come with a crowd of people coming to see the new member of the family.

In the Northern part of Nigeria, TBAs due to religious reasons are restricted to being females only, where as in other parts of the country both males and females are involved (Abdulhamid, et al., 2017). In Nigeria as well, TBAs are known to have a rich knowledge of herbal plants and educate women on the appropriate diet. They also speak on pregnancy-related taboos. However, some of the taboos may be today interpreted to have negative aspects on the health of the mother.

The husband is also noted as a passive yet important factor in the situation of things. In Nigeria, it is noted that the husband's occupation has also been identified as an important predictor for the utilization of TBAs, through antenatal and postnatal periods. The husband's unemployment is a cause for the low utilization of skilled care during childbirth. TBAs also prepare pregnant women and new mothers to also think about their husbands (Adewemimo, Msuya, Olaniyan, & Adegoke, 2013). A study focused on the Sikhunyani Village in the Limpopo Province of South Africa showed that the man's clothes must be washed properly hence women are not allowed to wash their husband's clothes just after delivery and she will not be able to wash them well. It is also shown that the woman should not have sex until she stops breastfeeding to avoid killing her husband (Ngunyulu & Mulaudzi, 2009).

A major difference between TBAs in South Africa and Nigeria is that, South African TBAs are more geared and trained to be extra careful because of the risks of contracting the HIV Virus. TBAs are trained to conduct prenatal checkups, assess the baby's position in the uterus, and deliver human immunodeficiency virus/acquired immunodeficiency syndrome care and services (Ebuehi & Akintujoye, 2012). Peltzer & Henda, 2006, a South African study showed that Most TBAs knew where to obtain voluntary counselling and testing (VCT), approved of distributing condoms, and were involved in HIV/STI management such as risk assessment, risk reduction counselling, distribution of condoms, community education and home-based care.

Most TBAs were found to be skilled to handle the rigors of pregnancy care and could identify the risks involved. They had extensive knowledge on delivery and even used traditional procedures to perform modern medicinal tasks. However, it was noted that both TBAs in Nigeria and South Africa are in need of more training (Peltzer & Henda, 2006; Ebuehi & Akintujoye, 2012). This would equip them to handle common obstetric problems, pregnancy complications and sexually transmitted diseases including HIV.

SUMMARY OF FINDINGS

- Most of the research work poses that Traditional Attendants should be embraced and combined with modern medicine
- Most TBAs use some form traditional ritual or practice
- TBAs are usually elderly women in the society and often revered
- TBAs also use natural herbs
- The research showed a preference for a qualitative form of research
- Father figures in Nigeria seem to have more presence in the lives of the pregnant women
- The Nigerian studies have shown that the northern part of Nigeria is more at risk; the pregnant women are more prone to infections.

- Studies in South Africa show TBAs as very capable when complications arise in pregnant women unlike their Nigerian counterparts
- A major problem in South Africa is the prevalence of HIV/AIDS and the risks it might pose for TBAs
- Not many available health care systems in Nigeria

CONCLUSION

After careful review of the studies, it is shown that TBA's in both Nigeria and South Africa assist pregnant women based on their religious or traditional beliefs (Makoe, 2000; PATH, 2010). TBA's act according to their knowledge on pregnancy related taboos and restrict pregnant women from committing such said taboos (Kayombo, 2013). There are also several traditional beliefs that TBA's practice in which they believe would aid childbirth. In South Africa, TBA's expected to be presented with a bundle of wood upon arriving. The bundle would be untied and this is said to help loosen up everything in the woman so that she gives birth effortlessly (Shangase, et al.). Some other beliefs include that the women should not have sex until she stops breastfeeding to avoid killing her husband. It is also believed that the placenta and bloodstained cloths, and the soil the woman bled on should be buried so that dogs can't eat them. This can result in the woman not conceiving anymore (Ngunyulu & Mulaudzi, 2009). Many of these mystic sanctions are not considered particularly bad, as long as they do not directly harm the mother or the baby (Shangase, et al.).

Furthermore, TBA's are known to have extensive knowledge on herbs appropriate for pregnant women and necessary to achieve a safe delivery (Kayombo, 2013; Abdulhamid, Lawal, Tahir, Harande, & Usman, 2017). Some of these herbs are derived from the roots, barks and leaves of local plants. Herbal medicines serve several purposes. It is known to help treat abdominal pain, guaranteeing safe pregnancy, giving strength to the pregnant woman, and increasing stronger contractions during labor (Makoe, 2000).

Pregnant women seek out TBAs for local herbs, concoctions and prayers given to them before and during delivery. The studies originating from Nigeria also highlight TBA's as herbalists or sometimes traditional healers (Inyang & Anuncha, 2015). Ebuehi & Akintujoye 2012, also derived from their study that TBA's are known to give herbal concoctions to make the baby strong. However, these herbs are known to be not entirely safe. Some TBAs use herbs during delivery to help in dilation but this may worsen issues by causing infections for the mother and baby. It could cause an infection called pelvic sepsis which leads to infertility, menstrual disorders and other complications (Inyang & Anuncha, 2015; Kayombo, 2013). The studies have shown that herbal treatments come hand in hand with the TBA practice. These herbs are known to have its benefits, however there are still risks involved with using such herbs.

The traditional birth attendants make great impact in the rural community, they are very close to the people and the rural women believe and have trust on them so much that they cannot be easily abolished in the community. To this effect, measures should be carried out to improve their skills for example giving them health education, training, organizing seminars and the need for referral of complicated cases to hospitals. There is need for the various Governments to improve access to and reduce cost of maternity services. There is also a need to adequately train TBAs, supervise their operations and possibly collaborate with them.

RECOMMENDATION

The researchers align with Shaikh, Khan, Maab & Amjad (2014) that training of TBAs not only enhances their knowledge and skills on obstetric care and referral mechanism, but also leads to greater community acceptance and a greater consumer satisfaction. They can play a vital role in birth preparedness and identification of danger signs. Training of TBAs has shown an impact on perinatal and neonatal deaths which can be significantly reduced. Moreover, TBAs have been a critical contributor in providing skilled maternal, newborn and child health (MNCH) care in the rural population of developing countries due to inadequate numbers of human resource for service delivery. And so there is a need for a health policy in actualizing this.

There must be a serious systematic approach for the transition of the TBAs to SBAs, with a well mapped out plan to inculcate the traditional birth attendance into modern health care services as they keep their form of lively hood. This is because they have become part of the people they render service to, in terms of culture and way of life.

The need to provide modern health care to the rural areas is very urgent, even if it is not so big but there should community health centers that will carter for maternal health care and train the TBAs. There must situated in such a way that the people, especially women can easily access with 10 minutes.

Those who patronize the TBAs are sometimes mostly the poor, who will need economic empowerment to get out of poverty, which will enable them to seek better health services. So the to create the atmosphere for economic development in the rural areas and among the poor in the society is very important.

Education is very important both for the TBAs and those who patronize them, it was found that in the study conducted in Akwa Ibom and Funtua Local government area, that women with low or without formal education at all, accounted for the high numbers who use the services of the TBAs. The need for education of everyone even as highlighted by the UN must be paramount in order to overcome these challenges that have continued to result in the loss of children every year.

The different religious bodies must play their role in convincing the people of some of the dangers that some cultural practices portrays and the need to completely do away with them. Because in times of pregnancy complications, the TBAs who are believed to be spiritual and know a lot, always become confused and cannot handle such medical complications which leads to death of mother and child many times.

Interventions to help nations to change from TBAs to SBAs are especially significant in light of need systems to expand SBAs and the human asset challenges in accomplishing this objective. Late undertaking moving work has concentrated on the jobs lay health laborers including TBAs can expect. As noted above, intercessions of enthusiasm for motivations behind this audit were those where TBAs were suppliers of labor care and endeavors were made to expand labor with a SBA. This included mediations where TBAs were connected with formal health administrations to raise SBA/office births; intercessions to expand organizations or cooperation with TBAs; or to discover new jobs for TBAs inside the proper health framework.

FUTURE RESEARCH DIRECTIONS

Since this chapter is an empirical review of literature on the indigenous communication role of Traditional Birth Attendants in Maternal Health Practices, it will be interesting to do empirical studies that employ different research methods on the role of Traditional Birth Attendants and Skilled Birth Attendants in maternal health practices through different media platforms.

REFERENCES

Abdulhamid, Z., Lawal, U. S., Tahir, A. A., Harande, M. M., Usman, H., & Nuhu, A. (2017). Perceptions of Hausa and Fulani Tribes on Traditional Birth Attendants in Zaria Local Government Area, Kaduna State, Nigeria. *Journal of Complementary and Alternative Medical*, *2*(2), 1–7. doi:10.9734/JOCAMR/2017/27773

Abrahams, N., Jewkes, R., & Mvo, Z. (2002). Indigenous healing practices and self-medication amongst pregnant women in Cape Town, South Africa. [PubMed]. *African Journal of Reproductive Health*, *6*(2), 79–86. doi:10.2307/3583133 PMID:12476719

Adatara, P., Afya, A., Baku, E. A., Salia, S. M., & Asempah, A. (2018) Perspective of Traditional Birth Attendants on Their Experiences and Roles in Maternal Health Care in Rural Areas of Northern Ghana. *International Journal of Reproductive Medicine*, 2018. doi:10.1155/2018/2165627

Adewemimo, A. W., Msuya, S. E., Olaniyan, C. T., & Adegoke, A. A. (2014). Utilisation of skilled birth attendance in Northern Nigeria: A cross-sectional survey: Contents lists available at *Science Direct Journal* homepage: www.elsevier.com/midw

Amutah-Onukagha, N., Gardner, M., & Pierre, K. (2017). Progresses and challenges of utilizing traditional birth attendants in maternal and child health in Nigeria. *International Journal of MCH and AIDS*, *6*(2), 130–138. doi:10.21106/ijma.216 PMID:29367889

Baggaley, R., Sulwe, J., Burnett, A., & Ndovi, M. (1996). Forging links between the formal and traditional in Zambia. Special report: *Traditional healers*. [PubMed]. *AIDS Analysis Africa*, *6*, 12–13. PMID:12290767

Berger, M. (2003). Traditional birth attendants in developing countries cannot be expected to carry out HIV/AIDS prevention and treatment activities. [PubMed]. *Reproductive Health Matters*, *11*(22), 36–40. doi:10.1016/S0968-8080(03)02286-9 PMID:14708396

Bland, R. M., Rollins, N. C., Van den Broeck, J., & Coovadia, H. M. (2004). Child Health Group, author. The use of non-prescribed medication in the first 3 months of life in rural South Africa. [PubMed]. *Tropical Medicine & International Health*, *9*(1), 118–124. doi:10.1046/j.1365-3156.2003.01148.x PMID:14728615

Bodeker, G., Carter, G., Burford, G., & Dvorak-Little, M. (2006). HIV/AIDS: Traditional system of health care in the management of a global epidemic. [PubMed]. *Journal of Alternative and Complementary Medicine (New York, N.Y.)*, *12*(6), 563–576. doi:10.1089/acm.2006.12.563 PMID:16884348

Bulterys, M., Fowler, G. M., Shaffer, N., Tih, P., Greenberg, A., Karita, E., ... De Cock, K. (2002). Role of traditional birth attendants in preventing perinatal transmission of HIV. [PMC free article] [PubMed]. *BMJ (Clinical Research Ed.)*, *324*(7331), 222–225. doi:10.1136/bmj.324.7331.222 PMID:11809647

Burnett, A., Baggaley, N., Ndovi-Macmillan, M., & Sulwe, J. (1999). *Hang'Omba B*. Bennett J.

Burnett, A., Baggaley, R., Ndovi-Macmillan, M., Sulwe, J., Hang'Omba, B., & Bennett, J. (1999, August). Caring for people with HIV in Zambia: Are traditional healers and formal health workers willing to work together. [PubMed]. *AIDS Care, 11*(4), 481–491. doi:10.1080/09540129947875 PMID:10533542

Ebuehi, O. M., & Akintujoye, I. (2012). Perception and utilization of traditional birth attendants by pregnant women attending primary health care clinics in a rural Local Government Area in Ogun State, Nigeria. *International Journal of Women's Health, 4*, 25–34. doi:10.2147/IJWH.S23173 PMID:22371657

Falle, T. Y., & Mullany, L. C. (2019) Potential Role of Traditional Birth Attendants in Neonatal Healthcare in Rural Southern Nepal. *J Health Population and Nutrition, 2009 Feb; 27*(1), 53–61.

Gaedei, B., & Versteegii, M. (2011). *The state of the right to health in rural South Africa* (p. 2011). Department of Rural Health, University of KwaZulu-Natal.

Inyang, M. P., & Anuncha, O. U. (2015). Traditional Birth Attendants and Maternal Mortality. *IOSR Journal of Dental and Medical Sciences, 12*(2), 21–26.

Jepson, A. P., & MacDonald, L. D. (1988). The practice of traditional birth attendants in Zululand. [PubMed]. *Tropical Doctor, 18*(4), 177–179. doi:10.1177/004947558801800413 PMID:3194950

Kayombo, E. J. (2013). Impact of Training traditional birth attendants on maternal mortality and morbidity in Sub-Saharan African countries. *Tanzania Journal of Health Research, 15*(2), 1–11. doi:10.4314/thrb.v15i2.7 PMID:26591718

Khambule, N. Z. (2016). *Experiences of pregnant women from a rural community regarding antenatal care services in ethekwini district, kwazulu-natal*. Durban University of Technology.

Lindsey, S. (2016). *Training Traditional Birth Attendants in Sub-Saharan Africa*. Liberty University.

Makoe, L. N. (2000). *The role of traditional birth attendants in the provision of mayterrnal health in lesotho*. University Of South Africa.

Mfrekemfon, P. I., & Okere, U. A. (2015) Traditional Birth Attendants and Maternal Mortality: IOSR *Journal of Dental and Medical Sciences (IOSR-JDMS) 14*(2) Ver. III (Feb. 2015), pp. 21-26. Retrieved from www.iosrjournals.org

Miller, T., & Smith, H. (2017). Establishing Partnership With Traditional Birth Attendants For Improved Maternal And Newborn Health: A Review Of Factors Influencing Implementation. *Miller And Smith Bmc Pregnancy And Childbirth, 17*(365), 1–10. PMID:29052533

Ngunyulu, R., & Mulaudzi, F. (2009). Indigenous practices regarding postnatal care at Sikhunyani Village in the Limpopo Province of South Africa. *Africa Journal of Nursing and Midwifery, 11*(1), 48–64.

Nolte, A. (1998). Traditional birth attendants in South Africa: Professional midwives' beliefs and myths. [PubMed]. *Curationis, 21*, 59–66. PMID:11040590

Ofili, A. N., & Okojie, O. H. (2005, June). Assessment of the role of traditional birth attendants in maternal health care in Oredo Local Government Area, Edo State, Nigeria. *Journal of Community Medicine and Primary Health Care, 17*(1), 55–60. doi:10.4314/jcmphc.v17i1.32428

Oyero, O. S., Oyesomi, K. O., Abioye, T., Ajiboye, E., & Kayode-Adedeji, K. T. (2018). Strategic communication for climate change awareness and behavioural change in Ado-Odo/Ota Local Government of Ogun State. African Population Studies, 32(1), (Supp.), 2018.

Oyesomi, K. O., & Salawu, A. (2019). Assessing the Uniqueness of Indigenous Language in Advertising: Analysis of Figurative Language Used in Selected Telecommunication Yoruba Advertisement in Nigeria. *Qualitative Report, 24*(10), 2574–2591. Retrieved from https://nsuworks.nova.edu/tqr/vol24/iss10/12

Oyesomi, K. O., Salawu, A., & Olorunyomi, B. (2017). Indigenous Communication: Socio- Economic Characteristics Influencing Contemporary Female Political Participation. [JIWS]. *Journal of International Women's Studies, 18*(4), 164–181.

Oyesomi, K. O., Salawu, A., & Onyenankeya, K. (2019, March). Newspapers' Compliance with the Code of Election Coverage of the 2015 Elections and citizens participation: Implication for Journalism Education and Professionalism. *African Rennaisance, 16*(1), 41–64. doi:10.31920/2516-5305/2019/V16n1a3

PATH. (2010). *Improving maternal and child health in South Africa.* Johannesburg, South Africa: www.path.org

Peltzer, K., & Henda, N. (2006). Traditional birth attendants, HIV/AIDS and safe delivery in the Eastern Cape, South Africa - evaluation of a training programme. *SAJOG, 12*(3), 140–145.

Sarmento, D. R. (2014). Traditional Birth Attendance (TBA) in a health system: what are the roles, benefits and challenges: A case study of incorporated TBA in Timor Leste. *Asia Pacific Family Medicine, 13*(1), 12. doi:10.118612930-014-0012-1 PMID:25469105

Shaikh, T. B., Khan, S., Maab, A., & Amjad, S. (2014) Emerging role of traditional birth attendants in mountainous terrain: a qualitative exploratory study from Chitral District, *Pakistan. BMJ Journals, 4*(11).

Shangase, M., Pengpid, S., Peltzer, K., Henda, N., Mosala, T., Dlamini, N., & ... . (n.d.). Traditional Birth Attendants and HIV/AIDS in South Africa: A Trainer's Manual. *Department of Health: Republic of South Africa.*

Sibeko, L., Dhansay, M. A., Charlton, K. E., Johns, T., & Gray-Donald, K. (2005). Beliefs, attitudes, and practices of breastfeeding mothers from a periurban community in South Africa. [PubMed]. *Journal of Human Lactation, 21*(1), 31–38. doi:10.1177/0890334404272388 PMID:15681633

Smith, L. (2016). *Training Traditional Birth Attendants in Sub-Saharan Africa.* Liberty University.

Troskie, T. R. (1997). The importance of traditional midwives in the delivery of health care in the Republic of South Africa. [PubMed]. *Curationis, 20,* 15–20. PMID:9287548

Ugboaja, J. O., Oguejiofor, C. B., Oranu, E. O., & Igwegbe, A. O. (2018) Factors associated with the use of traditional birth attendants in Nigeria: A secondary analysis of 2013 Nigeria national demography and health survey. *The Nigerian Journal of General Practice, 16*(2), 45.

Unyime, I. E., Idongesit, L. J., & Akpabio, E. A. (2016). High Patronage of Traditional Birth Homes: A Report from Akwa Ibom, Southern Nigeria. *AASCIT Journal of Health., 3*(1), 17–22.

Van der Kooi, R. (2006). Theobald S. Traditional medicine in late pregnancy and labour: Perceptions of Kgaba remedies amongst the Tswana in South Africa. *Afr J Trad CAM., 3*(1), 11–22.

World Health Organization. International Confederation of Midwives, & International Federation of Gynecology and Obstetrics. (2004). Making pregnancy safer: The critical role of the skilled attendant. *Bulletin of the World Health Organization.* Geneva. Retrieved from http://apps.who.int/iris/bitstream/10665/42955/1/9241591692.pdf

Chapter 2
Exploring the Use of Indigenous Languages in Antenatal Care Sessions Among Mothers in Lagos State

Oludare Ebenezer Ogunyombo
Olabisi Onabanjo University, Nigeria

Semiu Bello
Kwara State University, Nigeria

ABSTRACT

This chapter examines the use of indigenous languages during antenatal care (ANC) sessions among mothers in Lagos state. Authors investigate factors that influence the use of indigenous languages, the most preferred mode of presentation, and how the languages affect reception, participation, and knowledge of mothers on safe motherhood practices. Using in-depth interviews with nurses and observations during the ANC sessions, the study found that indigenous languages engender participation and are effective in building self-esteem, trust, and confidence of mothers. Songs in the indigenous language, particularly Yoruba language, help mothers retain and recall safe motherhood messages easily. Mothers generally demonstrate their understanding during the question and answer sessions, while also serving as agents of information reinforcement among themselves using indigenous languages. In view of the occasional need for interpreters, the study recommends that health workers should be encouraged to take courses in indigenous languages within their region as a second language.

DOI: 10.4018/978-1-7998-2091-8.ch002

INTRODUCTION

Since the 1990's, Nigeria has made efforts and recorded some progress at reducing maternal and child mortality. Nigeria's Maternal Mortality Ratio dropped from 1,200 deaths in 1990 to 540 deaths in 2013 per 100,000 live births. Similarly, under five Mortality Ratio dropped from 191 deaths in 1990 to 94 deaths in 2012 per 1,000 live births. Despite this progress, Nigeria still occupies the unenviable position as a leading contributor to the regional and global burden of women and children's death. Furthermore, child survival in Nigeria is threatened largely by nutritional deficiencies and illnesses, particularly malaria, diarrheal diseases, acute respiratory infections (ARI), and vaccine-preventable diseases (VPD), which account for the majority of morbidity and mortality in childhood (Society for Family Health, 2019).

In its bid to address this challenge, the Lagos State Government in 2008 inaugurated a committee to offer technical guidance on the various modalities needed for the reduction of the maternal mortality. The committee recommended a 5-year work-plan developed for the implementation of the Maternal and Child Mortality Reduction Programme (MCMR) to reduce the maternal and child mortality rates in line with the United Nations Millennium Development Goals 4, 5 and 6. An earlier study in the state gave the maternal mortality ratio in Lagos State as 555/100,000 live births. This figure was higher than the national average of 545/100,000 live births (Lagos State Ministry of Health, 2017). Hence, critical to safe motherhood is effective health communication, particularly during antenatal care sessions.

According to the World Health Organisation (2016), antenatal care (ANC) is the care provided by skilled health-care professionals to pregnant women and adolescent girls in order to ensure the best health conditions for both mother and baby during pregnancy. At the ANC, pregnant women want to have a "positive pregnancy experience". A positive pregnancy experience is defined as maintaining physical and sociocultural normality; maintaining a healthy pregnancy for mother and baby (including preventing and treating risks, illness and death); having an effective transition to positive labour and birth; and achieving positive motherhood (including maternal self-esteem, competence and autonomy). To achieve these, the midwives check the health of the pregnant mother and the baby; give the pregnant mother useful information to help her have a healthy pregnancy, including advice about healthy eating and exercise; discuss options and choices for care during pregnancy, labour and birth; and answer any other question which the pregnant mother may have. Thus, the components of ANC include risk identification; prevention and management of pregnancy-related or concurrent diseases; and health education and health promotion. (WHO, 2016; NHS, 2017)

Consequently, miscommunication in this regard can be life threatening. Essentially, effective health communication remains significant in mitigating mother and child morbidity and mortality because mothers must be able to understand what is being communicated. Amuseghan, Ayenigbara and Orimogunje (2010) agree that health communication has developed to turn its focus on enabling informed individual choice and reduce miscommunication or misrepresentation that could lead to morbidity or fatality. The need for such intervention crystallises the need to communicate in a language that would be easily understood by the mothers.

In agreement, Flood and Rohloff (2018) note that language is a key feature of models of health that is used by the indigenous people themselves. More so, global health programmes conceived and delivered using indigenous languages are likely to be successful. As an intervention, Mphasha and Lebese (2017) state that tackling health issues with the languages that people understand is essential in improving the lives and prospects of the people. In addition, Amery (2017) notes that "miscommunication is not just about languages, some of these difficulties also arise from the interface of communication and culture which are often derived from differences in world view". In effect, it is all about the totality of the presentations and approaches to how such indigenous languages are used by the health care providers when engaging with the mothers during antenatal services.

Interestingly, during antenatal sessions in Primary Healthcare Centres (PHC) and General Hospitals in Nigeria, it has been observed that healthcare providers, especially nurses, often deliver their health talks using indigenous languages. For instance, in some PHCs in Lagos, it has been observed that the healthcare providers speak the Yoruba language, which is a very common language spoken by people in Southwest Nigeria.

However, in view of Amery (2017) assertion that miscommunication can be subtle because parties in communication may come away with different understandings; this paper seeks to interrogate the approaches for engaging indigenous languages during antenatal sessions in PHC and hospitals in Lagos state. Although the authors admit that there may be other factors responsible for the not too encouraging state of maternal mortality in Nigeria, an attempt to establish the place of effective antenatal care session, using indigenous languages is what this paper seeks to address. Using observation and in-depth interviews as its method, this study specifically, examines the influence of indigenous languages on the reception, participation and knowledge of mothers on safe motherhood practices.

RESEARCH QUESTIONS

In view of the objectives of this study, the following are the research questions for investigation:

1. What factors influence the choice of indigenous languages by health workers during pre/antenatal sessions?
2. Which mode (talks, songs, drama) of indigenous language engagement do health workers and mothers found most effective during pre/antenatal sessions?
3. How do indigenous languages influence the reception of safe motherhood messages among mothers during pre/antenatal sessions?
4. How do mothers demonstrate their understanding of safe motherhood practices using indigenous languages during the pre/antenatal sessions?
5. What limitation do health workers and mothers encounter in using indigenous languages during pre/antenatal sessions?

LITERATURE REVIEW

Concept of Health Communication

Health communication is communication that relates to health matters. The common saying that health is wealth may sometimes, not be digested and understood to be non-negotiable until when individuals fall sick and require medical attention. The interchange of what eventually transpired in curing the deficient health state of such individuals may be found in health communication. The *Healthy People* (2010) states that health communication involves the study and use of communication strategies to inform and influence individual and community decisions that enhance health. It links the domains of communication and health and is increasingly recognized as a necessary element of efforts to improve personal and public health.

Health communication is an area of study that investigates and elucidates the many ways that human and mediated communication dramatically influences the outcomes of health-care and health-promotion efforts with research attempts dating back to the 1980s. The growth in health communication research has been necessitated by its potential to address complex and challenging healthcare demands across societies while guiding the promotion of public health (*Encyclopedia of Communication and Information*, 2002). Bello (2014) notes that health communication as a field of theory and practice involves interpersonal and mass communication programmes aimed at improving the health of individuals, organisations and larger populations through appropriate health information. At a broad level, this includes intrapersonal, interpersonal, group, organisational and societal communications (Ogundoyin and Soola, 2014).

Essentially, effective health communication can help raise awareness of health risks and solutions while providing the motivation and skills required to mitigate the threats associated with such health risk. It assists affected individuals to get succour from people with similar health issues, influence behaviours and reinforce healthy attitudes such as the demand for appropriate health services, selecting health plans, care providers and treatments. (*Healthy People*, 2010)

Notably, at the heart of healthcare and health-promotion efforts is communication. In order to gather relevant diagnostic information from their patients, healthcare providers are depending on their ability to communicate effectively by asking pertinent questions, interpreting responses, and probing for information that is more detailed. At the same time, patients depend on their own ability to communicate with healthcare providers when seeking help, identifying health problems, interpreting healthcare recommendations and treatment strategies, and negotiating their way when seeking health information.

On a wider scale, effective health communication engenders cooperation and coordination. For matters such as safe motherhood practices, health care givers must be able to communicate successfully with their audiences to achieve compliance. The messages must be well crafted, appropriate, compelling and delivered through the most appropriate communication channel and method to minimize wrong health choices and behaviours. (*Encyclopedia of Communication and Information*, 2002)

Espousing the principle of effective health communication to the wellbeing and survival of humans, Bello (2014) amplifies the essence of health literacy to complement health communication. He notes that health literacy denotes the application of literacy skill in the health context to enhance the healthy living of individuals and the general population. Invariably, low health literacy level may lead to frequent hospitalization and chronic health conditions. The World Health Organisation (2009) defines health literacy as the cognitive and social skills, which determine the motivation and ability of individuals to gain access, understand and use information in ways that promote and maintain good health. Health literacy is not only about the ability to read but involves improving people's access to health information and their capacity to use such information effectively to achieve health empowerment.

In this instance, if nursing mothers are unable to efficiently understand health talks and instructions given during their sessions with healthcare providers, then the consequence may not be palatable on the mothers and their children. Therefore, it may be concluded that health communication involves all communications and communication activities that are deliberately designed, reviewed and implemented among groups of people the purpose of providing, sharing, understanding and using health information in ways that promote and maintain good health.

Indigenous Language and Health Communication

Language is at the heart of every communication exchange. Language is a unique human endowment, which defines human's humanity. It is used as an instrument of communication as well as development in all spheres of life. Despite the status of English as a language spoken in quite a number of countries across the globe, to a large extent, Nigeria has effectively used most of its indigenous languages on its radio and television announcements and special programmes. About 450 indigenous languages have been used to reach Nigerians on health and political issues (Amuseghan *et al*, 2010).

Within the context of culture and the architecture of a given society, it important that health information such as safe motherhood practices uses the most appropriate language. Some dictionary definitions of language reflect the essence of appropriate use. The *Encyclopedia Britannica* defines language as a system of conventional spoken, manual, or written symbols by means of which human beings, as members of a social group and participants in its culture express themselves. The functions of language include communication, the expression of identity, play, imaginative expression and emotional release. According to *Collins English Dictionary*, language is a system of communication, which consists of a set of sounds and written symbols, which are used by the people of a particular country or region for talking or writing. By the definition of the *Oxford English Dictionary*, language is the method of human communication, either spoken or written, consisting of the use of words in a structured and conventional way. Oyero (2007) agrees that language does not exist without culture. It is situated within a socio-cultural setting or community as an integral part that can be facilitated or enhanced through direct or indirect context and acculturation.

Assertions from the foregoing show that members of a social group, which may be bound by country or region and tied by some cultural links to create an identity and express emotions, must speak language conventionally. More so, language is systematic and structured, which means it must follow a pattern of knowledge and presentation to convey the right meaning to the right people. Simply, every language is indigenous to a group of people within a society and the indigenousness largely facilitates the comprehension and assimilation of information disseminated within the group, or others who understand the language of the specific social group. In this instance, nursing mothers in Lagos state form a social group that such use of an indigenous language may be critical to their attitudes to safe motherhood practices.

Espousing this context, Maune (2017) describes indigenous language as a local means of communication between members of a people or community; it contains within it the essence of considerable information and knowledge and wisdom of the people or community. According to Oyesomi and Salawu (2019), Indigenous language is a language that is spoken by a group of people that resides in a locality or region. It is a language native to a country and spoken as a mother tongue by some of its indigenes (Olubode-Sawe, 2010). In terms of promoting developmental programmes, as it is in healthcare, Oyero (2007) notes that indigenous language has proved to be very potent in creating a critical mass of real communication for substantial change.

In health communication, researchers have established the value of indigenous languages. Meuter *et al* (2015) observe that understanding language in the context of a medical encounter is critical for understanding the problems that might result when patients and healthcare practitioners speak a different language. The study noted that miscommunication is more likely to occur when clinicians use an inadequately mastered language and cannot correctly convey certain nuances of risk and certainty. For instance, people from different cultural groups describe pain and distress quite differently. In addition, culturally specific terms, expressions, or metaphors can be difficult to navigate even when language competence is high. The situation could be worse when clinicians lack the linguistic and cultural skills needed and interpreters are not available to explain to the patients what they mean. In such cases, patients may have to rely on medically inexperienced, bilingual relatives or non-medical staff, which may result in poor health outcomes.

Amery (2017) in a study conducted on indigenous languages on the reception, choices and health behaviours among people in the Aboriginal region of Australia established that the communication gap between health professionals and indigenous Australians has a significant impact on health outcomes. The communication gap is most pronounced in remote areas where cultural and linguistic differences are greatest, therefore affirming the need for understanding the indigenous language to bridge the gap. This also became more important because more of the indigenes have difficulty with specialised language, with common terms such as infection, tumour, high blood pressure, stroke and bacteria often misunderstood. Consequently, the study concluded that a refusal to take Aboriginal languages seriously would result in less than optimal medical outcomes, mistrust and disengagement with the health sector and non-compliance with treatment regimens by the indigenes.

Examining the intersections between indigenous language, health and wellness, Van Beek (2016) notes that since values are important to emotional wellbeing and mental health, the language which contextualizes and holds those values must not disappear else, the community will become more vulnerable to stress and health challenges. Citing Reyhner (2010), Van Beek (2016) states that "the use of the native tongue is like therapy; specific native words express love and caring. Knowing the language presents one with a strong self-identity, a culture with which to identify and a sense of wellness". The study concluded that indigenous language goes beyond communication to connect people with their past. It involves situating them in their emotional and social vitality, involving them in their own identity and wellness as well as their connection to the community. Thus, indigenous language is vital to positive identity, relationships and health as a bond between self, the outside world and culture or community.

In another study conducted by Taff *et al* (2018), the impact of indigenous language use on wellness was examined. The findings revealed that using indigenous languages has beneficial effects on the health of descendant language users and if such use is suppressed, it may affect the well-being of the people. The study correlates indigenous language use with lower suicide rates, diabetes symptoms and reduction in risk factors for youth. The study concluded that being bi or multilingual in an ancestral/indigenous language appears to improve cognitive function throughout the life of an individual and delays ageing of the brain.

Despite the eulogy on indigenous language in healthcare activities, the findings of Paulino, Vázquez and Bolúmar (2018) showed a bit of a variation particularly in relation to ethnicity and inequities. In an Investigation on the indigenous language and inequitable maternal health care in Guatemala, Mexico, Peru and the Plurinational State of Bolivia, Paulino *et al* (2018) note that women who speak an indigenous language are less likely to have an institutional delivery and are more likely to attend fewer than four prenatal visits. In addition, the maternal mortality rate is higher in some areas where a large proportion of the population speaks an indigenous language, a finding that is consistent with the low level of coverage of maternal care services observed among indigenous women in the countries studied.

These findings are similar to that of Whalen, Moss, and Baldwin (2016) in their study on language maintenance and revitalization efforts on health-related benefits for Native Americans and other indigenous populations. Considering other studies on the subject matter, they concluded that speaking an indigenous language in itself may not be solely responsible for improved health status. Rather, community validation of the indigenous knowledge system, community-driven tribal education, comprehending indigenous medicine, and youth empowerment through language and culture identity formation all play significant roles in the ability of a minority language to thrive and for the community to experience healthy outcomes from the collective effort.

The assertions of Paulino *et al* (2018) and Whalen *et al* (2016) may be helped by health literacy as observed in an earlier study by Singleton and Krause (2009). Singleton *et al* (2009) examining the issues of language and culture on how nurses attend to their patients note that nurses are in an ideal position to facilitate the interconnections between patient's culture, language and health literacy in order to improve health outcomes. While acknowledging the challenges, the study concluded that nurses and indeed other healthcare service providers could make a difference by working to integrate cultural, linguistic and health literacy considerations into their activities to effectively communicate with culturally diverse patients. Day (2009) advises that such health literacy approach could be through storytelling, which allows hearers to reflect on the story told and actively apply it to their life situation, thus increasing health literacy across all ages.

Safe Motherhood: Issues and Perspectives

Ensuring safe motherhood has been a major concern across many countries in the world. Although quite a lot of effort has gone into several initiatives, issues still exist that make it apparent for countries to re-strategize. Observably, safe motherhood has taken a dimension of human rights for women's health. Several non-governmental organisations, community groups and associations have continually asked questions and demand for better health care delivery for pregnant and nursing mothers including their children. It is a great challenge for the whole world to make safe motherhood a reality.

According to *Vikaspedia* (2019), safe motherhood means ensuring that all women have access to the information and services they need to go safely through pregnancy and childbirth. It includes education on safe motherhood, prenatal care (care during pregnancy) and counselling with a focus on high-risk pregnancies. It also involves the promotion of maternal nutrition, adequate delivery assistance in all cases, provisions for obstetric emergencies including referral services for pregnancy, childbirth and abortion complications and postnatal care (care after childbirth). Critical to achieving safe motherhood is antenatal care (ANC) sessions.

AbouZahr (2003) notes that the consensus on the need to reduce maternal mortality expressed at international conferences of the 1990s laid the foundation for its inclusion among the health and development priorities that have emerged at the start of the new millennium. Particularly, safe motherhood got a significant attention in 1997 at the Sri Lanka meeting. At the meeting, there was a consensus that making motherhood safer requires a full display of interventions, which include health care for women throughout pregnancy and delivery and access to skilled medical care for complications. That means governments across the world have to intensify trainings, provide facilities and formulate policies that would enhance safe motherhood in their countries.

As a follow up, in December 2000, representatives of 189 countries collectively endorsed the Millennium Declaration, which explicitly calls for improvements in maternal health and reductions in levels of maternal mortality. This global commitment has been summarized in the Millennium Development Goals (MDGs), which have been commonly accepted as a framework for measuring development progress, focusing on efforts to achieve significant, measurable improvements in people's lives, especially for the poor (AbouZahr, 2003).

Generally, reasons for maternal and child mortality and morbidity could be divided into three major categories. They are social causes, medical causes and causes related to the availability of health care facilities. Social causes include early marriage and child sex preference while medical causes include obstructed labour and hemorrhage. Causes related to the availability of healthcare facilities include lack of essential supplies and trained health personnel at the health centres, the non-sympathetic attitude of health personnel, deficient medical treatment of complications and inadequate action taken by medical personnel (*Vikaspedia*, 2019).

Studies on safe motherhood practices across different regions reinforced the essence of effective health communication. Igbokwe *et al* (2013) studied safe motherhood practices among childbearing mothers (CBMs) in Nsukka Urban of Enugu State, Nigeria, discovered that there were inadequate nutritional practices (36.4%) among CBMs in Nsukka urban areas. They also noted that immunization practices among CBMs (52.1%) in Nsukka urban were fairly adequate while the personal hygiene practices among CBMs (69.0%) in Nsukka urban were adequate. They, however, recommended that health educators, institutions and other health professionals should design better educational strategies to improve health education practices among CBMs in the area of study.

Ochonogor and Ikems (2014) investigated the attainment of safe motherhood through communication campaigns in Obio-Akpor local government area in Rivers State Nigeria and found that majority of the respondents have heard about maternal mortality and safe motherhood although many of them do not fully understand all that is required to attain it. The study identified cultural limitations and poor access to healthcare facilities as major limitations to the use of communication to drive safe motherhood practices among women. Thus, the study recommended an intensified mass media campaign and interpersonal media to entrench save motherhood practices among women. In a similar study, Merenu *et al* (2017) assessed the utilization of safe motherhood practices among women in Umuna Orlu Local Government Area of Imo State Nigeria. Their study revealed that the level of awareness of safe motherhood practice was high (94.31%) among the women.

However, the experience in Bangladesh posed a mixed feeling on the safe motherhood practice in the country. In their study, Kamal and Islam (2012) examined the relationship between receiving antenatal care (ANC) service, seeking assistance from skilled birth attendants (SBA) and use of medical facility place for childbirth and socioeconomic and demographic factors in safe motherhood practices in Bangladesh. Using the Bangladesh Demographic and Health Surveys (BDHSs) conducted during

1993-2007; the study noted that there was a poor utilization of maternal health care services in Bangladesh. Half of the women still do not receive ANC services while they engaged in unsafe childbirth with unskilled and traditional birth attendance as they neglected the primary healthcare centres. The study thus recommended enhanced by information, education and communication (IEC) programme among the women to promote safe motherhood practices in Bangladesh.

In a related study on safe motherhood practices in Dalit, Nepal, Prasad (2012) found that illiteracy, low socioeconomic condition, lack of awareness about proper age of marriage and first pregnancy were major factors accountable for the poor safe motherhood practice in the Dalit community. Most of the respondents simply ignore safe motherhood practices like a proper antenatal checkup, administering T.T. vaccine and folic acid tablets during pregnancy despite being available at the health service facilities. Unsafe home delivery practice was prevalent in the community, which include the use of an unsterile instrument to cut the umbilical cord. Most of the respondents were not taking proper postnatal service and whereas most of the mothers stopped breastfeeding their babies within one year due to next pregnancy and insufficient milk production. Consequently, it was recommended that concerned authority and health service providers should be organized to espouse the dangers of these unsafe practices among the mothers to include pregnancy and childcare.

As a rule for safe motherhood practices, Gay *et al* (2003) stated that health education is effective in improving the numbers of women who seek skilled attendance with lower rates of stillbirths and neonatal deaths. In line with the principle of gender balance, the study proposed that both men women should be involved in education on safe motherhood practices to ensure full compliance. The authors posited that educating male partners and family members concerning safe motherhood improve ANC attendance and maternal health outcomes. Therefore, it may be concluded that safe motherhood has since seized to be an issue for women only but a socio-economic, socio-political and socio-cultural issue that must be focused by everyone that matters to achieve positive health behaviour in this regard.

METHOD

This paper adopted a qualitative method using an in-depth interview (IDI) with an interview guide and non-participant observation. An in-depth interview helps a researcher to deeply explore perspectives of respondents on a particular idea, programme or situation. It is useful in getting detailed information about a person's thoughts and behaviours, explore new issues in depth while creating a holistic understanding of the interviewee's point of view on such issues and identify interesting areas for further investigation (Ogunyombo and Azeez, 2018). In observation, the researcher is better able to understand and capture the context within which people interact, as the setting helps the researcher reduce guessing what the context is like. In observation, the researcher may see things that routinely escape awareness of the participant using a different method while there are chances to learn things that people may be unwilling to discuss in an interview (Bryant, 2015). Consequently, these two methods serve a complementary purpose in this study.

Due to the time constraint and the highly dispersed nature of the different general hospitals and primary health care centres, the convenience sampling technique was used in selecting the general hospitals and primary health care centres used in this study. Convenience sampling is a sampling technique for drawing representative data by selecting people because of the ease of their volunteering or selecting units because of their availability or easy access to help with the ease of data gathering (Business Dictionary, 2017). The hospitals selected for the study were: Ifako-Ijaye General Hospital, Meiran Flagship Primary Healthcare Centre, Asiwaju Bola Ahmed Tinubu Comprehensive Primary Healthcare Centre, Rauf Aregbesola Flagship Primary Healthcare Centre and the Orile Agege General Hospital.

In addition, purposive sampling was used in selecting the five (5) respondents for this study. Tongco, cited in Talabi, Ogundeji and Adedowole (2016) stated that purposive sampling is the most effective when studying certain cultural domain where knowledgeable experts are involved. By the nature of their training, nurses including midwives in general hospitals and primary health care centres are trained on providing health information to pregnant and nursing mothers during ante/prenatal sessions. They are trained in using appropriate mode and approaches in health communication particularly safe motherhood practices. The respondents have been pseudo named ANC1, ANC2, ANC3, ANC4 and ANC5.

In line with the research questions, thematic analysis was used in analysing the data generated from the respondents. In a thematic analysis, Anderson (cited in Meribe and Oke, 2017) stated that the researcher groups and distils from the texts a list of common themes in order to give expression to the community of voices across participants.

The purpose of thematic analysis is to identify patterns of meaning across a dataset that provide an answer to the research question being addressed. Patterns are identified through a rigorous process of data familiarisation, data coding, and theme development and revision. Thematic analysis is theoretically flexible. This means it can be used within different frameworks, to answer different types of research question. It suits questions related to people's experiences, or people's views and perceptions (The University of Auckland, 2018)

FINDINGS

The demographic analysis of the interviewees shows that all the respondents were females. They were all trained nurses. The average year of experience is 16, the highest been 34 while the lowest is 4 years.

Research Question 1: What factors influence the choice of indigenous languages by health workers during pre/antenatal sessions?

The language choice of the mothers and quest for understanding among them influences the use of indigenous language

All the respondents explained that in choosing the language of communication during the pre/antenatal sessions, they ask the mothers that are present to determine which language they want. Although the English language is the official language of communication, they sometimes still give the mothers options particularly when they observe the demography by registration and the common language of communication among the mothers. For instance, ANC1 stated that "the quest to have everyone understand the things we are saying makes us to use both languages (i.e. English and Yoruba). Our desire is for the mothers to practice whatever we told them to do to ensure safe delivery and good health for them and their children. Hence we must speak the language they understand". ANC2 added that "most times we ask about if they understand English or Yoruba. Most of them usually pick Yoruba. However, we sometimes speak the English language first and then translate into the Yoruba language. There is no way you will not have people with differences. So, we are compelled to drive at them understanding whatever we are saying because we need feedback from them. We recap in the Yoruba language for easy understanding." Where the concerned mothers do not understand the Yoruba language, the respondents stated that they seek for interpreters among the members of staff or they request that the husbands, who may understand a bit of English language to translate to the mothers.

As observed across the five healthcare centres, the claims of the nurses were reflected in their approaches to choosing the language of communication. For example, at Ifako-Ijaye General Hospital, the nurse after welcoming everyone in the English language switched to the Yoruba language with the introduction that "*fun awon ti ko gbo ede oyinbo ti a n so, …*" (meaning: for those who do not understand the English Language). At Meiran PHC, the nurse specifically asked: "*se e fe kin so ni ede Yoruba?*" (meaning: do you want me to explain in the Yoruba language?). It was observed that quite a number of the mothers said yes. At the Orile Agege General Hospital, it was observed that the request for the nurses to speak in the Yoruba language started like 'murmuring' which the mothers later voiced out that "*e ba wa so lede Yoruba ooo*" (meaning: please help us explain in the Yoruba language).

Thus, it may be concluded that the choice of indigenous languages is to serve as a compliment and drive understanding among the mothers on safe motherhood practices. However, the choice may be as decided by the healthcare providers or requested by the mothers at the ANC sessions.

Research Question 2: Which mode (talks, songs, drama) of indigenous language engagement do health workers and mothers found most effective during pre/antenatal sessions?

Songs are the most effective mode of indigenous language engagement during pre/antenatal sessions for the mothers and health workers.

Concerning the most effective mode of engagement using indigenous language during pre/antenatal, three (ANC1, ANC 3, and ANC5) out of the five respondents agreed that the use of songs has been the most effective when indigenous languages are been engaged during antenatal/prenatal sessions. They agreed that the songs help a lot with retention and recall because the mothers freely sing, even without been prompted. ANC2 stated that the talk is the most effective while ANC5 choose both the songs and talks. However, they all agreed that at some point, they mix the modes based on situations at hand.

On reasons they found the songs most effective, the respondents were unanimous on their assertion that the lyrics of the songs are usually words of prayers, which most times are better expressed in the Yoruba language. With the lyrics, the mothers are emotionally connected to the reality- that they would have a safe delivery. Some of the lyrics also include prayers for their husbands and the entire family for prosperity, good health and long life to take care of their children.

For instance, ANC1 stated that "Our mothers love the songs because the songs are very funny. Sometimes, they request for the songs themselves, particularly when they feel the talks are getting long, although such feelings have to do with their mood, which may be dictated by the pregnancy hormones. The songs help them retain some of the messages and they can easily remember the lyrics even when they cannot remember the main topic of discussion for the day". ANC3 agreed that "the song helps the mothers demonstrate, for instance, how they should carry their babies when feeding. The songs are also full of prayers that they all seek. The song really helps them to understand more and participate in ANC activities. We make deliberate efforts to embed quite a lot of safe motherhood messages in the songs". ANC4 added that "songs in the Yoruba language are more efficient although I inculcate the three modes. When singing, we demonstrate how to carry the baby. We make the "*shaky shaky mother*" (meaning: an apprehensive mother) jokes when singing so that we can allay the fears of mothers who might be worried on how to take care of their babies, particularly the first-timers. While singing, we also dramatise. So the most preferred are singing and dramatizing".

Songs serve as means of motivation and create emotional connections for the mothers

Still using the songs as a means of motivation, ANC5 explained "I encourage participation through songs. For instance, I reward any of the mothers that dance well by attending to them first. That makes them commit to listening to the songs and dramatise what we are discussing. The songs are sometimes in form of prayers, while others are messages, particularly on personal and environmental hygiene during pregnancy and after childbirth".

In addition, ANC4 gave an example of the song in the Yoruba language as follows:

"Maa f'omo mi lo yan mu, la siko. Ma f'omo mi loyan mu la si ko. Ee mi n'fa lafia f'omo mi, ma f'omo mi lo yan mu lasiko". (meaning: I will breastfeed my child on time. (x2) I want good health for my child so I will breastfeed my child at the right time)

As observed at the Rauf Aregbesola Flagship Primary Healthcare Centre, the mothers at the ANC session were very jubilant when singing the song expressed above. Mothers with their babies held them close very close to their bosom as if in unisons with the wordings of the songs. However, it was also observed that mothers who could not speak the Yoruba language make efforts to dance even with their limited knowledge of the language. In order to cater to this gap, nurses at the session gave a summary of the songs at the conclusion.

Consequently, it may be deduced that songs in indigenous languages help facilitate the participation of mothers during ANC sessions. Songs as a mode of indigenous language engagement motivate mothers to connect with the essence of safe motherhood during and after childbirth and the wordings of the songs creates emotional connections, most times inform of prayers, between the mother and the born or unborn child. Although talks and dramas are regularly mixed during the sessions, songs create more opportunities for participation during the ANC sessions.

Research Question 3: How do indigenous languages influence the reception of safe motherhood messages among mothers during pre/antenatal sessions?

Indigenous languages build self-esteem, trust, creates the spirit of inclusiveness and aid reception of safe motherhood messages among mothers during ANC sessions

Reviewing the influence of indigenous languages on the reception of safe motherhood messages during ANC sessions, the respondents agreed that indigenous languages aid the reception of health talks during the ANC sessions. They agreed that although the common indigenous language by territory in Lagos state is the Yoruba language, mothers who cannot speak the Yoruba language feel very comfortable and relaxed whenever they get to converse in their indigenous language. The use of indigenous language helps build self-esteem among mothers because they "feel among and honoured".

For instance, ANC2 stated that "speaking in their own (mothers) language makes them listen. When we speak in their indigenous languages, the mothers, particularly those that do not understand the English language, do not feel inferior because they can express themselves. Using the Yoruba language makes the mothers have high esteem and they feel good expressing themselves. This is particularly important to us because the feedback from the mothers are very essential in catering for their maternal health. Because we ask questions in the language they understand well, they always want to come back to us because we have established a relationship that is based on trust". ANC1 added that "They (mothers) love it (indigenous languages). They love the fact of inclusiveness that the Yoruba language brings. When we speak, they feel appreciated and they demonstrate their understanding by kind of questions that they ask". ANC4 reiterated that "we use the Yoruba language a lot for one-on-one counselling with mothers particularly those who come for family planning programmes. Because we discovered that at that time, the discussion needs to be sincere, even for those who understand the English language, we still use the Yoruba language to drive home certain points which we fill will help the mothers better in taking care of themselves and their children". Generally, ANC5 confirmed that with indigenous languages, "They (the mothers) understand your health talks because you have come down to their levels".

As observed during the ANC sessions, some of the mothers asked questions in the Yoruba language which the nurses answered. Among the mothers, it was also observed that they served as interpreters among themselves. For instance, when certain things are said in the English language, a mother who may not be paying attention or do not understand asked the person beside her, and she explains.

From these findings, it can be deduced that indigenous languages help to drive participation and reception of safe motherhood messages because it builds self-esteem among the mothers, in terms of opportunities to express themselves during the ANC sessions. The use of indigenous reduces the inferior complex among mothers, breaking the 'elitist boundaries' because the safe motherhood messages have been brought to the level of all the mothers present.

Research Question 4: How do mothers demonstrate their understanding of safe motherhood practices using indigenous languages during the pre/antenatal sessions?

Mothers show understanding of safe motherhood through questions, answers and demonstration of lessons learnt

Respondents in the study explained that they deliberately devise a monitoring and assessment mechanism largely in the form of question and answer sessions. They also sometimes use the mothers as agents of information reinforcement among themselves. For instance, when a particular mother asks a question based on the health talks, they ask another mother who understand the language to explain what has been said to the person who asks the questions. Based on the answers provided by the identified mother, the nurses provide clarifications where necessary and ensure that the right information is passed.

Mothers demonstrate their knowledge by serving as agents of information reinforcement among themselves

Explaining the process, ANC1 said that "we ask questions after talks in both indigenous language and English language. Most of the mothers get the questions right because the sessions are usually lively. We are very concerned about how the pregnant women conduct themselves when they get to the labour room, hence, we sometimes tell them to demonstrate positions and actions and they do so". ANC3 added that "when the mothers come in for ANC sessions, we first ask them to do a recap of the last session. To this end, we encourage the mothers to be regular as the ANC sessions. When a mother fails to remember what was discussed, any of her colleagues will be asked to explain thereby serving as an agent of information reinforcement. This is done both in indigenous languages and the English language".

Observations at Rauf Aregbesola Flagship PHC and Ifako Ijaye General Hospital reflected the assertions of the respondents. For instance, when the nurses asked questions in the English language, some of the mothers who answered chose to answer in the Yoruba language. It may be assumed that the mothers simply feel that expressing themselves in the Yoruba language will help them to adequately and sufficiently convey their understanding of the subject matter. A mother at the Orile-Agege General Hospital was asked to explain a term in the Yoruba language to her colleague who appears "nonchalant" about the health talk as given earlier. Afterwards, the nurses asked the defaulting mother to repeat what the other person said to serve as confirmation. Thus, it can be concluded that questions, answers and practical demonstration of aspects of the health talks during ANC sessions reflect the level of knowledge of mothers on safe motherhood practices.

Research Question 5: What limitation do health workers and mothers encounter in using indigenous languages during pre/antenatal sessions?

The inability of nurses to speak more than one indigenous language is a major challenge during ANC sessions

Assessing the challenges with indigenous languages during ANC sessions, the respondents agreed the inability to speak other indigenous languages aside the Yoruba language presents some challenges. Ironically, where the nurse-in-charge speaks another language aside the Yoruba language, she may be challenged with explaining the talk because of the obvious majority been Yorubas.

However, the centres to some extent adopted Pidgin English in explaining the terms to the affected mothers. ANC2 confirmed that "when the person does not understand the Yoruba language or Pidgin English, we get an interpreter which most times are their husbands. A lot of time we demonstrate and breakdown the words so they can understand very well".

DISCUSSION

This study set out to explore the use of indigenous languages during pre/antenatal sessions on safe motherhood practices among mothers in general hospitals and primary healthcare centres in Lagos state. Findings from the study showed that despite the fact the hospitals are based in Lagos state, whereas the Yoruba language is the major language in the state, the use of indigenous language is not automatic during ANC sessions. At the centres visited, English language remains the primary language, however, indigenous language, particularly the Yoruba language play a major support role in delivering health talks towards safe motherhood.

The engagement of an indigenous language, particularly the Yoruba language helped the nurses at the centre address issues noticed among mothers and women. In a study conducted by Amery (2017), he discovered that the communication gap created that the lack of understanding of some terms by the indigenes resulted in poor health outcomes. For instance, the indigenes have difficulty with terms such as infection, tumour, high blood pressure, stroke and bacteria, which are often misunderstood.

General observations from the respondents and centres visited in this study demonstrated an understanding of this gap in explaining the signs of labour to the mothers. For instance, the true sign of labour called "show" or "mucus" was explained as *"ikun bii kata to wa darapo mo eje..."* (Transliteration: mucus mixed with blood). The membrane rupture (water break) was explained as *"omi ara"*. In a general discussion with some of the nursing mothers, they explained that such words and explanations sing indigenous language help them remember the signs easily.

The study also revealed that songs are a very effective mode of engaging mothers using indigenous languages. Majorly, the mothers are enticed by the words of the songs which most times are words of prayers and reassurance which to a large extent serve as a source of encouragement for the mothers to see through the process of childbearing despite the challenges. These findings are consistent with the assertions of Van Beek (2016) that the use of the native tongue is like therapy because specific native words express love and caring. Again, knowing the language presents the mothers with a strong self-identity, a culture with which they identify and a sense of wellness. This sense of self-awareness and self-esteem, influence safe motherhood practices in both the short and long term among the mothers.

Regarding the influence of indigenous languages on the reception of safe motherhood messages, it was discovered that using indigenous languages builds self-esteem, trust, creates the spirit of inclusiveness and aid reception of the messages among mothers during ANC sessions. This finding is contrary to the observations of Paulino *et al* (2018) that women who speak an indigenous language are less likely to have an institutional delivery and are more likely to attend fewer than four prenatal visits resulting into poor health outcomes. Apparently, that the nurses at the PHCs visited, brought the health talks to the "level" of the women using indigenous language may be responsible for the success, which has resulted into high self-esteem among the women. This approach is consistent with Meuter *et al* (2015) observation that clinicians should endeavour to communicate in the language that the patients understand to grow the confidence of the patients and significantly reduce the reliance of the patients on non-medical staff- a situation that may result in poor health outcomes.

In the study, songs were found to be the most effective mode of engaging with indigenous language during ANC sessions. Because the lyrics of the song confer prayers and creates an emotional connection between the mothers and the babies, most of the mothers preferred that the nurses sing songs. It was also discovered that the songs help with retention and recall of the safe motherhood message with such "inspirational" lyrics. The adoption of the songs could be regarded as an initiative to drive maternal health literacy among mothers. For example, Day (2009) advised that such health literacy approach could be through storytelling, which allows hearers to reflect on the story told and actively apply it to their life situation. While singing, the nurses dramatise the message and implored the mothers to do the same.

Generally, the knowledge of the mothers on safe motherhood is assessed during questions and answers session that takes place after the ANC talks and during one-on-one counselling between individual mothers and the nurses. Further assessment of the level of knowledge also takes place when the mothers serve as agents of information reinforcement among themselves. The nurses occasionally ask mothers to explain to each other in the language they most preferred and understand. Although the cosmopolitan nature of Lagos state meant that there is more than one language indigenous to different kind of people, the nurses make attempt to communicate effectively using indigenous languages they could communicate with, particularly the Yoruba language.

In summary, the prevalent themes as in the use of indigenous languages to safe motherhood in general hospitals and PHCs in Lagos state are that of trust, confidence, positive self-esteem and inclusiveness. The use of indigenous languages during ANC sessions encourage the participation of mothers during the sessions, knowledge sharing among mothers and serves as a solid support structure for the English language.

CONCLUSION AND RECOMMENDATIONS

It can be concluded from the study that despite the predominant nature of the Yoruba language as the indigenous language spoken in the Lagos state, the use of the language during ANC sessions is not automatic. However, when used, indigenous language, Yoruba language in this case, has been very effective in delivering safe motherhood messages to mothers during pre/antenatal sessions. The use of indigenous languages has helped to create positive self-esteem among mothers because they are able to freely express themselves based on the trust and confidence they have in the nurses who speak at their level of literacy, using the indigenous languages. It can also be concluded that songs are most effective while using indigenous languages during ANC sessions in Lagos state because it facilitates the participation of the mothers in the session and helps them with retention and recall.

Based on the foregoing, the study recommends that:

1. Healthcare professionals, particularly those in ANC should make deliberate efforts to deliver their health talks in an indigenous language that may be peculiar to their region.
2. In cosmopolitan states like Lagos, a separate session should be organized for mothers who would prefer to speak their indigenous language for a more comprehensive session.
3. Since songs were found to be most effective and encourage mothers participation during ANC sessions, more songs should be composed with lyrics that could be easily retained and recalled.
4. In states where there may be difficulties in communicating safe motherhood messages during ANC sessions, deliberate efforts can be made to compose songs in the indigenous languages peculiar to mothers in the regions. This may facilitate mothers' participation as discovered in this study.
5. To cater to the deficiencies in language, medical training institution could make the study of an indigenous language as a second language compulsory for health officers. When health professionals understand some basics of a

second language, they can use them during their initial contact with patients, build a cordial relationship, trust, and engender positive outcomes.

6. Healthcare centres may also make a deliberate effort to employ people with bilingual experience to support during the sessions.

FURTHER RESEARCH DIRECTIONS

This study focused on health care centres in Southwest Nigeria using Lagos state as the catchment area. Future studies may be replicated in other parts of Nigeria, where other indigenous languages are spoken for the purpose of generalisability or otherwise of the findings from this study. Further studies may also be explored within the context of a communication theory.

CONFLICT OF INTEREST

The authors declare that there are no conflict of interest in conducting this study.

ETHICAL CONSIDERATIONS

The authors sought permission from the Heads of the Antenatal Units of the general hospitals and the primary health care centres used in this study. The unit heads gave their consents after the authors explained the purpose of the study albeit based on condition that the data will be used strictly for the purpose of an academic study. Therefore, the consent of the participants was self-determined for all the respondents based on their agreement to participate in the study. The identity of the respondents were also anonymised as agreed between the authors and the respondents although the name of the institutions were mentioned. The authors declare that there is no financial gratification for conducting this study from any sponsor.

ACKNOWLEDGEMENT

The authors appreciate the support of all the respondents in this study, particularly the heads of the antenatal units at the PHCs and General Hospitals that were visited.

REFERENCES

AbouZahr, C. (2003). Safe Motherhood: A brief history of the global movement 1947–2002. *British Medical Bulletin, 67*(1), 13–25. doi:10.1093/bmb/ldg014 PMID:14711751

Amery, R. (2017) Recognising the communication gap in Indigenous health care. *The Medical Journal of Australia 207*(1), pp. 13-15. doi:. doi:10.5694/mja17.00042

Amuseghan, S., Ayenigbara, G., & Orimogunje, T. (2010, May). Language and health communication strategies towards effective public health communication programmes in Nigeria. *Journal Media and Communication Studies, 2*(5), 111–117. https://academicjournals.org/article/article1380097791_Amuseghan%20et%20al.pdf

Bello, S. (2014). Interrelationship of health communication, health literacy, therapeutic communication and other related concepts. *Journal of Communication and Media Research, 6*(2), 175–194.

Bryant, M. (2015). *Conducting observational research*. Retrieved from: https://www.deakin.edu.au/__data/assets/pdf_file/0004/681025/Participant-observation.pdf

Business Dictionary. (2017) *Convenience sampling*. Retrieved from: http://www.businessdictionary.com/definition/convenience-sampling.html 3/5/2017

Collins English Dictionary. *Language*. Retrieved from: https://www.collinsdictionary.com/dictionary/english/language

Day, V. (2009). Promoting health literacy through storytelling. *Online Journal of Issues in Nursing, 14*(3). Retrieved from http://ojin.nursingworld.org/MainMenuCategories/ANAMarketplace/ANAPeriodicals/OJIN/TableofContents/Vol142009/No3Sept09/Health-Literacy-Through-Storytelling.html

Encyclopedia Britannica. *Language*. Retrieved from: https://www.britannica.com/topic/language/Meaning-and-style-in-language

Encyclopedia of Communication and Information. (2002) *Health communication*. The Gale Group Inc. Retrieved from: https://www.encyclopedia.com/media/encyclopedias-almanacs-transcripts-and-maps/health-communication

Ensuring safe motherhood. (2019, April 22). *Vikaspedia*. Retrieved from: http://*Vikaspedia*.in/health/women-health/pregnancy-health-1/ensuring-safe-motherhood

European Centre for Disease Prevention and Control. (2019) *What is health communication?* Retrieved from: https://ecdc.europa.eu/en/health-communication/facts

Gay, J., Hardee, K., Judice, N., Agarwal, K., Fleming, K., Hairston, A., ... Wood, M. (2003). *What works: A policy and program guide to the evidence on family planning, safe motherhood, and STI/HIV/AIDS interventions— Module 1 Safe Motherhood.* Washington: Policy Project; Retrieved from http://www.policyproject.com/pubs/generalreport/SM_WhatWorksps2.pdf

Health communication. (2010). *Healthy People* (vol. 1). Retrieved from: https://www.healthypeople.gov/2010/document/HTML/Volume1/11HealthCom.htm

Igbokwe, C., Orji, O., & Igbokwe, B. (2013). Safe motherhood practices among childbearing mothers (CBMs) in Nsukka Urban of Enugu State, Nigeria. *Journal of Applied Information Science and Technology*, *6*, 27–33. Retrieved from https://www.jaistonline.org/IgbokweOrjiIgbokwe-2k13.pdf

Kamal, S., & Islam, M. (2012) Promoting safe motherhood practices in Bangladesh: Progress and challenges. *Geneva Health Forum Archive*. Retrieved from: http://ghf.g2hp.net/2012/11/12/promoting-safe-motherhood-practices-in-bangladesh-progress-and-challenges/

Lagos State Ministry of Health. (2017). *Lagos State maternal and child mortality reduction (MCMR) Program*. Retrieved from: https://health.lagosstate.gov.ng/lagos-state-maternal-and-child-mortality-reduction-mcmr-program/

Maune, A. (2017). Indigenous knowledge intelligence and African development, In P. Ngulube (Ed.), Handbook of research on theoretical perspectives on indigenous knowledge systems in developing countries (pp. 173-197). Hershey, PA: IGI Global. doi:10.4018/978-1-5225-0833-5.ch008

Merenu, I., Diwe, K., Uwakwe, K., Duru, C., Duru, C., Iwu, A., ... Ohale, I. (2017). To assess the utilization of safe motherhood practices among women in a rural community, in Nigeria. *Unique Research Journal of Medicine and Medical Sciences*, *5*(3), 17–24.

Meribe, N., & Oke, B. (2017). Climate change reporting in Nigeria: Challenges and implications for development. *The Nigerian Journal of Communication*, *14*(1), 133–162.

Meuter, R., Gallois, C., Segalowitz, N., Ryder, A., & Hocking, J. (2015). Overcoming language barriers in healthcare: A protocol for investigating safe and effective communication when patients or clinicians use a second language. *BMC Health Services Research, 15*(1), 371. Retrieved from https://www.ncbi.nlm.nih.gov/pmc/articles/PMC4566365/pdf/12913_2015_Article_1024.pdf. doi:10.118612913-015-1024-8 PMID:26357948

National Health Service. (2017) *Your antenatal care-Your pregnancy and baby guide.* Retrieved from: https://www.nhs.uk/conditions/pregnancy-and-baby/antenatal-midwife-care-pregnant/

Ochonogor, C., & Ikems, K. (2014). Attaining safe motherhood through communication campaigns in Rivers state Nigeria. *Journal of Communication and Media Research, 6*(2), 195–210.

Ogundoyin, O., & Soola, E. (2014). Trends in methodological and theoretical approaches to interpersonal health communication research. *Journal of Communication and Media Research, 6*(2), 163–174.

Ogunyombo, O., & Azeez, O. (2018). Exploring the perspectives of selected public relations professionals on the made-in-Nigeria campaign. *Media &Communication Currents, 2*(2), 1–20.

Olúbòdé-Sàwè, F. O. (2010). Digital communication in indigenous languages. In R. Taiwo (Ed.), *Handbook of research on discourse behaviour and digital communication: Language structures and social interaction* (pp. 564–578). Hershey, PA: IGI Global; doi:10.4018/978-1-61520-773-2.ch036

Oxford Living Dictionaries. *Language*. Retrieved from: https://en.oxforddictionaries.com/definition/language

Oyero, O. (2007). Dynamics of indigenous languages in environmental communication. In I. Nwosu, & O. Soola (Eds.), *Communication in global, ICTs, and ecosystem perspectives- Insights from Nigeria*. Enugu: Precisions Publishers.

Oyesomi, K. O., & Salawu, A. (2019). Assessing the Uniqueness of Indigenous Language in Advertising: Analysis of Figurative Language Used in Selected Telecommunication Yoruba Advertisement in Nigeria. *Qualitative Report, 24*(10), 2574–2591. Retrieved from https://nsuworks.nova.edu/tqr/vol24/iss10/12

Paulino, N., Vázquez, M. & Bolúmar, F. (2018). *Indigenous language and inequitable maternal health care, Guatemala, Mexico, Peru, and the Plurinational State of Bolivia.* Geneva: World Health Organization 97: 59-67. doi: . doi:10.2471/BLT.18.216184

Prasad, S. (2012) Safe motherhood practice in Dalit community. *Academic Voices, 2*(1). Retrieved from: https://www.nepjol.info/index.php/AV/article/view/8291/6759

Singleton, K., & Krause, E. (2009). Understanding cultural and linguistic barriers to health literacy. *Online Journal of Issues in Nursing, 14*(3). Retrieved from http://ojin.nursingworld.org/MainMenuCategories/ANAMarketplace/ANAPeriodicals/OJIN/TableofContents/Vol142009/No3Sept09/Cultural-and-Linguistic-Barriers-.html

Taff, A., Chee, M., Hall, J., Hall, M., Martin, K., & Johnston, A. (2018) Indigenous language use impacts wellness, In K. Rehg, & L. Campbell (Eds.), The Oxford Handbook on Endangered Languages. Doi:10.1093/oxfordhb/9780190610029.013.41

Talabi, F., Ogundeji, B., & Adedowole, F. (2016). Influence of online editions on newspaper readership in south-western Nigeria. *Journal of Communication and Media Research, 8*(2), 141–162.

The University of Auckland. (2018). *About thematic analysis*. Retrieved from: https://www.psych.auckland.ac.nz/en/about/our-research/research-groups/thematic-analysis/about-thematic-analysis.html 11/6/2018.

Van Beek, S. (2016) *Intersections: Indigenous language, health and wellness: First peoples' cultural council deliverable for FNIS UBC Practicum 2016*. Retrieved from: http://www.fpcc.ca/files/PDF/Language/Intersections_Indigenous_Language_Health_and_Wellness_WebVersion.pdf

Whalen, D., Moss, M., & Baldwin, D. (2016). Healing through language: Positive physical health effects of indigenous language use. *F1000 Research, 5*, 852. doi:10.12688/f1000research.8656.1

World Health Organisation. (2009). *Track2: Health literacy and health behavior.* Retrieved from: https://www.who.int/healthpromotion/conferences/7gchp/track2/en/

World Health Organisation. (2016) *WHO Recommendations on Antenatal Care for a Positive Pregnancy Experience*. Retrieved from: https://www.ncbi.nlm.nih.gov/books/NBK409110/

KEY TERMS AND DEFINITIONS

Child Morbidity: This refers to the state of illness in a child, which may be due to lack or poor pre/postnatal care, a congenital condition or an accident.

Child Mortality: This refers to the state of death of a child, which may be caused by an illness, lack or poor pre/postnatal care, a congenital condition or an accident.

Health Communication: All forms of messages, written, verbal or visual that are deliberately designed to influence and stimulate behaviours that will enhance healthy living and conditions in a society.

Health Literacy: It is the basic and extensive knowledge acquired by an individual on matters relating to healthy behaviours, making positive health choices and engendering healthy living.

Information Reinforcement: The process of sharing and strengthening health information among individuals to facilitate positive health decisions.

Nursing Mother: A woman who is breastfeeding a day to two-year old child, although such care may extend beyond two years in certain conditions.

Postnatal Care: It is the continuation of care given to pregnant women from pregnancy up until the first eight weeks after childbirth.

Pre/Antenatal Care: The care given to pregnant women during pregnancy by health care providers at a recognised health centre. It involves giving routine health talks, information, guidance and conducting routine health checks on the pregnant women to ensure that the mother and the unborn child are in good health, and mitigate or reduce potential medical challenges that may impede safe delivery for the mother and child.

Primary Healthcare Centres: These are healthcare facilities provided by the state and federal government to cater and provide quick and easy access to healthcare services for people at the grassroots.

Public Health: The organized efforts to achieve wellbeing among the people by promoting healthy living through health education and literacy largely facilitated by government regulations and policies.

Safe Motherhood: These are all activities, programmes, campaign and communication purposely designed to provide mothers with relevant information to guide them before pregnancy, during pregnancy and after childbirth and ensure the safety of the mother and child. They are all clinical activities and programmes targeted at reducing maternal and child morbidity and mortality in society.

Yoruba: A common indigenous language originally spoken by people living in south-west Nigeria.

Chapter 3
Indigenous Communication and Traditional Health Practices Among the Yoruba During Pregnancy, Child Delivery, and Baby Caring

Victor 'Tunji Taiwo
Lagos State University, Nigeria

ABSTRACT

Communication is a vital aspect of human existence. It pervades man's existence and society, forming an integral part of human life. Communication is the means through which human beings express their feelings. Indigenous communication serves as the traditional means of conveying messages, all social and value exchanges of indigenous practice like the health practices. Traditional health practices include the use of knowledge skills, practices based on indigenous belief, experiences of culture used in maintenance of health-prevention, treatment and diagnosis in traditional health practices. This chapter examines and documents traditional health practices on how Yorùbás care for pregnancy, child delivery, and their babies. Such traditional health practices have existed since before the advent of modern health practices, thereby using indigenous communication for preservation and dissemination of valuable information that is significant for Yorùbá generations.

DOI: 10.4018/978-1-7998-2091-8.ch003

INTRODUCTION

The Yoruba speaking group forms one of the prominent cultural heritage groups in present day Nigeria. As Oyesomi and Salawu (2019) note that Yoruba is one of the ethnic groups in Nigeria; it is a collection of people bound together by same language The Yoruba inhabit the south western part of Nigeria but has sizeable population in Benin Republic, Togo, Cuba, Brazil and some part of USA. They are also found in some parts of Kwara, Kogi, Edo, and Delta States within Nigeria in addition to the core Nigeria south western states like Ogun, Oyo, Osun, Ondo, Ekiti and Lagos. By virtue of its spread, the Yoruba speakers also settled in some parts of West Africa neighbouring countries like Republic of Benin, Togo, Ghana, Sierra Leone, Liberia, and Ivory Coast respectively. Speakers of the language could equally be found in places like Brazil, Cuba, United Kingdom, United States of America, Jamaica, Trinidad and Tobago (Olatunji, 2013; Makinde, 2004; Ogungbemi, 2017; Adedina and Taiwo, 2018). In this regard, the population of the Yoruba people as estimated "in West Africa is forty million. This makes them one of the largest groups in sub-Saharan Africa" (Ogungbemi, 2017, p. 309 quoted Abimbola, 2006). Nevertheless, one key feature that marks the Yoruba people is their culture and communication systems. The Yoruba people are prosperous and rich in culture and communication (Adédínà and Táíwò, 2018).

Culture is part and parcel of every individual and people in the world. Culture, according to Tylor cited in Adélékè (2003) is that complex whole which includes knowledge, belief, law, art, moral customs and other capabilities and habits acquired by man as a member of a society. Sewell Jr. (2005, p. 80) sees culture from social life perspective as the learned behaviour. In essence, it is the whole body of practices, beliefs, institutions, customs, habits, myths, and so on built up by humans and passed on from generation to generation. A fact Lewis (2012, p.34) supports when he opines that culture is the total way of a particular group of people that distinguishes them from other groups. It is the totality of what makes up the life and living styles of a group of people living in the same geographical area. Culture can be 'shared' and 'learnt' in a community as it serves as a communal property and gives its people peculiar identity (Adélékè, 2003).

Culture could be adjudged from two aspects, tangible and intangible. The tangible includes the concrete materials like wood or artefacts, tools, shelter, dress: clothing, make-up, facial marks and food. The intangible culture comprises of the non-concretes like mythology, literature (both written and oral), 'the inner' culture or 'the sacred spirit' like religion, knowledge, philosophy or beliefs of the people which are values and norms like hardworking, honesty, greeting, interaction, respect, conjugal relations inherent in individual images with symbolic nature as communication within the community or society (Irele, 1991; Adélékè, 2003 and Lawal, 2015).

It is a way of sharing knowledge and schemes designed by a group of folks for interpreting, preserving, expressing and responding to the realities that emanated with their society. Dyslva (2006, p. 4) citing Hofstede (1997) describes culture as the collective programming of the mind that distinguished the member of an organisation or country from another. He further states that culture is the cumulative deposit of knowledge, experience, beliefs, values, attitudes, meanings, hierarchies, religion, notions of time, roles, spatial relations, concepts of the universe, and material objects and possessions acquired by a group of people in the course of generations from individual and the striving group striving. In other words, the ideas, meanings, values, beliefs that people learn as members of a society determines the culture of the people. In the view of Akangbe (2008, p. 6), culture is "the summation of both individual and collective life of a society which comprises its ideas, behaviours, social, religious and political peculiarities, sentiments and expressions." Culture is connected with human cognition, that is, what people's brain identifies as their culture is also their culture. These permeate through consciousness of the people about certain things about themselves, other people, or things that are common from generation to generation.

Culture is however linked with "ancient origin", connected with art, communication, language, tribes, individuals, transmission and interactions, (Danesi and Perro, 1999, p. 3). The authors further allude to the facts:

...in the sense of individuals living together, thinking and planning consciously, transmitting skills, and systems of social relationships to each other through language, and the working together to modify the environment, has become the defining attribute of the human species. (p. 3).

Perhaps, human being is not only a cultured being, but also as a social animal. Culture has made human life possible, thereby raising human being from levels higher than animal. This means, human being cannot survive as a being without culture, because, culture is a representation of the totality of success and achievement recorded by mankind. Ultimately, culture determines the quality of a society and the inhabitant of that society as what they learn like the arts, language and manners as expressed through communication in their daily routines, particularly, through indigenous representations as form of communication.

Communication therefore becomes a vital aspect of human existence, an idea that pervades man's existence and society, which forms an integral part of human life and through which human beings express their feelings, facts, opinions, views, fears, aspirations and thoughts. Through communication, the philosophies, beliefs, cultures, value systems and societal norms are preserved, shared and transferred from generation to generation. This implies that, without communication, human beings would have experienced a lonely existence without the radiance of embellishments, and lives would have become grey without any colour. Thus, Ugboaja, (1985, p. 1) captures the essence of communication by asserting that to be is to communicate, in the absence of communication man is not different from animal that is less high in position. He further maintains that outside communication men will cease to exist as social creatures because communication is a social relations affair. In consonance with the assertion, communication serves as one of those everyday activities that human beings engage in for societal development through social interactions. It is linked closely with all of human life so complex that we sometimes overlook its perverseness, importance, and complexity." Communication is central to human life. Every aspect of our daily lives is affected by our communication with others, as well as by messages from people we don't even know, people near and far, living and dead" (Littlejohn & Fuson, 2008; p. 2). In this way, Ọlábímtán, (1999) also stated that "communication itself is terminus," that is, there cannot be meaningful life without communication. Apparently, communication involves interactions between two or more people, animate or inanimate and systems. The perception from the foregoing indicates that communication is a process, particularly, indigenous communication. This chapter centres on indigenous communication and traditional health practices among the Yoruba during pregnancy caring, child delivery and baby caring before contemporary period.

CONCEPTUAL CLARIFICATIONS

Indigenous Communication

Indigenous communication refers to the informal means of disseminating or transferring indigenous practices, entertainment, persuasion, announcement, news, and social exchange of all kinds like health issues (Kiptiness, 2019; Agyepong, 2017). It is also an essential facet of culture and mode communication through which a culture is safeguarded, transformed, and passed down from one generation to the other. Oyèsomí, Sàláwù and Ọlọ́runyọmí (2017) posit that "indigenous communication enjoys high credibility because it is familiar and controlled locally" (p. 165). Hence, indigenous communications become basic needed components of the socio-cultural tradition peculiar to the people of Africa. It serves the purpose of transferring information and effective messages clearly to a group of people who reside in the within the locality. It is simplistic and basic in nature with the use of indigenous language. Events on situations as emotional appeals can be communicated to the people living in a particular local society using traditional communication system in line with their beliefs for them to have better understanding.

In addition, indigenous communication system in local areas can be used to convey positive messages as well as communicate more serious issues, such as problems that exist in the locality. Indigenous communication system is sometimes used to provide local populations with a source of entertainment, but it is also used as a tool to encourage people to examine their personal behaviours and make changes to their behaviours and attitudes as necessary, particularly as it concerns their health practices. Regardless of whether they are sad, funny, long, short or dramatic, indigenous communication systems are generally used to create popular events for people of the community or society, these events typically attracts no financial benefits, because of the their culture. It also reflects on their traditional health practices such.

Health Practices and Traditional Health Practices

Conventionally, health means the state of being free from illness or injury. This is in accordance with the position of the World Health Organisation (WHO) (1948) in which it describes health as the state of complete physical, mental, and social well-being and not merely the absence of diseases or infirmly. Svalastog, Donev and Gajovic (2017) capture the essence of health by asserting that health is a relative state in which an individual is to function well physically, mentally, socially and spiritually. The authors add that health could also be a means of expressing one's unique potential within the environment in which one lives. Therefore, this chapter, while aligning with the above submissions, notes that health could be referred to as the ability to adapt and manage physical, mental, and social challenges through life. In order words, the ability to manage the state or situation of health of every individual or group depends solely on the level of health practices put in place.

Health practice rest mainly on personal ability with coping skills involving series of actions taking by every person to prevent diseases and promote self-care, cope with challenges, and develop self-reliance, solve problems and make choices that enhances health. This can also influence the social, economic and environmental factors that inform any health decision. However, the positive achievements recorded through health practices depend on the degree of health communication. Health communication brings the patient and the health experts together. It serves as a link, thereby sensitising the patient (public). It equally fosters on the relationship between the health professionals and the patients regarding health information.

At the local level, indigenous communication becomes more essential as a means of relating and conveying health information to the people of a particular community or society. Indigenous/traditional health practice is the overall of the skills and knowledge, involving the practices based on the theories, beliefs, philosophies and cultural experiences, whether understandable or not, utilized for the upkeep and nurturing of one's health (WHO, 2008). Its use also entails diagnosis, prevention, treatment or improvement of mental and physical sickness. The traditional beliefs of the community members have deep-rooted in traditional health practices. Such traditional beliefs also have control over the kinds of food they eat and the medicines taking when experiencing any form of ill-health.

The Encyclopaedia of Public Health (2002) identifies three categories of traditional health practices that are typical to every local community. These include the beliefs that result in no harmful health effects; the beliefs that may produce beneficial health outcomes; and the beliefs and traditions, which have serious harmful health outcomes. Virtually every society engages in traditional health practices. For instance, acupuncture has been proof effective in relieving all kinds of pain disorders, high blood pressure, depression and morning indisposition. Same way the traditional Chinese herb *Artemisia annua* has been tested to be efficacious for the cure of malaria. In Yorùbá socio-cultural context, there exist traditional health practices.

Yorùbá Traditional Health Practices and Its Distinctive Identity

Yorùbá traditional health practice involves the use of native knowledge, and skills which entails traditional philosophies, belief system and indigenous experiences for the maintenance of the ill-health. The Yorùbá traditional health practices further include the use of traditional *ifá* geomantic codes to diagnose the nature of the sickness which may involve atonement *(ètùtù)*, certain sacrifices *(ẹbọ),* as may be directed by the *ifá* oracle through a diviner *(babaláwo)* (Jẹ́gẹ́dẹ́, 2002), herbalist *(oníṣègùn ìbílẹ̀)* or native doctor *(oníṣègùn agbẹ̀bí)*. In essence, these traditional practices are used to prevent and treat any form of sickness and improve the state of health of the patients within the Yorùbá milieu.

Yorùbá traditional health practice involves the use of native knowledge, and skills which entails traditional philosophies, belief system and indigenous experiences for the maintenance of the ill-health. According to Bọ̀rọ̀kìní and Lawal (2014) traditional medicine referrers as the alternative or non-conventional modes of treatment often involving the use of herbs in non-orthodox manner as well as consulting herbalists, medium, priests, witch doctors, and various local deities when seeking solution to divers' illnesses. In this regard, series of indigenous herbal medicine adopted for traditional health practices comprises of spiritual therapies, bone settings, psychiatric care, music therapy, massage therapy, circumcision care, maternity care and pregnancy care as the focus of this chapter to mention few. The traditional health professional within the Yorùbá society are recognised by the dwellers of the Yorùbá community. They utilize animals and their parts, leafs and roots of various kinds, natural resources of various substances and some other methodology associated with socio-religious, cultural knowledge, beliefs, skills and attitudes that are popular within the milieu.

From time immemorial, the Yorùbá had put in place a well-defined structure of indigenous communication that enhances traditional health practices system through which they were able to take good care of themselves. They also use this structure to create good co-existence among themselves regarding cultural values and relationship that exist between them and the traditional health healers or professionals. Before now, these acts were put to play at local levels, particularly, during pregnancy period, child delivery and baby caring as practices that were prevalent in time past (Bọ̀rọ̀kìní and Lawal, 2014).

Uses of Indigenous Communication During Pregnancy Caring: Yoruba Traditional Practices

Confirmation that a woman is pregnant can be ascertained when such woman misses her menstruation *(nǹkan oṣù)*. Menstruation being the period or monthly health practices of activities peculiar to women involves the process of regular discharge of blood and other materials from the inner lining of uterus via the female organ, the vagina. It is also the preparation of woman's body for pregnancy (Mtawali, Pina, Angle and Murphy, 1997). In essence, this makes pregnancy possible throughout the course of the woman's reproductive period, that is, from puberty to menopause stages. In order words, when such woman observes sexual intercourse with her male counterparts, she will be pregnant. This act is prevalent in every society.

In Yoruba society in time past, before a woman conceives, the husband did search for a native herbalist *(oníṣègùn ìbílẹ̀/agbẹ̀bí)*. This enhanced the curiosity and agitation during delivery. Early in the morning, the husband to the pregnant woman did visit the *(oníṣègùn ìbìlẹ̀/agbẹ̀bí)* with wrapped parcel of colanut *(obì)* and a full gourd of palmwine *(akeègbè ẹmu kan)*. These items were used to appease the gods as the pregnant woman would be handed over to the herbalist for intensive caring until she delivers. The reason for this act mainly was to help in tying the pregnancy *(dide oyun)* traditionally as a way of preventing miscarriage. The *(oníṣègùn ìbílẹ̀/agbẹ̀bí)* will assure the husband of the pregnant woman, and then communicate through prayers in indigenous language, thereby using the items – *(obì)* colanut and *(ẹmu)* palmwine - as symbolic traditional significations. The *(oníṣègùn ìbílẹ̀/agbẹ̀bí)* further refers to *Ọ̀sanyìn* the gods as a way of invocation for spiritual involvement to succeed. The herbalist will divide a colanut *(obì)* into four pieces. He then dialled the colanut as *ifá* geomantic code of ritual expression. If two out of the four pieces of the colanut face upwardly and the other two downwardly, traditionally, it signifies that there wouldn't be any form of problem. On the contrary, if the dialled colanuts fail to turn appropriately, even after several efforts, the *oníṣègùn ìbílẹ̀/agbẹ̀bí* would try to find out the likely root course before embarking on the pregnancy caring process. In doing so, some indigenous rituals *(ètò)* of sacrifice *(ẹbọ)* and atonements *(ètùtù)* would be carried out to appease the possible angry spirit and to avert any negative affliction on the pregnant woman as part of indigenous and traditional health practices.

In addition, tying of pregnancy *(díde oyún)* becomes another significant indigenous/ traditional health practices in Yoruba society before this contemporary time. It is evident in Yorùbá beliefs that until the Due Date of Delivery (DDD), and untied the pregnancy, the pregnant woman would not experience any form of miscarriage or premature. On this note, the *onísègùn ìbílẹ̀* could confidently communicate in indigenous language that *"bí àfọ̀n kò bá gbó, kì í wọ̀"* meaning that "if the 'treculia' African breadfruit does not reach the period of endowment, it does not fall from the tree". Indigenous/traditional health practices of tying of pregnancy can be done in three interrelated ways (Dáramọ̀lá and Jẹ̀jẹ̀, 1975; Ọlájùbù, 1978). It is pertinent to point out that this particular way of indigenous tying of pregnancy from which an aspect is being analysed is only one out of other ways. There are other indigenous ways of tying pregnancy, but in this chapter, we shall limit our discussion to one out of three ways. Below is a sample of indigenous/traditional health practice of tying pregnancy.

Indigenously, the *onísègùn ìbílẹ̀* will get a raw egg of local fowl *(ẹyin adìẹ ìbílẹ̀)*, with some other necessary roots of trees, pounded. He then rubs the pounded roots of trees round the raw egg and allows it to dry. After that, the pregnant woman would appear naked as the *onísègùn ìbílẹ̀* will rub the pregnancy from downward abdomen side of the pregnant woman upward. The *onísègùn ìbílẹ̀* did then dig a small hole closed to the wall of the house and gently put the egg inside the hole and cover it up. It then becomes important for the *onísègùn ìbílẹ̀* to put a sign to indicate the exact point with canwood *osùn* or local chalk *ẹ́fun*. The reason for this was to avoid any form of mistake of identity because the *onísègùn ìbílẹ̀* could be having more patients that he was attending to at the same time as he begins to count months. In the process, the pregnant woman begins to tell the *onísègùn ìbílẹ̀* as she observes any strange feelings as the native herbalist diagnosis by consulting *ifa* divination for solutions. When the month completes, the *onísègùn ìbílẹ̀* goes to the point where he kept the egg, brings it out and rubs it from the upper part of the pregnancy downward to the abdomen of the pregnant woman. Shortly, the pregnant woman begins to labour and eventually delivers the child (Dáramọ̀lá and Jẹ̀jẹ̀, 1975).

Uses of Indigenous Communication During Child Delivery: Yoruba Traditional Practices

Indigenous rite of passage involves the transformation from one situation to another, particularly, child delivery. Child delivery marks the end of pregnancy period experienced or carried by a woman. It is a passage of transformation when a baby leaves the woman's uterus thereby passing through the female organ, the vagina.

Sometimes, it could be through caesareans section. Caesarean section is such a contemporary health practice that involves surgery to deliver the baby. In addition, referral to as caesarean delivery occurs when the female organ, the vagina would cause danger to the life of the baby or the mother.

In Yoruba socio-cultural society, such indigenous communication and traditional health practices of child delivery differ. The moment the pregnant woman begins to observe the feelings of labour, thereby feeling pains below her abdomen, stomach and back pains, she voices out to the older women around her or to the *oníṣègùn ìbílẹ̀/agbẹ̀bí*. At that moment, the older women will confirm from her to know whether the pregnancy was tied and the exact point where it was kept. In the case of the *oníṣègùn ìbílẹ̀/agbẹ̀bí* being the one who is handling it directly, will go straight to where the items used in tying the pregnancy (raw egg) prepared with other traditional herbal medicines were kept. The reason for this was to first untie the traditionally tied pregnancy before embarking of the delivery process. Having done this, the women will position themselves, one of the women at the head side and one at the leg side expecting the sign of water in a skinning intestine sack to break through the female organ. However, in the case of complication that could delay a woman during child delivery, there could be use of indigenous communication of verbal arts like *ọfọ̀* (incantation). At this point, seven seeds of *ataare* (alligator pepper) would be chewed by the *oníṣègùn ìbílẹ̀/agbẹ̀bí* or the traditional midwife nurse, sprinkle on the woman's head, with one of her legs raised.

In addition, *àwẹ̀bí* the spiritual bathing of delivery is equally an essential indigenous/traditional health practices in Yoruba context of pregnancy caring. When the native doctor *oníṣègùn ìbílẹ̀/agbẹ̀bí* realises that the child delivery was taking longer than expected, he engages in preparation of traditional herbs that include roots of trees and a raw egg of local fowl boiled together. Having boiled these items, the *oníṣègùn ìbílẹ̀/agbẹ̀bí* will dig a hole of about 3feet by 3width at a secluded place or the back of the house that could accommodate human being in standing position. The pregnant woman will stand in the hole as directed by the *oníṣègùn ìbílẹ̀/agbẹ̀bí*, while the boiled egg will be unshelled for her to eat. After this, the pregnant woman will carry an empty basket on her head, and the *oníṣègùn ìbílẹ̀/agbẹ̀bí* begins to purr the boiled liquid herb into the basket for the pregnant woman to bath. This signifies the removal of unclean stigmatisation on the body of the pregnant woman. The remnant from the boiled roots of trees and the shell of the egg will be kept safe for further use. In a short time after all this traditional rituals, the pregnant woman begins to labour. The first thing that comes out of the pregnant woman's body will be water (known as rupture of the membrane of water break), followed by blood. At that point, the pregnant woman begins panting from lower concentration to the higher concentration, heavily. By so doing, the baby begins to come out gradually with the head. In some cases, a child under delivery may come with the hand or leg which is dangerous to the life of the mother. In a situation like that, the *onísègùn ìbílè/agbèbí* will embark on traditional use of indigenous power of incantation *(ọfọ̀)*, the power of words will put the baby in appropriate position. This signifies efficacy in the act of indigenous beliefs.

Uses of Indigenous Communication During Baby Caring Period: Yoruba Traditional Practices

Caring for new born baby is referred to as care that is given to the newborn infant immediately after delivery. In traditional context, particularly, Yoruba socio-cultural setting, the indigenous practices for taking care of a newborn baby begins the moment the baby is delivered. When a baby is delivered, instantly, the *oníṣègùn ìbílẹ̀/agbẹ̀bí* sprinkles palmoil *(epo-pupa)* on the floor of the delivery portion as part of the traditional health practices and belief systems. This signifies *ẹ̀rọ̀* (a traditional first aid to counter any misfortune that might have come suddenly).

More so, expectations will be high when the placenta of the baby is yet to come out after delivery. In a situation of such difficulties, the *oníṣègùn ìbílẹ̀/agbẹ̀bí* begins to incarnate *(p'ọfọ)*`in order to command it out. When the placenta comes out, it will be promptly taken care of, and ensure that it is not eaten by a dog. It is traditionally believed that if a dog have access to a placenta and probably eats it, the child who owns the placenta may be afflicted with lifelong misfortunes.

In Yorùbá health practices, the use of hot water from boiled herbs becomes necessary for bathing the baby with black soap and sponge being the first bathing. The bathing would have to be done by an elderly woman who will bath the baby very well and wash any form of mucus on the baby's body to avoid unpleasant odour in future. Táíwò (2019) refers to such significant bathing as a ritual bathing/washing of removing the spiritual blemishes or stigmatisations that would hinder the baby's fortunes in life. Therefore, bathing of the newborn baby is a symbolic signification of acceptance into the family and freshness after birth. The baby is rubbed with canwood *(osùn)* (local cream) and wrapped with wool clothing to keep the body warm as part of indigenous adornment associated with traditional health practices.

Similarly, indigenous/traditional health practices in line with the Yoruba beliefs take the issues of navel caring seriously. Immediately the baby is delivered and placenta is removed, the *oníṣègùn ìbílẹ̀/agbẹ̀bí* will cut the umbilical cord binding the baby and placenta together. After cutting, the navel of the new baby will be wrapped with cotton-wool as they begin to press it every day with pieces of cloth placed on broken pieces of local clay pot. This is done by placing it on the lump of clay set to support a vessel over a fire. The heat energy derived from the cloth is used to press the navel *(tẹ ìwọ́)*. Seven days of consistent pressing of the navel, the remaining small cord attached to the navel will fall off and will be buried. At this point, the mother of the baby will have to continue to press the navel to enable it heal very well. Failure to do so may lead to serious danger in future.

The Yoruba traditional health practices uphold indigenous belief and philosophy of feeding a baby with local herbs. Such practices were prevalent in Yoruba society with various traditional herbs for use. Dáramọ̀lá and Jẹ́jẹ́ (1975) identify such indigenous/traditional herbs that are essential for treating baby's sickness as parts of traditional health practices among the Yorubas. These include:

- **Àgbo Jẹ̀díjẹ̀dí (A Phytomedicine for Dysentery):** An infection of the intestines resulting in severe diarrhoea with possible presence of blood and mucus in the faeces. It occurs when faeces from the baby seized and the baby begins to fart at frequent intervals. Such baby will be given the herb for dysentery.
- **Àgbo Joríjorí/Làpálàpá (A Phytomedicine for Ringworm):** It is a contagious itching skin/head disease caused by any of a number of fungi affecting the scalp of the head or other part of the body. In this situation, when a baby is experiencing such disease that affects the hair, head and body, thereby putting division of mark lines on the baby's head, itching and others, the Yoruba traditional health practice permits preparation of special herbs for such disease. As the baby feeds on the herb by drinking and bathing, the disease will be cleared and the baby's body will be refreshed.
- **Àgbo Gìrì (A Phytomedicine for Convulsion):** It is a sudden or irregular movement of the body, cause by involuntary contradiction of muscles like epilepsy or fever in children. They begin to attack these diseases from childhood by preparing traditional herbs to cure it as part of Yoruba traditional health practices.
- **Àgbo Ehín (A Phytomedicine for Teething):** Teething is the process of growing or cutting milk teeth. In this regard, when a baby clocks two or three months, the mother begins to feed the infant with phytomedicine for teething. It also involves the use of traditional teething soap for bathing the baby to manage the challenges such as fever, stooling etc by the bay while growing the teeth.

Virtually all diseases that affect a baby involve traditional healing with the use of herbs for curing illnesses like cough, fever, stomach upset, and diarrhoea to mention few.

CONCLUSION

This chapter has been able to take a look at indigenous communication and traditional health practices that is prevalent among the Yorùbás in South-West Nigeria before modern medicine. It explores the existing traditional beliefs and philosophies in the Yorùbá environment concerning the use of indigenous language for effective communication. It places premium on the nature of Yorùbá culture and communication; its distinctive identities with utmost concentrations on the uses of indigenous communication during pregnancy, during child delivery and caring for the baby after birth.

DIRECTIONS FOR FURTHER STUDIES

Since the present article has established the interest of indigenous communication and traditional health practices, with focus on Yoruba society during pregnancy, child delivery and baby caring, it will be interesting if further researchers in this field concentrate on indigenous communication and traditional health practices and possibly carry out a study on existence of such practices in this contemporary time.

CONFLICT OF INTEREST

The author make known that this paper does not have any form of conflict of interest.

ACKNOWLEDGEMENT

The author acknowledges the intellectual works of the authors used and cited in this article as their input and involvement towards socio-cultural development of the people.

REFERENCES

Abimbola, K. (2006). *Yoruba Culture: A Philosophical Account*. Birmingham: Iroko Academic Publishers.

Adedina, F., & Taiwo, V. (2018). Ẹkun-ìyàwo: An Aesthetical Appraisal of Nuptial Chants in Yoruba Folklore. *Journal of Communication and Media Research, 10*(2), 161–173.

Adeleke, D. A. (2003). Culture, Art and Film in an African Society: An Evaluation. *Nordic Journal of African Studies, 12*(1), 49–56.

Agyepong, A. O. (2017). "International Communication: A Narrative of Selected Indigenous Practices of the Akan Group of Ghana" in Handbook of Research on Theoretical Perspectives on Indigenous Knowledge Systems in Developing Countries.

Borokini, T. I., & Lawal, I. O. (2014). Traditional Medicine Practices among the Yoruba People of Nigeria: A Historical Perspective. *Journal of Medicinal Plants Studies, 2*(6), 20–33.

Daramola, O., & Jeje, A. (1976). *Awon Asa ati Orisa Ile Yoruba*. Ibadan: Onibon Oje Press.

Encyclopaedia of Public Health. (2002). "Traditional Health Beliefs, Practices" The Gale Group Inc.

Irele, A. (1991). Culture and the Arts. In L. Thompson & ... (Eds.), *Culture and Civilisation* (pp. 52–57). Ibadan: Afrika–Link Books.

Kiptiness, E. M. (2019). Indigenous Communication Practices and Myths. Available at:https://www.slideshare.net/EvonneMwangaleKiptin/indigenous-communication-practices-and-myths

Lawal, H. O. (2015). 'Cultural Aesthetics in Nigerian Video Films: A Critical Reading of Sikiru Adesina's Ogunmola – Basorun Ibadan'. In *Repositioning Nollywood for the Promotion of Nigeria's Cultural Diplomacy & National Security*. In B. F. Ayankoroma, & A. D. Akoh (Eds.), *Book of Proceedings of the Int'l Conference of SONTA*.

Littlejohn, S. W., & Fuson, K. A. (2008). *Theories of Human Communication* (9th ed.). U.S.A: Thomson Wadsworth.

Makinde, T. (2004). Motherhood as a Source of Employment of Women in Yoruba Culture. *Nordic Journal of African Studies, 13*(2), 164–174.

Mtawasli, G., Pina, M., Angle, M., & Murphy, C. (1997). *The Menstrual Cycle and Its Relation to Contraceptive Methods: A Reference for Reproductive Health Trainers. United State of America: INTRAH Publication*. University of North Carolina.

Ogungbemi, S. (2017). Traditional Religious Belief System. In T. Falola, & A. Akinyemi (Eds.), *Culture and Customs of Yoruba* (pp. 309–324). Austin, TX: Pan-African University Press.

Olabimtan, A. (1999). The Relevance of Yoruba Communication Arts to National Development in the Twenty-First Century. Lecture Delivered on May 1, 1999, Lagos State University, Ojo, Lagos.

Olajubu, O. (1978). *Ìwé Àṣà Ìbílẹ̀ Yorùbá*. Lagos: Longman Nigeria Ltd.

Olatunji, R. W. (2013). *"Uses of Semiotics in Periods of Hostilities, Armed Conflicts and Peace Building among the Yoruba, South-West Nigeria." An International Journal of Arts and Humanities*. Ethiopia: Bahir Dar.

Oyesomi, K., Salawu, A., & Olorunyomi, B. (2017). Indigenous Communication: Socio-Economic Characteristics Influencing Contemporary Female Political Participation. *Journal of International Women's Studies, 18*(4), 164–181. Available at http://vc.bridgew.edu/jiws/vol18/iss4/12

Oyesomi, K. O., & Salawu, A. (2019). Assessing the Uniqueness of Indigenous Language in Advertising: Analysis of Figurative Language Used in Selected Telecommunication Yoruba Advertisement in Nigeria. *Qualitative Report, 24*(10), 2574–2591. Retrieved from https://nsuworks.nova.edu/tqr/vol24/iss10/12

Sewell, W. H. Jr. (2005). The Concept(s) of Culture. In G. M. Spiegel (Ed.), *Practicing History: New Directions in Historical Writing after the Linguistic Turn*. UK: Routledge Publishing.

Svalastog, A. L., Donev, D., & Gajovic, S. (2017). Concept and Definition of Health and Health Related Values in the Knowledge Landscape of the Digital Society. *Croatian Medical Journal, 58*(6), 432–435. doi:10.3325/cmj.2017.58.431 PMID:29308835

Swallow, D. (2010). Meaning of Colours Across Cultures. Online Material. Retrieved from June 17, 2017: http://www.deborahswallow.com/2010/02/20/meaning-of-colours-across-cultures/

Tylor, E. B. (1871). *Primitive Culture*. London, UK: John Murray.

Ugboaja, F. (1985). *Communication: An Overview* (p. 1). International Keynotes.

Ugboaja, F. (2000). Communication for Social Change Anthology: Historical and Contemporary Readings.

World Health Organization. (2008). "Traditional Medicine: Definitions".

ADDITIONAL READING

Abubakar, A., Baar, A. V., Fischer, R., Bomu, G., Goma, J. K., & Newton, C. R. (2013). *Socio-Cultural Determinants of Health-Seeking Behaviour on the Kenyan Coast: A Qualitative Study*. Published; doi:10.1371/journal.pone.0071998

Jimoh, A. O., Adaji, S. E., Adelaiye, H., Olorukooba, A. A., Bawa, U., Ibrahim, I. H., . . . Shittu, O. S. (2018). "A Cross-Sectional Study of Traditional Practices Affecting Maternal and Newborn Health in Rural Nigeria" in The Pan African Medical Journal. doi:10.11604/pamj.2018.31.64.15880

Lawal, I. O. (2014). Traditional Medicine Practices among the Yoruba People of Nigeria: A Historical Perspective. *Faslnamah-i Giyahan-i Daruyi*, *2*(6), 20–33.

Offiong, D. A. (1999, July). Traditional Healers in the Nigerian Health Care Delivery System and the Debate over Integrating Traditional and Scientific Medicine. *Journal of Anthropological Quarterly.*, *72*(3), 118–130. doi:10.2307/3317426

Chapter 4
Indigenous Language Media and Safe Motherhood Practices

Aloysius Chukwuebuka Ifeanyichukwu
Legacy University, Nigeria

ABSTRACT

The chapter focuses on safe motherhood practices in Africa and how indigenous language media can be utilized to achieve the prevalence of safe maternal health. While highlighting the deplorable state of maternal health in Africa, the chapter recognized that to a large extent the success of safe motherhood initiative depends on effective communication. It reiterated the fact that communication is said to have taken place only when the sender and receiver have understood each other, and in this case indigenous language appears to be the right fit for the less literate mothers in communicating the message of safe motherhood practice. The chapter adopted the health belief model to drive its point home while recommending intense government action to achieve safe maternal health. It concluded by adjudging indigenous language an effective means of achieving the goals of safe motherhood initiative.

INTRODUCTION

The safety and care of child-bearing women all over the world is currently a top priority focus of governments globally. This makes it a critical agenda in the Sustainable Development Goals (SDGs 1,2,3,4, and 5). Excellent safe motherhood practice has grown to become one of the globally accepted and coveted indices of development. The reason behind this development trend is not far-fetched. Ikhioya (2014) notes that nearly 600,000 women between the ages of 15 and 49 years die every year globally as a result of complications arising from pregnancy and

DOI: 10.4018/978-1-7998-2091-8.ch004

childbirth. More than half a million women and girls die each year as a result of pregnancy, childbirth, and related complications (United States Central Intelligence Agency (CIA), 2016; World Health Organization (WHO, 2010). A recent report on maternal mortality, jointly released by WHO, UNICEF, UNFPA, World Bank Group and the United Nations Population Division, estimates a worldwide number of 295 000 maternal deaths in 2017. This figure represents a 38% reduction since the year 2000 an average reduction of just fewer than 3% per year. For women, this means that the global lifetime risk of maternal mortality – the risk that a 15-year old girl will die eventually from a maternal cause –was approximately 1 in 190 for 2017, nearly half of the level of risk in 2000 (WHO 2019).

Even though, the United Nations International Children Emergency Funds (UNICEF, 2015), reported that from 1990 to 2015, the global maternal mortality ratio declined by 44 per cent – from 385 deaths to 216 deaths per 100,000 live births, according to UN inter-agency estimates, it is still less than half the 5.5 per cent annual rate needed to achieve the three-quarters reduction in maternal mortality targeted for 2015 in Millennium Development Goal 5. More worrisome is the report from International Planned Parenthood Federation (IPPF, 2019) that every day some 830 women die from causes related to pregnancy or childbirth. Many more have serious injuries or long-lasting consequences. Going further, reports from Society for Family Health (2019) confirms these worrisome statistics by holding that high unmet need for family planning contributes to maternal death as women are exposed to pregnancies:

- Too soon (early onset / adolescent pregnancy);
- Too frequent (lack of spacing)
- Too many (several children) and
- Too late (pregnancies in women of older age)

According to reports from WHO (2012) about 800,000 women in Nigeria are living with Vesico-Vagina Fistula (VVF), a disabling condition often caused by problems in childbirth; the number grows by 20,000 each year. While in Tanzania, about 9,000 women die annually of complications related to pregnancy. The country's maternal health facilities are often too far away and the women lack adequate transport.

The sad part of this unfortunate development is that maternal mortality can be avoided if concerted efforts are made by all including the woman, the man, the community and government. Nwokocha (2008) cited in Olonade, Alabi, and Imhonopi (2019) reechoed this fact by holding that maternal mortality, known to be the loss of lives of women in their maternity stage due to pregnancy complication, is classified among preventable deaths. Thus, it is more of negligence and the non-application of the right attitude towards maternal health that results to maternal mortality.

It is therefore in response to this recurring global tragedy that Safe Motherhood Initiative was launched in 1987 to tackle the challenge of maternal and infant mortality which has been hitherto largely ignored. According to World Health Organization – WHO (2000) safe motherhood is a worldwide initiative aimed at reducing maternal morbidity and infant mortality and to improve women's reproductive health. Safe motherhood is the concept or initiatives founded to ensure that women receive high quality care in order to achieve the optimum level of health of mother and infant. It is designed in a way that the women is ensured of high-quality gynecological, family planning, prenatal, delivery and postpartum care (Adhikari, 2018). Thankfully, the adoption of the MDGs between the years 2000 and 2015 and the subsequent introduction of Sustainable Development Goals (SDGs) saw to a significant drop in the number of women dying during childbirth in the world each year from 543,000 to 287,000 (MDG Report' 2015). But this is nowhere close to the three-quarter reduction targeted by the MDGs from 1990 to 2015.

Buttressing, the idea behind the birthing of safe motherhood initiative, Fathalla (2006) blames the problem of rising maternal mortality rate on the society by holding that women are not dying because of disease that cannot be treated, but because societies in which they live are yet to make the decision that their lives are worth saving. Regrettably, the developing countries account for about 99% of an estimated half a million maternal deaths that occur each year. A review of the Millennium Development Goals (MDGs) by Okereke, Aradeon, Akerele, Tanko, Yisa, & Obonyo (2013), shows that for reasons bordering on negligence and poor implementation plans; limited progress is being made to reduce maternal mortality across developing countries especially in Africa. While the remote cause of persistence of maternal mortality in Africa may be ascribed to her governments' unwillingness to prioritize the health of mothers as done by the developed worlds, an immediate cause of this persistence is simple – inadequate communication.

The indigenous language media promises an innovative opportunity to bridge this gap and achieve this goal under the current era of Sustainable Development Goals (SDG). The inability of some of the women in dire need of safe motherhood practices to access the mainstream media equally highlights the importance of propagating these messages through indigenous language media. With culture and religion as constant features of the African society, it is imperative to employ a system of communication that will understand these peculiarities and work through them to elicit desirable result. The indigenous language media stands the best chance of achieving this feat. In view of these, this study primarily focused on how to utilize the indigenous language media to promote safe motherhood practices. It sought to gain and deepen the understanding on how these media work; the rate of their acceptability among the target audience and their general prospects in keeping child-bearing mothers safer.

CONCEPTUAL OVERVIEW

Indigenous Language Media

Indigenous language media can either be in the form conventional mass media or local media of communication peculiar to a people. According to Ansu – yeremeh (1998:68) any form of endogenous communication system which by virtue of its origin from, and integration into a specific culture, serves as a channel for messages in a way and manner that requires the utilization of values, symbols, institutions, and ethos of host culture through its unique qualities and attributes. The underlying fact regardless of which applies is that the media particularly transmit information using the indigenous language of the target audience. The idea behind indigenous language media to some extent stems from the desire of the developing world to evolve their own media through which they can tell their story by themselves and thus avoid misrepresentation. This move apparently tallies with the recommendations of the New World Information and Communication Order (NWICO) and that of development communication scholars like Ekeanyanwu (2015) that developing nations must rise above complaints and begin to evolve standard media system that will enable them become major players in the global information flow.

The multilingual nature of the African society makes the discourse of indigenous language media most cogent. Presently, Africa as a continent is said to have about 2000 languages and from these 2000 languages the number of individual languages listed for Nigeria alone is 525. Of these, 517 are living and 8 are extinct. Of the living languages, 507 are indigenous and 10 are non-indigenous. Furthermore, 19 are institutional, 76 are developing, 299 are vigorous, 81 are endangered, and 42 are dying (Eberhard, Simons, and Fennigs, 2019). Consequent upon this unique and enormous linguistic diversity of Africa, some scholars claim that Africans cannot share or work in their own languages (Prah, 1999: 3). This submission so far has been clearly refuted by Egbokhare, (2004) and Prah (2001) who agrees that the real problem of African linguistic diversity lies in the criteria with which African languages are counted. According to Egbokhare, Oyetade, Eno-Abasi, and Ahmed (2001), a good understanding of African languages reveals that about 80 percent Africans speak not more than 12 key languages: Fulfulde, Hausa, Swahili; Nguni, Sotho-Tswana, Western Inter-Lacustrine Bentu, Amharic, Yoruba, Igbo, Bamsara, Oromo and Luo. They there suggest for the harmonization of these diverse languages into language clusters and through that means sort out the challenge of linguistic diversity in Africa. Equally these cluster arrangements can be replicated within nations and in all make mediating using indigenous languages possible and in turn carry the indigenes along. The evolution of indigenous language media is only necessary to reflect the unique global diversity of humanity. Salawu (2006 p.88) buttresses this by holding that no region of the world is linguistically monolithic, which means there is diversity in the modes of communication used in different regions of the world. And, despite the dominance of some languages, the smaller languages continue to exist and are spoken with relish by their native speakers and used to varying degrees in the media.

Indigenous language media takes into account the cultural peculiarities of the host language and brings messages to the audience in a manner that they would understand. The radio, television, newspaper or magazine can all serve as indigenous language media. Rev. Henry Townsend was the first to explore this idea in Africa when he founded the first vernacular newspaper in Africa- "Iwe Irohin Fun Awon Ara Egba Ati Yoruba" which in English language means "Newspaper in Yoruba for the Egba and Yoruba people." Though Townsend added English language later on, Iwe Irohin as an indigenous newspaper became very popular especially among elderly indigenes whom it gave huge sense of belonging reading in their own language. Today the indigenous language media has grown to include outlets like, Ogene newspaper, Okun Radio, Ogene Fm, Ogbako BBC, Unwana Efik, Alaroye, Abawole BBC, Labaran, Aminiya, BBC Hausa Service, Igbo Area TV etc. While it may be argued that the indigenous language media are less popular than their English or French counterparts, a glaring fact remains that they are more trusted and accepted among the communities for whom they are targeted at.

Safe Motherhood Practices

The Safe Motherhood Programme is an intervention initiative launched in 1987 by WHO and other concerned international agencies in Nairobi, Kenya. The cardinal aim of this initiative according to WHO (2000) is to promote global efforts that will lead to drastic reduction of maternal mortality and morbidity in the world especially in the developing nations. Simply put, it is a situation in which a woman going through physiological processes of pregnancy and child birth does not suffer any injury or lose her life or that of the baby (Action Health, 1999). Other varied definitions of safe motherhood practice abound; Ikhioya (2010) defines it as the ability of a woman to have a healthy pregnancy and delivery. As for Partnership for Transforming Health Care System – PATHS (2005) safe motherhood practice concerned efforts by a pregnant woman herself, her family members (immediate and extended), her community and all health personnel at the three tiers of health care system to ensure that safety of a pregnant woman and her baby during pregnancy, delivery and after delivery. According to Adesokan (2010) safe motherhood encompasses a broad range of direct and indirect efforts to reduce deaths and disabilities resulting from pregnancy and childbirth and also to improve women's reproductive health. Since the official launch of this programme, many countries have keyed into the initiative by inaugurating their own National Safe Motherhood Programme. Accordingly, the global community has adopted May 8th of every year as the International Safe Motherhood Day.

Evidently, the need for safe motherhood practice is heightened by the frightening rate at which women die during childbirth and pregnancy. Some of the causes of maternal mortality and morbidity include; illiteracy, poverty, rural-urban differences, under-reporting and poor record keeping of cases. Safe motherhood practices seek to correct these anomalies through its varied programme options. Olise (2007) marshaled out some of these corrective programme options to include:

- Providing family planning.
- Improve socio-economic status.
- Provide safe, legal abortion services.
- Improve emergency obstetric care.
- Train traditional birth attendants.
- Inform and mobilize the community.

Through these programmes, efforts are made to tackle the challenge of maternal mortality and morbidity to a significant level.

Effective Communication Approach and Successful Safe Motherhood Practices: The Nexus

Indeed the importance of communication in achieving global spread and implementation of safe motherhood practices cannot be overstated. That which is expected to be practicalised must first be communicated and communicated in a manner that the target audiences will understand. The idea of communication fidelity as commonly held in the parlance of communication entails that before communication is said to have taken place, both the sender of the message and the receiver must have well understood each other. It is premised on this great essence of communication that scholars formed a branch of study known as health communication. The study of communication in relation to health evidently reechoes the critical role of effective communication in delivery effective health services.

Accordingly, communication is the first step towards achieving standard maternal health in that safe motherhood practices must be successfully communicated to the women in need of it first before they are expected to uphold the practices. Effective communication is employed at various level of safe motherhood campaign. It plays a role when convincing mothers and their husbands, or adults at the level of community to embrace the practice of safe motherhood. Proactively children can also be taught at school or at home on the essence of safe motherhood; all through effective communication. During pregnancy and labour, care givers are equally expected to be armed with effective communication skills in dealing with mothers and their families.

Effective mass communication is equally very vital in delivering the gains of safe motherhood initiative. However, while the contemporary mass media has played vital roles in seeing to the achievement of significant result so far in the promotion of excellent maternal health, a lot still needs to be done with the rate of the decline; falling far less than half of what was needed to achieve the MDGs' target of a three quarters reduction in the mortality ratio between 1990 and 2015 (Maternity worldwide 2015).

A major reason the message of safe motherhood practices is yet to fully permeate the developing world in dire need of it may be attributed to the suitability of media with which the mothers are exposed to those messages. Since the populations of mothers who are yet to embrace safe motherhood practices are concentrated in the rural areas, it follows that they are more likely to embrace the messages if presented to them in the language and through the media they can trust. While the use of mainstream media and popular languages may be convenient, it is imperative to carry everyone along regardless of social stratifications; thus the need for indigenous language media.

THEORETICAL FRAMEWORK

Since this study recommends certain behavioural and attitudinal change for mothers, a communication model is deemed important to explain the communication process that should lead to the expected behavioural change. In this case, the health belief model which is a sub-classification of the behaviour change communication model is considered suitable. Behaviour Change Communication (BCC) could be seen as an interactive process with communities geared towards developing tailored messages and approaches using a variety of communication channels to develop positive behaviours; promote and sustain individual, community and societal behaviour change; and maintain appropriate behaviours.

The Health Belief Model (HBM) is the most widely used theory in health education and promotion. This model was first developed in the 1950s by social psychologists working in the U.S. Public Health Services (Ngigi & Busolo, 2018). The model was developed in response to the failure of a free tuberculosis (TB) health screening program. Since then, the HBM has been adapted to explore a variety of long and short-term health behaviors, including sexual risk behaviors and the transmission of HIV/AIDS. The HBM holds that individual behavior depends on a number of beliefs about threats to an individual's wellbeing and the effectiveness and outcomes of particular actions or behaviors (University of Twente 2017).

Essentially, The Health Belief Model (HBM) posits that messages will achieve optimal behavior change if they successfully target perceived barriers, benefits, self-efficacy, and threat (Jones, Jensen, Scherr, Brown, Christy, & Weaver 2015) . Perceived threat is at the core of the HBM as it is linked to a person's 'readiness' to take action. The health belief model suggests that people's beliefs about health problems, perceived benefits of action and barriers to action, and self-efficacy explain engagement, or lack of it, in health-promoting behavior (University of Twente 2017).

At the heart of this model is a constant variable- belief. Ngigi and Busolo (2018) further noted that the perceived susceptibility is about a person's subjective perception of the risk of acquiring an illness or disease. Here a person nurses a feeling that he or she is vulnerable to a disease if a given health action is not taken. Perceived severity on the other hand refers to the feeling or fear that a given sickness when contracted as a result of not taking a particular action would be so severe. There is wide variation in a person's feelings of severity. Often, a person considers the medical consequences, such as death or disability, and social consequences, including family life and social relationships, when evaluating the severity (Ngigi & Busolo 2018).

Perceived benefits are about individual's perception of the effectiveness of various actions available to reduce the threat of illness or disease. The course of action a person takes in preventing or curing illness or disease relies on consideration and evaluation of both perceived susceptibility and perceived benefit, such that the person would accept the recommended health action if it was perceived as beneficial (University of Twente, 2017).

In the case of perceived barriers, the individual dwells more on hindrances that prevents him or her from taken a particular health action. The person weighs the effectiveness of the actions against the perceptions that it may be painful, time consuming expensive etc. Due to this the individual is likely to take action commonly known as cue to action. However, this needs stimulation to trigger the decision-making process to accept a recommended health action (Ngigi & Busolo). In the case of self-efficacy an individual relies on his or her to successfully achieve a given health behavior.

With HBM, the prevalence of safe motherhood practices can easily be realized. To achieve this emphasis will simply be placed on the risk and benefit of safe motherhood practice. Like earlier held, the success of safe motherhood campaign depends to a greater extent on the content and how the messages are communicated to the mothers. There are proven dangers associated with ignoring safe motherhood habits and also there are risks associated. Communicating these risks and benefits properly to the mothers in the language they can perfectly understand is crucial to achieving the global maternal health objective. The indigenous language in this case is deemed vital to reach the mainly less literate mothers who are likely victims of unsafe motherhood practices. Once the rewards of safe motherhood practices and the risk of neglect becomes a belief for the mothers, they will certainly change their behaviours.

Good Governance and Promotion of Safe Motherhood Practices in Africa

At the level of society, it is the onus of the government to ensure the protection of mothers through well thought out health policies and incentives. While childbearing women retain significant responsibilities in ensuring their safety and the safety of their unborn child, it is factual that government retains the bigger responsibilities. Statistically, sub-Saharan Africa continues to possess the highest rates of maternal mortality across the globe. In recent years, it was estimated that almost half of all global maternal fatalities from pregnancy-related complications occurred in Sub-Saharan Africa (Batista 2019). Going further, Batista (2019) traced the problem of maternal mortality within Sub-Saharan Africa to three major human rights issue: gender, education and literacy, and economic factors. The implication thus being that Africa is holding herself in advancing the status of her maternal health.

At the social level, gender has a major hand in the status maternal mortality in Sub-Saharan Africa. Incidences of gender biases are still on the high and remain linked to the many cases of premature death of mothers during pregnancy. This bias is often evidenced in how the distribution of health services is conducted in these African communities. A

high correlation between maternal mortality ratios (MMRs)- the number of maternal deaths per 100 000 live births- and gender inequalities as it relates to the accessibility of health services has been found in Angola, Botswana, Malawi, Mozambique, South Africa, Zambia and Zimbabwe (WHO & UNICEF, 2015). Scholars have equally investigated the systemic gender inequalities embedded within the fabric of many Sub-Saharan African countries, including Nigeria, Tanzania, and Kenya, where male-dominated social ideals and systemic mores continue to silence and marginalize African women (Chirowa, Atwood, Van der Putten, 2013).

Education and literacy serves as another important social determinant of maternal mortality in Sub-Saharan Africa. Studies have found an inverse correlation between a populace's level of education, particularly women's education, and the country's maternal mortality ratio. For example, in one analysis Mauritius demonstrated relatively high levels of education among women and therefore a relatively lower maternal mortality ratio (Alvarez, Gil, Hernández, Gil. (2009)

Economic factors serve as significant determinants of maternal mortality in Sub-Saharan Africa. Researchers in the field posit a highly significant correlation between Sub-Saharan African countries Gross National Products (GNP) per capita and health status as indicated by the incidence of maternal morbidity and mortality (Alvarez, Gil, Hernández, and Gil. (2009). Scholars have found that economic factors, such as per-capita government expenditure on health and Gross National Income (GNI) per capita, purveyed an inverse relationship with the nation's MMR in Sub-Saharan Africa (Buor, & Bream, 2004)

Aside from formulating sound government policies which will ensure the achievement of high safe motherhood status, government of African countries must sit up to address these three determinant factors mentioned amongst others. It is evident that gender equality in Africa is far from being realized with religo-cultural sentiments which relegate women to the background still thriving. Brain drain is reality fueled by the failed standard of education in greater parts of Africa. The state of education in Africa is poor while lack of educational facilities has become common. The economic situation of Africa is deplorable with inflations and depressions hitting every facet of most African economy. This heightened economic downturn has seen governments of most African nations depend heavily on foreign aid and grant to run their nation. For instance a country like Nigeria borrowed morning to fund its annual budget and still find it impossible to implement the workers' new minimum wage.

To ensure the prevalence of safe maternal health, true democracy must be instituted in these developing nations, to ensure only leaders with vision and sincerity of purpose are elected. Incidences of corruption, terrorism, and tribalism must be eschewed. To realize the objectives of safe motherhood initiative, government must in reality function in service of the people.

Media Trends in Coverage of Safe Motherhood Campaigns

Indeed, significant efforts have been made by the media worldwide towards promoting the discourse and accessibility of safe motherhood. The tenth year anniversary of Safe Motherhood Initiative in 1997 provided an opportunity for a global media campaign in both donour and developing countries (Safe Motherhood Review, 2007). Sequel to this, a Technical Consultation was launched in October 1997 with the following tasks;

- Development of story ideas, press releases, and features;
- Media training for potential safe
- Motherhood spokespeople in both developed and developing countries;

- Identification of a “circle” of 100 journalists from important print and broadcast outlets;
- A media-only Web site for information (also called a virtual press office);
- event-related press relations;
- A master press kit to help partners in developing countries extend the media attention on key safe motherhood issues; and
- Development and distribution of public service announcements (PSAs).

The Safe Motherhood Review (2007) furthered that the anniversary programme drew extensive media coverage from over 350 television and 200 radio outlets in more than 80 countries. The PSAs were frequently relayed by such outlets as CNN International, CNBC Europe, Star TV, and MTV (North and South), as well as national television stations in Malaysia, Bangladesh, the Czech Republic, Lesotho, Pakistan, Zimbabwe, and Uganda. In a survey of country-level participants conducted by the Committee on Technical Consultation, it was revealed that 70% of respondents felt that local media coverage about safe motherhood had increased during the campaign, though no formal country-by-country evaluation was conducted. A media analysis of the press coverage of World Health Day 1998 events in Washington, DC and around the world with focus on Safe Motherhood reveals that: countries like United States, India, Sri Lanka, Malaysia and South Africa paid noticeable media attention to safe motherhood programmes most than others. The impact of news agencies like Associated Press, PressWire, Agence France Presse, and Reuters were noticed too.

Seventy-four of the published articles analyzed were news items, 36 were opinion pieces, three were editorials, and one was a letter. The source of the coverage was broken down as follows: interviews or press briefings (62%); third party (i.e., WHO, unicef) (19%); press releases (11%); and spontaneous coverage 3% (Safe Motherhood Review, 2007). It was further noticed that the emergence of Millennium Development Goals (MDGs) accounted for increased attention to scholarly discourses in maternal health and safe motherhood.

The Need for Indigenous Language Media in the Implementation of Safe Motherhood Initiative

A sad fact evident in the above enumerated media coverage statistics from Safe Motherhood Review 2007 is that the developing world which harbours more cases of maternal mortality and morbidity is lagging behind in terms of media coverage. Specifically, the statistics show that Africa which has the highest cases maternal death is discussing less the solution to these problems than United States of America. Aside from poverty, distance, inadequate services, cultural and religious practices, a major cause of the persistence of maternal mortality is inadequate information. This problem of inadequate information here may be discussed as dearth of information or inability of the media used to penetrate the target society and effect desired social change. Admittedly, several health programmes abound in various national and State media supported by international organizations like Department for International Development (DFID) and Society for Family Health to promote safe motherhood practices. The reality however remains that notwithstanding these media efforts, maternal mortality is still prevalent in the developing world.

The idea of an indigenous language media presents an opportunity of exploring more effective communication strategy to aid the achievement of safe motherhood targets. An indigenous language medium is situated closer to the people in order to enhance better understanding and thus effect desired social change. This principle is in line with the views of Lasswell (1960) who asserts that a function of mass media is transmission of cultural heritage for social continuity. He furthered that African media will be fulfilling this function if they are actively involved in the promotion of African languages. On the essence and impact of indigenous language media with focus on Nigerian media, Omoloso and Abdulrauf-Salau (2014, p.12) elaborated that:

Indigenous languages through the use of the Nigerian mass media can be used to bring about sustainable development in Nigeria. There is no gainsaying in the fact that the language (and culture) of development is the mother tongue or a language(s) rooted in the people's culture and tradition. With the use of indigenous languages in the media, information is brought closer to more people, the non-literate inclusive. This consequently makes development more broad based.

The simple logic therefore is that since the problem of maternal mortality is more among the rural dwellers who may be regarded as indigenous people. It follows that the best medium to reach them and get them to embrace a given social change is through indigenous language media. The indigenous language media takes the cultural and religious standing of the people into account and through this means mediates messages to the target audiences not just in the language but in the manner they will understand. Salawu (2006) passed a vote of confidence in the use of the indigenous language media in Africa by describing them as local agenda setters and pace-setters, reflecting the original essence of African languages. A better compliance with the tenets of safe motherhood initiative may thus be achieved using the indigenous language media.

Reflecting on the significant rise of indigenous media in today's communication world, Meadows (2009, p. 119) noted that a key influence on the quest by indigenous people for empowerment at various levels —including media empowerment — is a continuing failure by the broader public sphere to account for Indigenous cultural needs. This has played a central role in the development of alternative media systems and alternative public spheres, including Indigenous public spheres. Africa as a society has its own peculiarities distinct from those of the West. Problem arises when these peculiarities are seen as inferiority markers rather than differences. Thus, any campaign carried out based on this manner of relationship is bound to fail. Similarly, Molnar and Meadows (2001) bemoaned this manner of relationship when they noted that indigenous voices remain suppressed in mainstream news coverage of events in which they are deeply implicated; notwithstanding these bottlenecks, the indigenous agency has been a crucial element of a global push for media access.

1. It is also important to note that the messages of safe motherhood are not meant for women alone. Men must also play critical roles in the diffusion and implementation of these messages. In societies like Africa where patriarchal norms are dominant, men are often major decision-makers for the family, hence decisions around when, where and even if a woman should have access to healthcare often are made by men (Ganle, Otupiri, Parker, Fitpatrick, 2015). The use of indigenous language media is therefore necessary to avoid needless misunderstanding and get the men to support their wives in the quest for better health. In such patriarchal societies which may be rural, the conventional media is often adjudged to be instrument of evil and cultural pollution. In this case the local indigenous media like town-criers, venue-oriented media, dance, folklores may apply. However, the conventional mass media may apply in so far as the indigenous is used as the programme language.

The "Story Story" BBC World Service radio drama is a good example of an indigenous language programme through which messages of safe motherhood are transmitted. The programme in Nigeria mainly adopts pigeon English as its programme language but have the cast speak the language with accents of the three major languages in Nigeria- Hausa, Igbo and Yoruba. There is Wazazi Nipendeni an all-round media safe motherhood media campaign in Tanzania. Other forms of safe motherhood campaigns may be obtained all-round Africa including handbills and posters containing safe motherhood information posted at hospitals or rural clinics. The underlying fact thus is that while the mainstream media programme continues to run, the indigenous media must equally function to complement its effort towards achieving prevalence of safe motherhood practice in Africa.

CONCLUSION

Clearly, the era of neglecting the potency and role of indigenous language media in delivering effecting campaign or programme messages is gone, considering that mainstream media cannot be fully accessible and comprehensible to all audiences. The extent of diffusion of safe motherhood messages has clearly exposed this deficiency. Hence, it is advocated here that the best way forward is the adoption of a synergistic option which will ensure cooperation between the mainstream and the indigenous language media. The essential purpose of communication is to ensure transfer of meaning and not reverence for language. Currently the international community has adopted the Sustainable Development Goals (SDGs) as a follow up from the Millennium Development Goals (MDGs) which got terminated in 2015. The adoption and effective utilization of indigenous language media will essentially prove useful in the implementation of this development plan in Africa and the world at large.

RECOMMENDATIONS

Specifically, this study suggests the following as recommendations towards achieving prevalence of safe motherhood practice through indigenous language media:

1. Intense government action through the Ministry of Health is needed to ensure that expectant mothers especially in the rural areas are adequately informed about safe motherhood habits through their indigenous language media.
2. Outdoor advertorials on safe motherhood habits using indigenous languages should continuously be utilized to reach expectant mothers. For instance, posters and handbills.
3. The message of safe motherhood habit must not only be spread on the conventional media and in the hospitals, venue oriented traditional media, like market, funerals, riverside, etc should all be utilized to adequately inform expectant mothers on the need to observe safe motherhood habits.
4. Conventional media like radio and television must never fail to utilize indigenous languages in their various safe motherhood practices programmes.
5. A proactive approach must be adopted by parents especially mothers also to informally teach their female children about safe motherhood practices ahead of time. In this way they would internalize the attitude even before becoming mothers.

FUTURE RESEARCH DIRECTIONS

A direction for future research could be to examine the role of men in promoting safe motherhood habit in societies. While it is natural that only women become mothers, the men especially in traditional societies assumes perhaps for patriarchal reasons that they have no hand in helping their wives and daughters maintain safe motherhood habits; a future research may attempt to ascertain the merits and demerits of this position.

REFERENCES

Action Health. (1999). *Meeting the sexual and reproductive health needs of young people in Nigeria: A Guide for Action.* Lagos.

Adesokan, F. O. D. (2010). *Reproductive health for all ages*: Ekiti State: Sammy prints.

Adhikari, S. (2018). Pillars of safe motherhood, Retrieved on September 25, 2019 from www. Publichealthnotes.com

Alvarez, J. L., Gil, R., Hernández, V., & Gil, A. (2009). Factors associated with maternal mortality in Sub-Saharan Africa: An ecological study. *BMC Public Health, 9*(1), 462. doi:10.1186/1471-2458-9-462 PMID:20003411

Batista, J. (2019). *An intersectional analysis of maternal mortality in Sub-Saharan Africa: a human rights issue.* Retrieved from www.jogh.org • doi: Accessed September 25, 2019 doi:10.7189/jogh.09.01032

Buor, D., & Bream, K. (2004). An analysis of the determinants of maternal mortality in sub-Saharan Africa. *Journal of Women's Health, 13*(8), 926–938. doi:10.1089/jwh.2004.13.926 PMID:15671708

CDC. (2018). *Health Communication Strategies*: Available at www.npin.cdc.gov. Accessed on 25th September 2019

Champion, V., & Skinner, C. S. (2008). The Health Belief Model. In K. Glanz, B. Rimer, & K. Viswanath (Eds.), *Health behavior and health education, 4* (pp. 45–65). San Francisco, CA: Jossey-Bass.

Chirowa, F., Atwood, S., & Van der Putten, M. (2013). Gender inequality, health expenditure and maternal mortality in sub-Saharan Africa: A secondary data analysis. *African Journal of Primary Health Care & Family Medicine, 5*(1), 1–5. doi:10.4102/phcfm.v5i1.471

Eberhard, D. M., Simons, G. F., & Fennig, C. D. (2019) *Ethnologue: languages of the world.* Dallas, Texas: SIL International. Retrieved from http://www.ethnologue.com. Accessed on May 14, 2019.

Egbokhare, F. O., Oyetade, S. O., Eno-Abasi, U., & Ahmed, H. A. (2001). Language clusters in Nigeria. CASAS Monograph Series, No. 12. Cape Town, South Africa.

Ekeanyanwu, N. T. (2015). *International Communication.* Ibadan: Stirling-Horden Publishers.

Fathalla, M. F. (2006). Human Rights aspects of safe motherhood. *Best Practice & Research. Clinical Obstetrics & Gynaecology, 20*(3), 409–419. doi:10.1016/j.bpobgyn.2005.11.004 PMID:16469542

FHI, & USAID. (2002). *Behaviour Change Communication (BCC) for HIV/AIDS a Strategic Framework.* Available at www.hivpolicy.org. Accessed on 25 September 2019.

Ganle, J., Otupiri, E., Parker, M., & Fitpatrick, R. (2015). Socio-cultural barriers to accessibility and utilization of maternal and newborn healthcare services in Ghana after user-fee abolition. *International Journal of Maternal Child Health, 3*(1), 1–14.

Ikhioya, G. O. (2010). Maternal mortality and the safe motherhood programme in Nigeria: Implication for Reproductive Health. *International Journal of Education and Research, 2*(10). IPPF Factsheet 2019.

Jones, C. L., Jensen, J. D., Scherr, C. L., Brown, N. R., Christy, K., & Weaver, J. (2015). The Health Belief Model as an explanatory framework in communication research: Exploring parallel, serial, and moderated mediation. *Health Communication, 30*(6), 566–576. doi:10.1080/10410236.2013.873363 PMID:25010519

Meadows, M. (2009). Walking the talk: Reflections on indigenous media audience research methods. *Journal of Audience and Reception Studies, 6*(1).

Meadows, M., & Molnar, H. (2002). Bridging the gaps: Towards a history of Indigenous media in Australia. *Media History, 8*(1), 9–20. doi:10.1080/13688800220134473

Ngigi, S., & Busolo, D. (2018). Behaviour Change Communication in Health Promotion: Appropriate Practices and Promising Approaches. *International Journal of Innovative Research and Development,* (7), 9.

Okereke, E., Aradeon, S., Akerele, A., Tanko, M., Yisa, I., & Obonyo, B. (2013). Knowledge of safe motherhood among women in rural communities in northern Nigeria: Implications for maternal mortality reduction. *Reproductive Health, 10*(1), 57. doi:10.1186/1742-4755-10-57 PMID:24160692

Olise, P. (2007). *Primary health care for sustainable development*. Ibadan, Nigeria: Omoade Printing Press.

Olonade, O., Olawande, T. I., Alabi, O. J., & Imhonopi, D. (2019). Maternal Mortality and Maternal Health Care in Nigeria: Implications for Socio-Economic Development. *Open Access Macedonian Journal of Medical Sciences*, *7*(5), 849–855. doi:10.3889/oamjms.2019.041 PMID:30962850

PATHS. (2005). Maternal and child health. *Journal of World Health Forum*, *7*(21), 11–21.

Prah, K. K. (1999) *Workshop working paper on the harmonization and standardization of Nigerian languages*. Lagos.

Prah, K. K. (2001) The idea of an African Renaissance, the languages of the Renaissance and the challenges of the 21st century. In E. Kurimoto (Ed.), *JCAS Symposium Series 14*. JCAS, Osaka, Japan.

Salawu, A. (2006). Indigenous language media: A veritable tool for African language learning. *Journal of Multicultural Discourses*, *1*(1), 86–95. doi:10.1080/10382040608668533

United States Central Intelligence Agency (CIA). (2016). *World Fact Book[Online]*. Retrieved from https://www.cia.gov/library/publications/the-world-factbook/. Accessed September, 25 2019.

University of Twente. (2017). *Health Belief Model: Explaining Health Behaviors*. Available at www.utwente.nl. Accessed on September 25, 2019

WHO. (2000). *Strategies for promoting safe motherhood in Nigeria by the year 2010*. Abuja: The Author World Health Organization (WHO). (2010). Trends in Maternal Mortality: 1990 to 2008[Online]. https://www.who.int/reproductivehealth/publications/monitoring/9789241500265/en/. Accessed September 25 2019

World Health Organization. Fact sheets. (2012).

World Health Organization. Fact sheets. (2019).

World Health Organization & UNICEF. (2015). Trends in maternal mortality: 1990 to 2013: estimates by WHO, UNICEF, UNFPA, The World Bank and the United Nations Population Division. Retrieved from http://apps.who.int/iris/bitstream/.

KEY TERMS AND DEFINITIONS

Communication: is the process of passing information and understanding from one person to another with a feedback.

Cultural Peculiarities: is conceived as a people's way of life and behaviour which only belongs to that given people or society. Such peculiarities like language, dance, dressing, food etc is used to denote people from that area.

Indigenous Language: An *indigenous language* is a *language* that is native to a region and spoken by *indigenous* people, often reduced to the status of a minority *language*. This *language* would be from a linguistically distinct community that has been settled in the area for many generations.

Mass Media: Mass media are channels of communication which aid the transfer of meaning from a sender to heterogenous audiences simultaneously. It refers to a varied range of media technologies that reach a large audience through mass communication. Examples include; television, radio, newspapers, magazines, motion pictures.

Maternal Health: refers to the health of women during pregnancy, childbirth and the postpartum period and maternal health care services are antenatal care (ANC), delivery care and postnatal care (PNC) services.

Maternal Mortality: is defined by the World Health Organization (WHO) as "the death of a woman while pregnant or within 42 days of termination of pregnancy, irrespective of the duration and site of the pregnancy, from any cause related to or aggravated by the pregnancy or its management but not from accidental or incidental causes.

Pregnancy: The state of carrying a developing embryo or fetus within the female body. This condition can be indicated by positive results on an over-the-counter urine test, and confirmed through a blood test, ultrasound, detection of fetal heartbeat, or an X-ray.

Safe Motherhood: Safe motherhood involves series of initiatives, practices, protocols and service delivery guidelines structured to give mothers high-quality gynecological, family planning, prenatal, delivery and postpartum care, in order to achieve optimal health for the mother, fetus and infant during pregnancy, childbirth and postpartum.

Safety: the condition of being protected from or unlikely to cause danger, risk, or injury. It is the absence of threat to life or properties.

Chapter 5
Impact of Indigenous Language Media on Safe Motherhood Practices

Funmi Falobi
Yaba College of Technology, Nigeria

ABSTRACT

This chapter examines the role of indigenous language media and how it has impacted safe motherhood practices in Lagos State. The objectives are to know how the media using indigenous languages have been able to reach more women and inform them on best practices on safe motherhood practices and whether professional health providers communicate in indigenous language to women during ante natal sessions. A questionnaire was administered on pregnant women and nursing mothers at a public general hospital in the state while nurses were interviewed on the use of indigenous language. The research was also carried out in three indigenous radio stations in Lagos. The study found that for Nigeria in general, and Lagos State in particular, to reduce maternal mortality rate and advance in safe motherhood practices, involvement of indigenous language media is imperative in giving women necessary information. The majority of the respondents answered that they would prefer health workers to speak in the local language.

INTRODUCTION

Globally, there is a serious concern on safe motherhood practices and the need to address women's reproductive health challenges. Many women are still losing their lives during childbirth in spite of advances in the field of health. As part of efforts

DOI: 10.4018/978-1-7998-2091-8.ch005

in addressing the issue, the World Health Organisation (WHO) came up with the Safe Motherhood Initiatives (SMI) at how communication could be a veritable tool in bridging the gap especially in the rural areas.

There is no doubt that safe motherhood decreases maternal and infant mortality and morbidity. Although, most maternal and infant deaths can be prevented through safe motherhood practices, millions of women worldwide are affected by maternal mortality and morbidity from preventable causes. Every day, 830 women die from preventable causes related to pregnancy and childbirth around the world. Globally, that amounted to about 303,000 women in 2015 (Stanton, Kwast, Shaver, McCallon, Koblinsky, 2018).

After the 30th anniversary of the launch of the global Safe Motherhood Initiative, it became imperative for the world to renew its visionary goal of ending preventable maternal mortality. Progress toward that aspiration is often equated with the 44% reduction in global maternal mortality between 1990 and 2015. Yet this reduction was still far from achieving Millennium Development Goal (MDG) 5 of reducing the maternal mortality ratio (MMR) by three-quarters between 1990 and 2015, and it is even farther from achieving Sustainable Development Goal (SDG) 3, which aims to attain a global MMR of less than 70 deaths per 100,000 live births by 2030.

Study indicates that when women have greater knowledge through education, there is greater likelihood that they will have better pregnancy and delivery outcomes. However, communication plays a very crucial role in educational and information dissemination. It is of essence that for any policy education programme or information dissemination activity to be a success, there must be in place effective communication. One of the pillars of an effective communication process is audience-based communication that is carried out to reach target audience in their indigenous language.

This paper looked at the role of indigenous language media and how it has impacted safe motherhood practices in Nigeria, using Lagos State as a study. It reviewed how the media, using the indigenous language has been able to reach women and inform them on best practices on safe motherhood practices, service delivery, and training and how to access information using indigenous language. It also looked at the role of professional health providers, traditional birth attendants, policy-makers, and community members in improving reproductive health and reducing maternal deaths, from a communication perspective. This paper equally discussed how indigenous language media has been able to reduce maternal mortality rate among women and how women have been able to access information, thereby leading to quality service delivery on the part of service providers.

The researcher argued that while indigenous language has been able to impact safe motherhood practices, there is need for policymakers to encourage health personnel to address women in indigenous language. Also, the media in using indigenous language have a lot to do in dissemination of information to the target audience towards the success of the SDG3 goal.

BACKGROUND

Safe motherhood reduces maternal and child mortality and morbidity. It includes initiatives and service delivery that provide quality healthcare for women in order to attain ideal health for the mother, fetus and infant during pregnancy. Overview of the Sustainable Development Goal, SDG 3, shows that significant reductions in maternal mortality are possible, and they are taking place. The global maternal mortality ratio has reduced from 342 maternal deaths per 100,000 live births in 2000 to 211 deaths per 100,000 live births in 2017. In many countries, maternal deaths have fallen as women have gained access to family planning and skilled birth attendance with backup emergency obstetric care. Some countries have halved their maternal deaths in the space of a decade (UNFPA, 2019).

However, there is still much more to be done. The United Nations Population Fund, UNFPA, declares that high rates of maternal mortality persist, particularly in impoverished communities. Of the hundreds of thousands of women who died during pregnancy or childbirth in 2017, approximately 86 per cent lived in sub-Saharan Africa and Southern Asia.

Nigeria, Africa's most populous country with a population of about 200 million people has women as half of the population. The nation has one of the highest maternal mortality ratios in the world and maternal mortality is estimated to be more than twice as high in the rural areas than in the urban areas. Newly revised estimates of the World Health Organisation (WHO) indicate that there are 1,100 maternal deaths for every 100,000 live births in the country and that a woman's lifetime chance of dying during pregnancy, childbirth or the postpartum period is one in 18. (Bankole A et al, 2009).

Regional variations abound in maternal mortality figures across Nigeria. Evidence suggests that maternal mortality rates (MMR) are significantly higher in northern Nigeria compared to the southern part of the country. The North East and North West zones with MMR of 1,549 deaths per 100,000 live births and 1,025 deaths per 100, 000 live births respectively have rates about ten and six times higher than in the South West (165 deaths per 100,000 live births). High MMRs in the northern part of the country significantly impacts on the national MMR, estimated at 545 deaths per 100, 000 live births which are among the highest in the world. (Okereke, Aradeon, Akerele et al., 2013).

Ogundipe (2013) citing (Onah, Ikeako, and Iloabachi, 2006) noted that most women in Nigeria live below the poverty level and lack access to comprehensive antenatal and delivery services. Infant mortality figure is also staggering; Child mortality rate under age 5 years was 143 per 1,000 births in 2010 compared with 5 per 1,000 for United Kingdom (World Bank, 2011).The Nigerian government has adopted several policies aimed at reducing maternal mortality by 75% by 2015. However, they lack effective implementation, largely because of the very low level of government spending on health care. Most programming on safe motherhood has been initiated by non-governmental organisations working with funding from international donors. (Bankole, Sedgh, Okonofua, Imarhiagbe, Hussain and Wulf, 2009).

Ample evidence indicates that when women have greater knowledge through education, there is greater likelihood that they will have better pregnancy and delivery outcomes. This is likely because acquiring knowledge through education equips women to make appropriate decisions about their health including during pregnancy and childbirth. (Okereke, E., Aradeon, S., Akerele, A. et al, 2013).

The researcher believes that for Nigeria to join the rest of the world that has made headway in SDG3 and have been able to halve maternal mortality and child morbidity there must be political will power on the part of the government to overhaul the healthcare delivery system in the country. And as (Stanton, Kwast, Shaver, McCallon, Koblinsky, 2018) put it:

Success will require that ending preventable mortality remains a political priority. This will necessitate strengthening of networks, individuals, and organisations to keep up the pressure, push for investment in what works, be bold in tackling new challenges, and ultimately support nations to have resilient health systems to meet the needs of all people.

One of the essential components of national programmes is communication for safer motherhood. Studies show that women especially those in the rural areas are more comfortable with health service providers that could relate with them in their local language and this is one of the reasons for high patronage of the traditional birth attendants.

Safe motherhood communication intervention, if well designed and properly implemented, can impact this needless combination of ignorance, misconception and neglect, and overcome longstanding resistances at policy, facility and household level. (Mona Moore, Independent Consultant, Reproductive Health communication).

The objective of this paper is to look at the role of indigenous language media and how it has imparted safe motherhood practices in Nigeria using Lagos State as a case-study.

RESEARCH QUESTIONS

In view of the objectives of this study, the following are the research questions for investigation:

1. Does indigenous language radio station broadcast programmes on safe motherhood practices?
2. Do women get adequate information on safe motherhood practices from indigenous language radio station?
3. How relevant is the information given out to women on safe motherhood practices?
4. How frequent are the information on safe motherhood practices disseminated on indigenous language radio station?

CONCEPTUAL CLARIFICATION

Indigenous Language Media

There is no doubt that indigenous language media are veritable tools for development in any society. Indigenous media is the vehicle the common people or rural farmers employ for the delivery of their messages N'gombe (2000). Indigenous communication, according to Wang (1982:3) cited by Mundy and Compton opines that indigenous communication is the communication system which existed before the arrival of (contemporary) mass media and formerly organised bureaucratic systems, and is still existing today despite changes. The fact that indigenous communication is appropriate for rural population is demonstrated more in their functions which, according to Ojebode (2002), are not universal. First of these is that indigenous communication media practitioners - poets, musicians, theatrical performers, orators, carvers – constitute a formidable agency of opinion moulding. They not only feel the pulse of the society, they as well shape it. They educate people on correct social behaviour. Higher (1990:46-158) gives examples of Kwagh Hir puppet plays aimed at moulding the opinion of people in areas of social conduct. Such plays condemned prostitution, encouraged good home-making and women virtues, condemn laziness and educated people on the values of good health care.

Closely linked to the above is the role of being the voice of the people. Olabimtan (1981:157) quoted by Ojebode (2002:93) observed that "in traditional Yoruba society, the poet seemed to have no personal voice. He usually expressed the voice of his society which was largely ruled by custom in which the elements of individual judgment and initiative was small."

In addition, indigenous media also serve as custodians of the people's history, culture and values this Kidd (1992) calls the function of recovery, revival and reassertion. Hove (1997) calls the traditional poet "the memory bank of the community." Furthermore, indigenous media educate by teaching people informally and through entertainment, the norms, mores and standards of the society. It may also be through direct instructions from experts (Ojebode, 2002). Finally, a very important role of traditional media, as stated by Ojebode "is their use in development efforts."

Relating indigenous communication to the field or rural development and utilization of innovation, Soola (1984) observed that, traditional media forms have been successfully utilized for non-formal, broad-based, out-of classroom education. It has been used to teach such themes as environmental sanitation, family planning, rural cooperatives, nutrition and scientific methods of farming. It has also been employed to wage war on social maladies as corruption, indolence, ignorance, disease, greed and avarice as well as various form of indiscipline (Soola, 1984; WAI, 1984).

Salawu (2006) explained that the mass media, because of their general accessibility, are said to be veritable tools in popularising the use and learning of African languages that are, presently, being threatened out of existence by the European languages foisted on the African peoples through the advent of colonialism. For the mass media to achieve this task, the media using African languages must be encouraged and sustained. He appreciates indigenous language media as extending African language literacy. Mberia, (2015) argues that promoting indigenous languages in media sustains and promotes regional and national cultural identities stressing that indigenous language media are essential tools for conveying communication for development. Accordingly, the use of indigenous languages enhances the media's informative function and audience participation (Kupe 2016).

Salawu (2006) argued convincingly about the capacity of the indigenous language media (including, notably radio) to promote indigenous language learning, Akinleye and Ojebode (2004) focused on news content, Brieger (1990) worked on frequency of listening to radio programmes in general, and Adekunle et al. (2004) focused on family planning radio programmes in an urban setting, Consequently, the researcher posits that indigenous language media is a veritable tool in promoting safe motherhood practices in Nigeria, especially in the rural areas to reach the larger number of women in informing them of best practices and gaining access to information that would aid safe delivery and reduce the maternal mortality rate.

Indigenous Language Media in Nigeria

The origin of the African language press is usually associated with Christian missionaries. They chose to establish a press in the local language for their evangelical activities (Akinfeleye, 1985; Tsumba, 2002; Salawu, 2003, 2007). They understood that in order to convey their messages to the natives, effective communication in the indigenous languages became imperative. In Nigeria, the first newspaper, Iwe Iroyin Fun Awon Ara Egba ati Yoruba was established in 1859 using the indigenous language, Yoruba, to disseminate information. After Iwe Iroyin, many newspapers also came on board using the indigenous languages. Today, after over a decade from the establishment of the first newspaper, incidentally an indigenous language publication, many indigenous publications in Nigeria are still faced with problems of irregularity while some are not even known. Many others have also gone extinct. In fact today, Nigerian newspaper industry has the publications in English language as the mainstream newspapers while the few published in local languages are more or less supplements (Omoloso, Abdulrauf-Salau, 2014).

As reported by Wikipedia (www.edutech402.blogspot.in/20) of 2012, radio started in Nigeria with the introduction of Radio Distribution System in 1933 in Lagos by the British colonial government under the Department of Post and Telegraphs (P & T). In 1935, the Radio Distribution System (RDS) was changed to Radio Diffusion System (RDS). The aim was to spread the efforts of Britain and her allies during the Second World War through the BBC. The Ibadan station was commissioned in 1939, followed by the Kano station in 1944. Later, a re-appraisal of radio broadcast objectives gave birth to the establishment in 1950 of the Nigerian Broadcasting Service (NBS). The NBS began broadcast in Lagos, Ibadan, Kaduna, Kano and Enugu on short wave and medium wave transmitters.

Through a Bill by the House of Representatives, the Nigerian Broadcasting Corporation (NBC) was established in 1956. The NBC took up the responsibilities of radio broadcast in Nigeria. The Federal Radio Corporation of Nigeria (FRCN) was established in 1978. The Voice of Nigeria (VON) which served as the external service was established in 1990. With the creation of more states and each state wanting to propagate its people and culture, the pace for radio broadcast began in Nigeria and has spread fast across the length and breadth of the nation However, as many radio stations there are in Nigeria, the major medium of communication is only English Akanbi, T. A., & Aladesanmi, O. A. (2014).

At the inception of modern television broadcasting system in Nigeria, the system was lauded in the area of education while cultural transmission suffered setback. This was because the country greatly relied on foreign imported programmes. UNESCO (1974) noted that only 25% of the programmes were produced within the nation; the rest were foreign.

Initially, radio and television stations used to be owned by the government but licenses have been granted to private broadcasters as well. Today, there are so many radio and television stations both private and state-owned stations all over the country providing information, news, sports and entertainment to people. Though there are programmes aired in the various surrounding indigenous language(s), such programmes occupy a lesser percentage when compared with the totality of the programmes rendered or aired in English (Akanbi, T. A., & Aladesanmi, O. A, 2014).

Indigenous Language and Health Promotion

World Health Organisation defines health promotion as: "The process of enabling people to increase control over, and to improve, their health. It moves beyond a focus on individual behaviour towards a wide range of social and environmental interventions."

The importance of indigenous language in health promotion cannot be overemphasised. Language of communication has been identified as one of the barriers to effective communication (Oyesomi, Salawu & Olorunyomi, 2017, Oyesomi & Salawu, 2019). In a country like Nigeria with diverse cultural, socio-economic and religious orientation, health communication must be properly planned.

The development media theory lays emphasis on the use of indigenous language in media text to reduce ambiguity and this implies that the impact of indigenous language on safe motherhood practices is sacrosanct to attain the 2030 sustainable development goal 3 to halve maternal and child mortality rate.

Through advocacy for health, health promotion aims to make political, economic, social, cultural, environmental, behavioural and biological factors favour health. However, the use of indigenous language and involvement of indigenous language media in health campaigns would help greatly in communicating safe motherhood practices among the rural dwellers. Nevertheless, health communicators and practitioners require the understanding of how effective is the indigenous media in planning public health messages and its interventions (Dooley, Jones and Desmarais 2009),

THEORETICAL FRAMEWORK

Social Cognitive Theory

The theory posits that learning occurs in a social context with a dynamic and reciprocal interaction of the person, environment, and behavior. The unique feature of SCT is the emphasis on social influence and its emphasis on external and internal social reinforcement.

Developed by the renowned Stanford psychology professor, Albert Bandura, the theory provides a framework for understanding how people actively shape and are shaped by their environment. In particular, the theory details the processes of observational learning and modeling, and the influence of self-efficacy on the production of behavior.

The theory views people as active agents who both influence and are influenced by their environment. This implies that for indigenous language media to impact safe motherhood practices among the people, the media as well as health professionals must be able to influence the populace by identifying with their culture. Invariably, the media must communicate in the local language while the health professionals must speak the people language for effective health advocacy and campaign.

A major component of the theory is observational learning: the process of learning desirable and undesirable behaviours by observing others, then reproducing learned behaviors in order to maximize rewards.

To Leitner (2000), events would not happen the way they do nor would they have the same impact as they have without language. They (i.e. events) are in themselves mirrors of reality while they inform, interpret, entertain, and educate.

In all, Leitner examined the different levels, domains and audience design of the mass media. Looking at the impact the media ought to have on recipients, he said, "To gain and maintain a stable audience, communication media must include recipients' needs and expectations early on in message production."

METHOD

As parts of the methodology adopted in carrying out this research, this paper focuses on the impact of indigenous language media on safe motherhood practices using Lagos State as a case study.

Lagos State is the commercial nerve of Nigeria and former capital of the country. While the state is essentially a Yoruba-speaking environment, it is a socio-cultural melting pot attracting both Nigerians and foreigners alike. Since December 2007, Yoruba has been the second official language of debate and discussion for the House of Assembly after English. However, maternal mortality rate is still an issue in the state.

This study utilised survey analysis in the form of questionnaire, interview and personal observations. The population comprised all pregnant women and nursing mothers at a public general hospital in Lagos State. A sample size of 42 respondents was selected for the study. Questionnaire was used for data collection. The research is carried out in three indigenous radio stations – Radio Lagos -*Tiwan Tiwa*, *Faaji* FM and *Wazobia* FM. Radio Lagos is owned by the Lagos State Government and predominantly a Yoruba speaking station. *Faaji* FM is a privately owned station and Yoruba speaking while *Wazobia* FM, a privately owned station uses pidgin communication language to reach its audience. Radio Lagos programme is "*Se'rigbo,*"

Table 1. Age of respondents

Age	Respondents	%
Below 20	2	4.8%
20-30	11	26%
30-40	12	28.6%
40 and above	17	40.5%
Total	42	100%

Table 2. Status of respondents

Status	Respondents	%
First time Pregnancy	19	45.24%
Others (More than once)	23	54.76%
Total	42	100%

a sponsored programme that focuses mainly on family planning aspect of the safe motherhood practices. *Faaji* FM has "*E Gbe Yewo,*" a current affairs programme that focuses on family while *Wazobia* FM programme is "*Kulele* Zone" a health programme that brings a guest health expert on board.

Data Analysis

Age of respondents: The total number of respondents to the questionnaire is 42 women who have experienced childbirth at one stage or the other. Of the 42 respondents, 11 women fall between the ages of 20-29, the age range of 12 women fall between the age of 30-39 while 17 women were age 40 and above.

Status: Of the 42 women, 17 of them are first time pregnancy, 20 have given birth more than once and 5 respondents did not answer the question on the questionnaire.

Q1. Which of the following radio stations do you listen to?

Twenty-one 21 respondents listened to *Tiwan Tiwa,* 11 respondents are loyal listeners of *Faaji* FM and 7 respondents listen to *Wazobia* FM while only 3 contenders indicated that they listened to more than one radio stations.

Table 3. Respondents preferred radio stations

Medium	Respondents that listen to:	%
Radio Lagos	22	52.38%
WAZOBIA	08	19.02%
FAAJI	12	28.6%
Total	42	100%

Table 4. Radio information on health

Medium	No of Respondents who receive information on health, antenatal or safe motherhood practices	%
Yes	29	69.05%
No	13	30.95%
Total	42	100%

Table 5. **Frequency of health information received**

How often is information on health received	Radio Lagos	%	%	Wazobia	%	Faaji	%
Everyday	-	-		1	25%	0	0
2-3 times per week	6	50%	50%	1	25%	2	15.38%
Once in a week	0	-		0	0	4	30.77%
Once in a while	6	50%	50%	2	50%	7	53.85%
Total	12	100%	100%	4	100%	13	100%

Q3. Do you listen or receive information on health, ante natal or safe motherhood practices from any programme from the above radio stations?

Twenty-nine respondents listen to information about health from the above radio station, while 13 respondents do not listen to information about their health from the above radio stations.

Q4. If yes, how often do you listen to, or receive information from the programme?

Twenty-nine respondents said they often received information on health on radio. In specific term, only one of the respondents listened to the health information on the radio every day. 11 respondents listen to health information on the radio 2 or 3 times a week, 8 respondents listen once a week, while only 14 listened to health

Table 6. Quality of information

Quality Ratings of Health Information	Radio Lagos	%	Wazobia	%	Faaji	%
Very Good	5	41.67	1	25	6	46.15
Good	7	58.33	3	75	7	53.85
Average	0	0	0	0	0	0
Total	12	100%	4	100%	13	100%

Table 7. Relevance of information

Relevance of the info to respondents	Radio Lagos	%		Wazobia	%	Faaji	%
Very Useful	10	83.33		2	50	12	92.13
Somehow Useful	2	16.67		2	50	1	7.7
Not really Useful	0	0		0	0	0	0
Total	12	100%		4	100%	13	100%

information on the radio once in a while. Of the 42 members only 8 did not respond to the question.

Q5. How will you rate the quality of information given out?

Twelve respondents classified the information received as very good, while 20 classified this information as good and only one respondent felt the information received was average. Nine respondents did not respond to this question at all.

Q6. How relevant is the information to you and your health?

Twenty-six respondents consider the information received as very useful, 6 respondents feel the information received is somehow useful and zero respondent thinks the information is not really useful.

Q7. When you go for ante-natal, do health providers (in hospital) speak your language (e.g. Yoruba) to explain things to you during ante natal?

Twenty-five Respondents answered yes, meaning that the health provider speaks its language; while 2 answered no. 13 respondents did not answer this question at all.

Q8. Would you have preferred health workers explain things to you in your language rather than in English?

Nine respondents said they preferred their mother tongue from health workers, while 7 respondents said they preferred English, while 24 of the respondents said they preferred both languages. Two candidates did not respond to this question.

Q9. Have you ever visited or consulted a traditional birth attendant (Agbebi)

Table 8. Usage of local language by health providers

Respondents that got Info in Local Language	Radio Lagos	%	Wazobia	%	Faaji	%
Yes	10	83.33	1	25	9	69.23
No	1	8.333	0	0	0	0
Not really	1	8.333	3	75	4	30.77
Total	12	100%	4	100%	13	100%

Table 9. Language preference by respondents

Respondents that will prefer Local Language	Radio Lagos	%	Wazobia	%	Faaji	%
Yes	4	33.333	0	0	3	23.077
No	1	8.333	3	75	0	0
Both	7	58.333	1	25	10	76.92
Total	12	100%	4	100%	13	100%

Table 10. Visitation to traditional birth attendants

Respondents that have consulted Native Doctors (TBA)	Radio Lagos	%	Wazobia	%	Faaji	%
Yes	0	0	1	25	0	0
No	12	100	3	75	13	100
Total	12	100%	4	100%	13	100%

Of 29 of respondents, 28 said they have never visited traditional birth attendants, one responded in the affirmative, while 3 respondents were undecided

DISCUSSION

The data reveal that women listen to indigenous radio disseminating information in local language to get information either for health or entertainment especially music. Radio Lagos (*Tiwa n Tiwa*) with 52.38% has the highest number of women listening to it for health information. In rating the quality of information on safe motherhood practices on the radio stations, 41.67% goes to very good while good has 58.33%. And looking at how useful the information has been to the target audience, very useful has 83.33% for Radio Lagos, 92.31% for *Faaji* FM and 50% for *Wazobia*FM. This shows that for Nigeria in general and Lagos State in particular to reduce maternal mortality rate and advance in safe motherhood practices, involvement of indigenous language media is imperative in giving women necessary information.

Personal observation during the clinic day at the public general hospital revealed that the nurses engaged the pregnant and nursing mothers through local languages – Yoruba and Pidgin. After speaking in English, they interpreted in Yoruba and pidgin for non-Yoruba speaking women. Interacting with the Assistant Chief Nursing Officer, Mabel Omorokpe, affirmed that indigenous language has impacted safe motherhood practices among women in the state. "We speak Yoruba and pidgin to the women when they come for ante and post-natal treatment. Indigenous language has impacted and improved safe motherhood practices among women in the state. Speaking the local languages has made the women to know that they can get what they want here instead of embracing unsafe practices. They now know that they can get safe motherhood practices and this has reduced mortality to some extent."

It was also learnt that for those from the northern part of Nigeria that reside in Lagos, the women are encouraged to come with their husbands who serve as interpreters during the ante natal sessions,

This therefore highlights the importance of local language by health providers to women especially in rural areas. Majority of the respondents answered that they would prefer health workers to speak in local language. This invariably means that, for the non-Yoruba speaking women, aside pidgin, there should be provision for interpretation especially for people from the Northern part of the country.

Development communication has to do with the mobilisation of a people to have a positive change in their living conditions. Through it, people are provided with adequate knowledge and information so that they are persuaded, through sound reasoning to change in a predetermined direction (Oyero, 2003). This implies that the objective to reduce maternal mortality and child morbidity rate can be achieved.

Indigenous language media propagate indigenous knowledge, experiences and culture; and when creatively used, they enhance development ideas and messages to the people. And utilization of the mass media of communication, which de-emphasizes the use of indigenous media therefore, constitutes a threat to development (Oyero, 2003; FAO, 1998; Soola, 1984).

Several other scholars have called to the importance of indigenous language in mobilizing the people development. Soola (1998) as quoted also by Oyero (2003:111), while discussing the family planning information dissemination methods, notes that the success of such messages will be determined by the extent to which such communication is "predicated on an understanding of the society's culture, its peculiar system of values and attitudes". Oyero (2003) also quoted by Burnay

(1997) "as saying that indigenous has been proven to be very potent in creating a critical mass of real communication for substantial change."

CONCLUSION

Media is a veritable tool in promoting health development both at national and regional levels. The outcome of the research shows that the indigenous radio stations are not doing enough in disseminating information on safe motherhood practices to the target audience. Radio Lagos is constant on the *Se'rigbo* programme in divulging information on family planning, but the question is: after the expiration of the sponsored programme, what next?

Faaji FM on its own does not have any health programme, its *E Gbe Yewo* is a current affairs programme which could deal with health issues as the challenge presents itself and its family belt on the programme is not specifically for health. *Wazobia* FM on its own sometimes might not air the *KuleleZone* programme as a result of structural adjustment in the organisation thereby preventing the target audience from gaining access to information. The stations however aired trending health issues in the society in their news hour.

The result shows that more than half of the respondents are benefiting from the programme while others listened to the radio stations for entertainment especially music. This reveals that indigenous language radio could reach large number of women thereby leading to greater knowledge on safe motherhood practices and accessing information that would aid safe delivery. The survey also underscores the importance of indigenous language among the women. Many of them are at home when they listen to information in the indigenous language and more comfortable when health providers speak in the local language to them. This is one of the reasons some women patronise traditional birth attendants.

In interview with health providers in general hospitals across the state, it is discovered that they communicate in indigenous languages –Yoruba and pidgin due to the cultural diversity in Lagos. They declared that communicating in indigenous language has improved safe motherhood practices in the state and has helped the women to know they can get what they want in general hospitals. However, the study reveals that there is no legislation in the state by the government in the use of local language to the target-audience but the health providers embarked on it to reach the women.

RECOMMENDATIONS

As a way of recommendations, there is a need for legislation of indigenous language as an alternate means of communication in the health sector by the state government in order to reach wider women and improve safe motherhood practices in Lagos. This will encourage women to use government health facilities. Also, the indigenous language media need to do more in the area of disseminating information through local programmes that would focus on safe motherhood. The state government could as well sponsor a health programme in that regards.

FUTURE RESEARCH DIRECTIONS

It is pertinent for future research direction to focus on the imperatives of having more indigenous language programming and productions as media content.

CONFLICT OF INTEREST

There is no conflict of interest regarding the paper.

ACKNOWLEDGEMENT

The author appreciates the staff of Orile Agege General Hospital, Lagos State especially the maternal section for their support. The author recognises Head of the nurses, Chief Matron, Mrs. Margret Agbeleke for permission to administer the questionnaire. The respondents are also commended for their responses which is contributing towards safe motherhood practices,

REFERENCES

Adeniyi, H., & Bello, R. (2006). *Nigerian Media, Indigenous Languages and Sustainable Development. Lagos*. Nigeria: Lagos State University; http://www.lingref.com/cpp/acal/36/paper1419.pdf

Bandura, A. (2012). Social Cognitive Theory. In P. A. M. Van Lange, A. W. Kruglanski, & E. T. Higgins (Eds.), Handbook of theories of social psychology (pp. 349-373). Thousand Oaks, CA: Sage. doi:10.4135/9781446249215.n18

Bankole, A., Sedgh, G., Okonofua, F., Imarhiagbe, C., Hussain, R., & Wulf, D. (2009). Barriers to Safe Motherhood in Nigeria, New York: Guttmacher Institute. Retrieved from https://www.guttmacher.org/sites/default/files/report_pdf/motherhoodnigeria.pdf

Dooley, J. A., Jones, S. C., & Desmarais, K. (2009). Strategic social marketing in Canada: Ten phases to planning and implementing cancer prevention and cancer screening campaigns. *Social Marketing Quarterly*, *15*(3), 33–48. doi:10.1080/15245000903144999

Health, P. S. U. The Public Health Bush Book Vol. 1. Strategies and Resources. Department of Health; Darwin, NT, Australia: 2007. [Google Scholar]

Itari, P. E., Beshel, C. A., & Okeme, I. (2015). Indigenous Communication Media and Utilization of Development Information in Rural Communities of South-South Nigeria. [IJEL]. *International Journal of English and Literature*, *5*(1), 85–96.

Moore, M. K. (n.d.). A literature review on behalf of and under the overall guidance of WHO'S Division of Reproductive Health. Retrieved from https://apps.who.int/iris/bitstream/handle/10665/69834/WHO_RHT_97.34_eng.pdf;jsessionid=F8AC617DE6A670C4BF5362D87EB1512E?sequence=1

Okereke, E., Aradeon, S., Akerele, A., Tanko, M., Yisa, I., & Obonyo, B. (2013). Knowledge of safe motherhood among women in rural communities in Northern Nigeria: Implications for maternal mortality reduction, licensee BioMed Central Ltd. doi:10.1186/1742-4755-10-57

Oye-Adeniran, B., Odeyemi, K., Gbadegesin, A., Akin-Adenekan, O., Akinsola, O., Ekanem, E., & Osilaja, O. (2019). Causes of maternal mortality in Lagos State, Nigeria. Ann Trop Med Public Health. Retrieved from http://www.atmph.org/text.asp?2014/7/3/177/149501

Oyesomi, K. O., & Salawu, A. (2019). Assessing the Uniqueness of Indigenous Language in Advertising: Analysis of Figurative Language Used in Selected Telecommunication Yoruba Advertisement in Nigeria. *Qualitative Report*, *24*(10), 2574–2591. Retrieved from https://nsuworks.nova.edu/tqr/vol24/iss10/12

Oyesomi, K. O., Salawu, A., & Olorunyomi, B. (2017). Indigenous Communication: Socio-Economic Characteristics Influencing Contemporary Female Political Participation. [JIWS]. *Journal of International Women's Studies*, *18*(4), 164–181.

Omoloso, I. A., & Abdu rauf-Salau, A. (2014). May Indigenous Language Newspapers in Nigeria from 1914-2013: Review, A. A Paper presented at the Amalgamation National Conference of the Department of Political Science & Department of History and International Studies. Ibrahim Badamasi Babangida University. Lapai, Niger State, Nigeria. Retrieved from: https://www.academia.edu/17562000/

Salawu, A. (2006). Indigenous Language Media: A Veritable Tool for African Language Learning, *Journal of Multicultural Discourses* doi:10.1080/10382040608668533

Salawu, A. (2016). Indigenous Language Media and Democracy in Africa. In A. Salawu, & M. B. Chibita (Ed.), Indigenous Language Media, Language Politics and Democracy in Africa (pp. 13-27), Palgrave Macmillan, UK doi:10.1057/9781137547309_2

KEY TERMS AND DEFINITIONS

General Hospital: A government secondary public health facility.

Health Communication: The process of enabling people to increase control over, and to improve, their health.

Health Provider: A person that provides a health care service.

Indigenous Language: language that is native to a region and spoken by indigenous people of the same cultural value and belief.

Indigenous Media: Forms of media expression conceptualized, produced and circulated by indigenous peoples around the globe as vehicles for communication.

Maternal Mortality: Death of a woman while pregnant or within 42 days of termination of pregnancy, irrespective of the duration and site of the pregnancy, from any cause related to or aggravated by the pregnancy or its management but not from accidental or incidental causes.

Nursing Mother: A mother who is breastfeeding her baby.

Radio: The transmission and reception of electromagnet waves of radio frequency, especially those carrying sound messages.

Safe Motherhood: Ensuring that all women receive the care they need to be safe and healthy throughout pregnancy and childbirth.

Yoruba: The language of the Yoruba, African people of south-western Nigeria and Benin.

Section 2

Indigenous Language Media/Communication and Health-Related Issues

Chapter 6
Indigenous Language Media, Communication, and Sickle Cell Disorder:
Peculiarities of Indigenous Language Media in Tackling Misconceptions of Sickle Cell Disorder

Opeyemi Olaoluwa Oredola
https://orcid.org/0000-0002-0361-3895
Covenant University, Nigeria

Kehinde Opeyemi Oyesomi
https://orcid.org/0000-0002-5318-0442
Covenant University, Nigeria

Ada Sonia Peter
Covenant University, Nigeria

ABSTRACT

The importance of health communication and information cannot be over emphasized especially with issues related to sickle cell disorder. Sickle cell disorder, common among Africans, has a lot of myths and misconceptions tied to it, so this chapter unearths and explores how indigenous communication can facilitate learning and understanding of the disorder majorly in rural areas and some urban areas where knowledge of the disorder is assessed low using the focus group discussion. It also reveals the importance of incorporating indigenous language and communication techniques in increasing awareness and eradicating stereotypes as regards sickle cell disorder. The findings of this chapter reflect that misinformation occurs due to lack of

DOI: 10.4018/978-1-7998-2091-8.ch006

proper understanding of language used in sickle cell health communication-related issues. Hence, this chapter proposes that health education about the concept of SCD should be executed majorly in indigenous languages and through the indigenous media platforms.

INTRODUCTION

There is no other known inherited disorder present at such high frequency in a large population and of comparable severity as sickle cell anemia in Africa. With rising standards of living and control of malaria, sickle cell anemia will become an immense medical, social and economic problem throughout the continent (Elguero, et. al, 2015, p. 3).

The World Health Organization projects that as many as 30% of Nigerians are carriers of the sickle cell trait. An estimated 150,000 children are born with the disease in Nigeria each year, in the absence of knowledge and how to manage the disease, many go in search of their own cures (Adegoke, Kuteyi 2012, p. 5). In order to increase the awareness, eradicate myths and misconceptions amongst Nigerians on the disorder, indigenous language media becomes a potent tool in communicating such.

In Nigeria, Sickle Cell Disorder and linked education is now being taught as part of social studies in colleges, consequently generating more awareness nonetheless, this is limited in rural areas (Olakunle, Kenneth, Olalekan, & Adenike, 2014, p. 13). However, this limitation can be curbed if the technique of indigenous language is employed in educating carriers and relations on issues related to the disorder.

This paper therefore examined the importance of incorporating Indigenous language and communication techniques in increasing awareness and eradicating stereotypes as regards sickle cell disorder. It is believed that the authenticity attached to indigenous communication techniques via indigenous language can be used effectively to teach the peculiarities of sickle cell disorder.

The study also seeks to find out how indigenous communication can facilitate learning and understanding of the disorder majorly in rural areas and some urban areas where knowledge of the disorder is assessed low. This study will employ the use of focus group discussions in analyzing the uniqueness of indigenous language media and communication techniques in creating and expanding knowledge as regards sickle cell disorder. Literature will also be reviewed to find out the research findings and positions of scholars and researchers on the subject matter.

The results of the study brought to fore the distinctive peculiarities in employing the indigenous language media and establish a high level of understanding of the disorder as opposed to modern and western communication techniques which had yielded little or minimal desired results. The researchers therefore argue the need to examine the use of indigenous language media and communication technique in tackling the misconceptions and eradicating the myths by educating the populace through the use of indigenous language media whose reliability has been proven by several authors over other media forms.

BACKGROUND TO THE STUDY

Sickle cell disease (SCD), also known as sickle cell anemia or sickle cell disorder is one of the most widespread inherited lethal diseases in the world; and was first described in 1910 (Herrick, 1910). It is a common genetic disorder caused by mutations in both copies of the β-globin gene, a major subunit of hemoglobin (Hb) which damages and deforms red blood cells. The clinical picture of the disease usually emerges after four months of age with highly phenotypically variable disease (Bunn, 1997). SCD affects millions of people worldwide. About 300, 000 children globally are born yearly with the disease (Okpala, Thomas, Westerdale, Jegede, Raj, Daley, & Abbs, 2002), whose origin is traceable to the people of Sub Saharan-Africa, Mediterranean, Middle Eastern, and Indian descent (Luzzatto, 1981). Amongst these groups, people of Sub-Saharan African are known to have the highest occurrence (Gubis, Ferster, Kentos, N'Gay Munungi, Cotton, & Vertonge, 2005; Creary, 2007). A plethora of major clinical symptoms are associated with SCD. Some of these include chronic pains, acute anemia, infection, and joint swelling and other idiosyncratic complications (Serjeant & Serjeant, 2001). These symptoms often require sufferers go to a variety of Specialists for management. It has been estimated that up to 90% of patients are admitted to hospitals at one time or the other for episodes of pain (Brozovic, Davies, & Brownell, 1987). Individuals with SCD are also at risk of academic failure, as well as psychosocial maladjustment (Brown, Armstrong, & Eckman, 1993).

Approximately three quarters of all new SCD births and 7.0% of the world's carrier population of the SCD gene are found in Africa (Weatherall, 2001). SCD is a key health problem in Nigeria, the most populous black nation in Africa, with a population of over 140 million. It is estimated that SCD affects about 2% of the general population in Nigeria, which is has the highest incidence of SCD patients than any other country in the world, with over 24% of the population being carriers of the muted gene (World Health Organization (WHO, 2006). The life expectancy of patients with SCD is reduced by 25-30 years compared to that of the general population (Platt, Brambilla, Rosse, Milner, Castro, & Klug, 1994).

Over the years, progress in scientific breakthrough has resulted to an increasing number of SCD Patients living longer, with fewer incidents of painful crises, and enhanced improved quality of lives. The most scientific breakthrough is the use of a drug called *hydroxyurea* which has reduced mortality dramatically in developed countries. Despite these scientific advances and breakthrough in ensuring SCD patients live longer, these advances and its applicability are still very scanty in poorer countries of the world. Patients with SCD are faced with the difficult challenges of having access to drugs and qualified doctors to provide them the latest advancement in the management of their condition.

The epidemiology of SCD has made it a global disease of public health importance that has been recognized by the WHO (Makano, Williams & Marsch, 2007). In fact, the UN-WHO resolution (22 December, 2008) declaring 19 June the World Day for Sickle Cell and Thalassemia underscores the global importance of the disorder. Mabayoje (1956) highlights the burden of the disorder is this way:

Sickle cell anemia is a major disease of West Africa. It is a cause of distress in many families. It therefore deserves much better recognition than it gets at present. It should be treated as a major disease in schools of tropical medicine, textbooks and in all medical schools in tropical Africa. (p. 196).

SCD is a serious disorder that needs close monitoring in the population (Michael, 1993). Its management is burdensome on sufferers, and it has been demonstrated to affect psychological well-being (Bamisaiye, Bakare, & Olatawura, 1974; Ohaeri, Sokunbi, & Akinlade, 1995). The Nigerian society, and by extension African societies, have an aberrant attitude towards people with various forms of illnesses in the form of stigma, rejection, and disrespect. It is thought that illnesses like SCD are caused by witchcraft, magical spells, curses, or water spirits. These misconceptions, according to Ugwuegbu (1994), may lead to negative attitudes towards SCD patients.

SCD symptomology compares in some respects with the *ogbanje (Igbo) or Abiku (Yoruba)* phenomenon (Nzewi, 2001) expressed in Wole Soyinka's (Soyinka, 1967) and J.P Clarke's (Clarke, 1967) *Abiku.* In the preternatural the *Abiku* is 'ageless' and lives on the baobab and other big trees from which s/he selects a mother from among humans and enter a continuous cycle of birth, death, and rebirth to the same woman, preventing the birth of more children to the home. Clarke expresses it thus...*Tired, her milk going sour, where many more mouths gladden the heart.* The *Abiku's* intention is assumed to be the punishment of the particular family that has been chosen. Thus, the following line written by Soyinka: *...Must I weep for goats and cowries, for palm oil and sprinkled ash? Mothers! I'll be the suppliant snake coiled on the doorstep, yours the killing cry.* Moreover, the child is thought to have the ability to either stay alive or die, and therefore are usually urged to 'step in and stay', and given reasons and promises to do so.

Negative attitudes to and stigma against people living with sickle cell disorder, emanate from a lack of knowledge of the nature of the disorder, and add up to the burden imposed on Patients and their families. They also influence the health-seeking behaviour of patients and their family members (Asakitipi, 2008). Families of SCD children may rather seek spiritual solution than medical counselling/intervention, especially in the rural areas. Although Onwubalili (1983) did suggest the decrease in belief in the *ogbanje* phenomenon due to advances in the medical science, supportive data to that effect is still lacking. To effectively manage, control, and prevent SCD the public needs must understand it properly.

The objective of this study therefore is to determine the impact of indigenous language media in increasing general knowledge and tackling misconception of SCD by University students. The level of awareness of etiological and possible interventions in SCD would be investigated in the study. Misconceptions, wrong attribution of causes and treatment would be investigated in the study. The study would similarly highlight areas of inadequate knowledge. It is hoped that the findings from this study would encourage the development of promotional and educational approaches that would enhance the understanding, management, and prevention of SCD.

RESEARCH QUESTIONS

In view of the objectives of this study, the following are the research questions for investigation:

1. How can indigenous communication facilitate learning and understanding of sickle cell disorder?
2. What are the importance of incorporating indigenous language and communication techniques in increasing awareness and eradicating stereotypes as regards sickle cell disorder?
3. How do indigenous languages influence the reception of information and messages as regards sickle cell disorder?
4. How can indigenous language communication be used to tackle myths and misconceptions as regards sickle cell disorder?

CONCEPTUAL CLARIFICATIONS

Indigenous Language Media

The exceptionality of indigenous language media for development purposes cannot be over emphasized as shown in previous studies (Oyesomi, Salawu & Olorunyomi, 2017, Oyesomi, Okorie, Ahmadu & Itsekor, 2014, Oyero, Oyesomi, Abioye, Ajiboye & Kayode Adedeji 2018, Oyesomi & Salawu, 2019). It is evident that the battle for the soul of African languages is not yet over. Rather than the languages becoming increasingly appreciated and embraced by the owners, there is evidently a decline (Eyoh, 1986 p. 112; Salawu, 2001). This worrisome decline is signposted by the advancement of technology and modernity. The explanation is that as Africans admire technology and crave modernity, they see everything African (language, culture) as primitive and ancient. It is apparent that originality and excellence in African languages and cultures are quickly vanishing, as there remains only a small remnant of that authentic tradition. Many of the old Africans who were well versed in the excellent use of African languages in all their ramifications (diction, idioms, proverbs, phonology) are no longer alive. Only a very negligible few young Africans can really boast of excellence and originality in the use of African languages.

In most developing countries, communication in indigenous languages has been adversely affected due to the fact of their colonisation. For instance, English is Nigeria's official language and the main medium of communication; therefore, indigenous languages are not highly esteemed. The structure that the colonialists handed down remains today, decades after they have left. In fact, it is even more strengthened as English (for instance) and Western education continues to be the language and education of power and progress in life. Therefore, there is understandably ever and fast-growing interest in both the language and the education. But by far the greatest problem militating against the survival of African languages is that of the attitude of most native speakers to their languages.

This was further explained by NgugWa Thiong'o, a foremost Kenyan writer, in an interview, who painted the picture thus: "Whereas you see today people identify themselves with that which is removed from them. That which is near them, they don't want to identify with". (Eyoh, 1986, p. 112). The elites are, however, the guiltiest of this. This is, equally, reflected in their attitude towards the patronage of indigenous language press, in terms of readership and advertisement placement (Salawu, 2004a, 2004b). For instance, Salawu (2004b p. 213) found that the higher the level of education, the lower the readership of Yoruba newspapers. This means that the more (Western) education a respondent acquires, the more likely he is not to be able to operate (speak or read) in the local languages; and, of course, the more his interest in local language and culture will wane. Similarly, the study revealed that the higher the level of education, the less regular the readership of Yoruba newspapers.

The study also revealed that people with a higher education level, who are most likely to be in the higher income level, read the Yoruba newspapers less and less regularly than the low-income earners. Already, some African languages have ceased to exist. Again, there are palpable and genuine fears that many more are on the verge of extinction. The disappearance seems only a matter of time now. For any African with a concern for the soul and survival of his language and culture, there must be a deliberate and sincere effort to learn and teach the language in its proper form (Adegbite, 2002). Alas, the situation with the learning, and by extension, the teaching of African languages is by no means cheerful.

Not many young Africans are interested in learning the languages, ether formally or normally. Akinleye (1988) discloses that nobody has studied Efik (a language in the South-eastern part of Nigeria) n the senor secondary schools in the past 14 years. The situation may just be a little better with the bigger African languages. Compared to the enrolments for the study of European languages (like English and French) n our universities, there is a lot to worry about n the enrolments for the study of African languages. In fact, many of the students of African languages in the universities carry on with diminished egos. At the school level, the performance in African languages is anything but excellent. Awoniyi (1995 p. 446) showed the failure rates in the Yoruba language at both the West African School Certificate and Primary School Leaving Certificate levels over a period of years. For instance, between 1983 and 1985, over 44% of the total number of candidates who sat for the Yoruba language at the WASC Examination failed. The important point to make here is that there is a problem with the teaching and learning of African languages.

Yet, the languages must be taught and learnt. This is because no group of human beings can afford to have its language discarded. It is only in teaching and learning the languages that the heritage will live on. Every language reflects the culture of a people. Thus, it is local to say that people would express themselves and their cultures better in the language of their own. Communication is better enhanced in a medium that expresses the totality of the culture of a given people (Broughton et al., 1978).

One of the arguments against the development and use of African languages as languages of the media is the multiplicity of the languages. It is claimed that linguistic diversity in Africa is of such proportion that Africans cannot share or work in their own languages (Prah, 1999 p. 3).

Africa is sad to have 2000 languages, 400 of which are found in Nigeria alone. For this reason, it is argued that it is too late for African languages to be developed. Africans should therefore carry on n the colonial languages' (Prah, 2001). Labeling the African language multiplicity as 'Tower of Babel myth' (Egbokhare, 2004 p. 8), Prah (2001 p. 188-189) pointed out that the real problem appeared to be the criteria used to count African languages. Eghokhare et al. (2001) contended that 80% of Africans speak no more than 12 key languages: Fulfulde, Hausa, Swahili; Nguni, Sotho-Tswana, Western Inter-Lacustrine Bentu, Amharic, Yoruba, Igbo, Bamsara, Oromo and Luo. They argued further that the so called 400 languages in Nigeria can be reduced to less than 100 mutual intelligibility clusters. Referring to the sad publication, Egbokhare (2004 p. 9) states: Besides, if we take the population of those who speak the 10 major and medium languages ether as first or second languages in Nigeria, we would cover close to 90% of the population. There is no reason for instance why Efik, Ibibio, Anang should be listed as different or why a large number of the Edoid languages are listed as separate autonomous languages (Egbokhare et. al 2001).

Prah (1999) sad that as far as African development is concerned, the upshots of these facts are that the harmonization of African languages which show high levels of mutual intelligibility would greatly facilitate the economics of scale in the development of educational, media and cultural materials which would go a long way in strengthening the bass of society for the cultural and social development of Africa.

It provides the key to the methodology of eradicating the stigma of inferiority, which the colonial experience has invested in African languages. No region of the world is linguistically monolithic, which means there is diversity in the modes of communication used in different regions of the world (Cheyney, 1992).

And, despite the dominance of some languages, the smaller languages continue to exist and are spoken with relish by their native speakers and used to varying degrees in the media (Lasswell, 1948; 1960 & 1989).

Indigenous Language Media in Nigeria

When the modern television broadcasting system came to Nigeria, the expectation was that t would provide adequate services in education, social and economic development (Emenyonu, 1982). The system was also expected to transmit the Nigerian and African cultures, tradition, politics, literature, drama and entertainment (UNESCO, 1974). As expected, the system, at its inception, did very well in the area of education. However, it left a big gap in the area of cultural transmission. Between 1959, when television came to Nigeria, and 1975, the nation heavily depended on foreign imported programmes.

UNESCO (1974) noted that only 25% of the programmes were produced within the nation; the rest were foreign. For this reason and also because of the frequency allocation problem (Eyoh, 1986), the Federal Government of Nigeria decided in 1975 to take over the administration of all television station in the country. While justifying the decision, the government sad it would like to see television 'highlight the way of life of Nigerians as against the present programmes whereby foreign films which have no relevance to our way of life dominate their dally events' (Folarin, 2000).

According to Oyetunde and Umolu (1991), this intervention appeared to have changed the tide for good for cultural transmission and the use of local languages on the nation's television. The radio system was also affected, as around this time, precisely n 1978, the Federal Radio Corporation of Nigeria (FRCN) Decree No. 8 was promulgated. Amongst other things, t restructured FRCN into four linguistic zones, namely: Kaduna: Hausa, Fulfulde, Kanuri, Nupe and English. Enugu: Igbo, Tiv, Izon, Efik and English. Ibadan: Yoruba, Edo, gala, Urhobo and English. Lagos: English. The local languages and English designated for various zones became each zone's languages of broadcasting. Radio stations across the country actually contributed to the promotion of a number of Nigerian languages through various message types and programmes: news, features, interviews, discussion programmes and chit-chats. The situation has, however, changed with some radio stations and some languages in Nigeria.

For instance, Onukaogu (2002) noted that the media in Cross River and Akwa Ibom States are no longer gang prominence to the local language known in that area, Efik. According to him, out of a total of 7560 minutes expended n broadcasting in the week, only a total of 425 minutes is allocated to the indigenous language, leaving a total of 7135 minutes for programmes in English. This translates to 5.6% for local language and 94.4% for English. Onukaogu remarked: The result is that the medium that should create awareness for the people in local language has little or no regard for the local language.

Consequently, publishers' audience size dwindles and the attraction to publish in these languages became inexistent. (Onukaogu, 2002 p.9). By and large, the print media seem more culpable than the electronic media in the use of local languages. This is probably accounted for by virtue of the broadcast media being principally an oral/aural medium.

Being oral, the indigenous language does not cost the broadcaster, who may not be able to write it, anything to broadcast n t (Osgood, 1954). Also, being aural, it does not cost the listener, who may not be able to read the language, anything to listen to it. In other words, the broadcast medium breaks the barrier of illiteracy. Added to this is the economic nonviability of publishing in indigenous languages. t has already been settled that Africans, especially the educated (Western), do not seem to appreciate their languages as being fit for serious matters of education, business, governance etc.; as such, they do not patronize it. Unlike the broadcast media, the print media require repeated purchase for use. So, if the educated, who are more likely to have the economic power to purchase, are not appreciative of their languages, then they cannot patronize the media ether in terms of copy purchase or placement of advertisements.

This, actually, is the reason why newspapers, especially those published in indigenous languages, have not been viable. Though it is true that the indigenous language press marked the beginning of the Nigerian press, the fact remains that despite this historical masterstroke, things have not been rosy for the indigenous language press (Salawu, 2001a, 2004b).

For instance, until the emergence of the Alaroye phenomenon on the scene of the Yoruba press in 1996, this section of the press had remained silent for a long time (Salawu, 2004c). The emergence of Alaroye newspaper in 1996 marked a milestone in the affairs of Yoruba and, indeed, the indigenous language press in Nigeria.

Within a short time, this newspaper became popular because of its arresting cover design and styles of headline-casting and story presentation. t actually popularized reading of Yoruba newspapers among the people. It is the largest local language newspaper, with a circulation figure of not less than 150,000 per week. It sells in Europe and several West African countries where the Yoruba reside. Its publishers, World information Agents, have also added other Yoruba publications to their titles. They include: Alaroye magazine, Atoka Alaroye, IririAye and Akede Agbaye. There is no doubt that with the tremendous patronage the Alaroye publications and similar others are enjoying, the appreciation and learning of the Yoruba language, for instance, will be fast tracked.

Indigenous Language and Health Promotion

As opined by Webster (2018), the dearth of health services and promotion rendered in Indigenous languages is hampering the delivery of care and information to Indigenous populations. In most scenario, health care personnel who do not speak or understand indigenous languages rely on patients and other staff as informal interpreters, although they have limited understanding of medical terminology.

Training health care workers who speak local languages can reduce linguistic barriers to receiving adequate health care. Furthermore, the existence of information from care givers and experts on sickle cell disorder in local languages will facilitate the reception and understanding of messages as regards the disorder.

Additionally, employing the use of indigenous language during health campaigns will aid understanding and reduce drastically myths and misconceptions amongst the people. A 2015 report by the Office of the Languages Commissioner of Nunavut found that language boundaries negatively affect access to medicinal services, understanding privacy, access to psychological wellness administrations, consistence to treatment plans and human services costs. It additionally influences nature of consideration, and can prompt misdiagnoses, medicinal mistakes and ill-advised drug, expresses the report.

Furthermore, Webster believes language is a good indicator of a person's "cultural connectedness," Indigenous patients and health care givers who speak their cultural tongue are more likely to be connected to their culture, which in turn improves their well-being. Likewise, being unable to speak their people's tongue is a red flag of cultural disconnection, which is linked to worse health outcomes. Regarding promoting health services, Oyero (2007) noticed that indigenous language has demonstrated to be intense in making a minimum amount of genuine communication for generous change.

Indigenous Communication Techniques

Indigenous information is preserved and adapted by being used and communicated to others. Just as the mass media and other external channels manly carry messages generated outside local communities, localized indigenous channels manly carry information about local issues. Understanding how such information is communicated could be an important key to identifying local technologies that can be adapted and used elsewhere. Indigenous communication can take many different forms. They are explained hereunder:

Folk media are the forerunners of mass media. Like the mass media they are used primarily for entertainment, but may also promote education, social values, and cultural practices (Schramm, 1954). Each culture has its own forms: song, dance, puppetry, festivals, plays, storytelling, debates, proverbs, parades, and so on. Up until very recently, Icelandic commutes passed the long hours of winter darkness entertaining each other by recounting the great sagas. The sagas were used to transmit information which both amused and educated and served to retain much indigenous knowledge in the commutes. Television, introduced only in the 1960s in that country, threatens to undermine this tradition. When development professionals talk of communicating with technology users, many are thinking of the mass media or extension agencies.

Vast amounts of money have been poured into building up these organizations and promoting messages through them, and a myriad of studies has looked at how they function and how effective they are (Severin & iTankard, i1992). i

Outside agencies have often adapted folk media to carry messages on topics such as family planning or politics. While such strategies can be very successful, they have two dangers: the implanted messages may not fit the chosen medium, and audiences may resent outsiders who tamper with the traditional form.

Deliberate Instruction. According to Uche (1989), parents teach children, craftspeople instruct apprentices, elders guide youths, and adolescents undergo initiation rites. Many societies have traditional, often religious, schools. Much of the information that is needed to survive is learned not through the occasional puppet show or even through schools or the mass media, but through deliberate instruction. This is just as true in the industrial world, yet deliberate instruction has received little attention from development specialists.

One way in which outsiders can make use of these channels is by training and learning from indigenous professionals, adding to instead of replacing the skills of traditional healers of both humans and livestock, blacksmiths, and midwives. These experts can then teach their new skills to their clients and apprentices. Tapping into and co-operating with the indigenous experts who already serve their communities avoids the costly training of new personnel from scratch, avoids creating tensions in the community by superimposing new people and staff where capacity already exists, and ensures that people in remote areas receive services that would be difficult to provide conventionally.

Informal channels carry perhaps the bulk of indigenous communication. At home, in the tea house, in the fields and on the road, in the chief's house and at the market - all are situations where technical information and skills can be communicated. Such communication is not orchestrated or controlled, but is spontaneous and informal.

Development professionals have tried to take advantage of informal channels by trying to place messages in the form of posters and radio programmes into areas where people gather, such as mosques, coffee shops, grinding mills, and wells. Outsiders often hope that these informal channels will take over and diffuse the message further once a few key opinion leaders have been informed. But this is not always the case. People must consider a message sufficiently 'newsworthy', and credible, before they pass it on to others in informal conversation. And what they do say is coloured by their own memory and interpretation, which can lead (in the eyes of project officials) to message distortion and loss. But in the eyes of local people, such selective communication can also lead to local innovations and cultural adaptations.

Records may take many forms. Balinese irrigation associations traditionally write land ownership records and tax obligations on palm leaves. Chinese libraries contain ancient works of immense current value - an example being the descriptions of medicinal plants that Chinese scientists have drawn on recently to discover the new anti-malarial drug, artemisinin. But records need not be written: African storytellers narrate memorized historical epics and genealogies in detail and at length.

Direct observation Communication does not have to be intentional - or even involve another person. Most learning during childhood and apprenticeships is a result of imitation. A farmer may see a neighbour's bumper crop and conclude that the variety or technique used is good.

THEORETICAL FRAMEWORK

Media Framing

Entman (2007 p. 168) defines framing as the process of gathering selected elements of a perceived reality and constructing a narrative that leads to a particular interpretation. Prominent media narratives shape attitudes about a chronic illness such as sickle cell disorder (Entman and Rojecki, 2001). Thus, in addition to direct personal encounters (e.g., knowing someone with sickle cell or learning about it in school), an individual's perceptual schema about the condition may be influenced by the information that she or he acquires through indigenous, modern or online media. This point is particularly relevant given the increased media visibility that sickle cell has received over the last decade.

A recent search of the LexisNexis Academic database revealed that more than 950 print articles about sickle cell disorder appeared in major American media outlets between 2007 and 2009. Beyond the surprisingly large number of media are the implicit frames communicated through them. Sickle cell-related media generally fall into two categories: (1) biomedical characteristics, where basic information about etiology or clinical treatment of the condition is provided (e.g., Weiss, 2007, p. 2); and (2) human interest aspects that highlight personal challenges and social implications of managing sickle cell disorder (Lee, 2007 and Lerner, 2007). 'Human interest' media frequently portray Blacks as subjects, while media describing biomedical aspects of sickle cell disorder rarely mention race or ethnicity (Bediako and Haywood, 2009). In addition, educational materials about sickle cell disorder often feature phenotypically dark-complexioned individuals. This is an important point because despite the global impact of sickle cell (and, concomitantly, its racial/ ethnic diversity), the almost exclusive pairing of the condition with darker-skinned individuals may reinforce the perception that people of colour (particularly Blacks) are prototypical exemplars for sickle cell (Wailoo, 2001, Bediako and Haywood, 2009, p. 1066). As we discuss later, this perception though usually unintended may have significant consequences.

Social Cognitive Theory

Theories that emerge from research on social cognition, or how people process, encode, and retrieve information and apply it to social situations (Higgins, 1996 p. 145) could also potentially inform a general conceptual framework for studies that investigate the influence of race on social attitudes toward sickle cell disorder. Social cognitive research describes the tendency for perceivers to use schemas, or mental shortcuts, to fill in the gaps when they are unsure about their observations of social phenomena (Fiske, 2010).

Implicit personality theories constitute one type of schema that individuals use to form judgments of what others are like (Asch, 1946 p. 246). Some researchers purport that individuals use implicit personality theories to organize various personality traits into meaningful categories that help them to efficiently make sense of others (Sedikides and Anderson, 1994, p. 298). This construct is particularly relevant to studies of social attitudes about sickle cell disorder for three key reasons. First, as previously noted, media invariably pair images of sickle cell disorder with that of Blacks. Second, research has shown that there are pejorative connotations associated with Black people and that these connotations are ubiquitous particularly in American society (Goff, Eberhardt, Williams & Jackson, 2008 p. 298). Third, the consistent portrayal of sickle cell as a Black disorder and the generally depreciatory social attitudes associated with Black people are expected to yield an implicit theory where the condition is not only perceived to be exclusively associated with Blacks, but also grouped with negative attitudes that exist about them. As a result, attitudes toward sickle cell disorder may not only be derived from illness-related perceptions, but might also reflect general social views grounded in subtexts related to race (Rouse, 2004). Consequently, it follows that perceivers who see sickle cell disorder as exclusively related to Blacks would also be more likely to utilize implicit theories that associate the condition with dominant cultural themes about Black people. We speculate that race-based views of sickle cell disorder, though most likely implicit, can shape attitudes among providers and the general public that influence clinical outcomes and public health efforts.

METHOD

This study adopted a focus group method in order to capture information regarding the subject from randomly selected 15 respondents above the age of 18 years. Three focus groups (FGA, FGB and FGC) of five people met on three occasions each. The focus group transcripts were analyzed using an open coding approach, staying close to the original testimonies by highlighting scripts in terms of descriptive, linguistic and conceptual comments, identifying emergent themes, and searching for cross-connections between themes. The coding process was iterative, involving reading emerging codes against the other transcripts, refining the coding scheme and re-reading these against the transcripts again until theoretical saturation was reached and the coding scheme mapped appropriately to material in all transcripts.

DISCUSSION

The first focus group in each series reiterated many themes from the individual focus group, as participants were introduced to one another for the first time and shared their challenging experiences of sickle cell disorder and the orientation about myths and misconceptions which they have heard from the society. Even in the first FGs complex exchanges suggested good rapport was established early between the participants.

During the course of the focus group discussion, the participants drew a reflection on the perception of people about sickle cell disorder in their communities. They further perceived the failure of the traditional and modern media in tackling the myths and misconceptions of sickle cell disorder. Hence, they suggested a need to use the indigenous language media techniques in tackling this myths and misconceptions.

Aderonke, Joke, Gbenga, Damilola, Comfort, Hannnah, Odekunle and Eniola hails from: Oyo, Ogun, Osun, Ekiti, Lagos, Lagos, Kwara and Ondo state respectively. These are the south-western states of Nigeria where cultural beliefs and traditions were held in highest esteem. The participants affirmed that their primary language was Yoruba which was their mother-tongue. They buttressed that quite a number of sickle cell patients are living in daily fear due to the stigmatization from the community. The stigma many at times, come in form of verbal abuses and misconceptions in the indigenous language of the community." Awon omo ti o pe, (incomplete children), Aisan foniku, fola dide, ogun idile lo ma n faa (Sickle cell diseases are orchestrated by family curses from the dieties), Awon omo ti won ti gbabode, agba naa ni won je (Sickle cell patient seen as evil obsessed individual and a black sheep of every family on a mission to bring setbacks to that family).

Furthermore, the participants identified during the course of the focused group discussions that people who have no genuine access to the sensitization and awareness regarding sickle cell disorder, hence the falsehood and misconceptions about sickle cell diseases. These findings were not quite surprising as these dogmatic views is equally obtained in most rural and countryside areas of the country.

The focused group discussions among the participants are summarized below:

Aderonke (Female, 26 Years): *Having sickle cell disorder is not a big deal as long as you love yourself and believe you can cope with all kinds of pain associated with sickle cell. Any pain that comes your way, you can cope better than someone that is not an SS patient. Each time I see this, I get stronger and stronger. It makes me feel that my blood is a wonderful blood regardless of societal perspective about me. When an SS patient, goes through pain, he would get up and move around, but some others when they go through that pain, that's the last of them. They will not make it; the next thing is they are in the mortuary. So that keeps me going. The pain*

I'm talking about is the shame and reproach of the society which you can term as myths and misconceptions about sickle cell. I come from a polygamous home in the south-western part of Nigeria (Yoruba tribe) where people tag sickle cell patients as 'Emere' (demon possessed). This is a big stigma, but I have decided to always encourage myself and not be deterred by the disposition of people around me.

In the focus groups, participants began to share information with one another, such as their perception about sickle cell

Joke: *I know of a sickle cell woman that pounds yam for seven people in the household to make them happy.*

Gbenga: *Ha! She wants to kill herself.*

Damilola: *There are some people who would like to show that they can meet up with responsibilities and would want to satisfy others to the disadvantage of themselves. I cannot do that.*

Comfort: *This is what I have been saying. We need to be our brother's keeper. I could imagine many persons with sickle cell trying to prove that they are strong and they kill themselves. We can save these persons as a group. When we talk on radio and television and any other means so that people know and understand what we can do and cannot do. When people know you have hypertension, they do not stress you. And the person with hypertension tells them and will not stress himself. Why can't they do same thing for people with sickle cell?*

Gbenga: *It is the person with sickle cell who is trying to prove what is not there. It is the person with sickle cell that needs to be taught on what to do and what not to do and to have our backing as a group. She is killing herself under pretense [FGB1: 13].*

The participants recognize a particular type of situation in which perceived pressure to meet societal expectations runs the risk of contravening good self-care, and that it falls to them, acting as group on the basis of shared group interests, to advocate on behalf of individuals. The focus groups also permitted the emergence of a collective challenge to the negative attitudes and reactions of others in society, and a group rejection of the myths and misconceptions that others attach to people living with SCD.

Damilola: *I don't even feel comfortable saying the word 'sickler'. It means I am known with sickness.*

Hannah: *Yes. That word should not even be used for us. It is not a good word.*

Joke: *It is not a good word ...*

Damilola: *I think people should know and respect us and give us the space and what we need. It is our nature and that is it.*

Gbenga: *Once people cannot come to meet me and tell me the rubbish, I am okay. If there is a law that prohibits them from saying that and it is enforced, I am happy. [FGB1: 11].*

Other ways in which they rejected the myths and misconceptions about sickle cell disorder included: challenging the attitudes of others who felt they had the right to pass opinions on those living with SCD; developing the resilience to challenge myths and misconceptions; conceiving the negative attitude/reaction of others as a form of violence against the person with SCD and challenging any individual who projected a negative image of people with SCD by use of disparaging labels especially to illiterates and unlearned individuals who may not understand the core of sickle cell disorder.

However, in the later focus groups, the emphasis moved beyond merely rejecting myths and misconceptions, to the realization that the genesis of such labels lies not in themselves but in wider society.

Odekunle: *We can then go on as a group to tell people about how to support us and not to exclude us from the society by giving us names that are not our parents' names. So, we need to work as a group to learn effective ways of responding individually to such persons and then learn how to address it as a group up to schools, and government levels. If we do it alone on the individual level, I know it is not as effective as when it is done on the group level but I think the group can teach individuals to be confident and be strong and then the group can also create awareness on a broad basis so that most people will know and support the individuals. [FGA3: 6]*

As Kitzinger (1994) has noted, an important feature of focus groups is the scope they provide for participants to interact, disagree and modify one another's opinions. In these series of focus groups, the participants were able to debate and challenge different proposed strategies for dealing with societal myths and misconceptions about SCD.

More so, in a bid to correct the societal anomaly of myths and misconceptions regarding sickle cell disorder using different languages, the participants, also have this to say:

Eniola: *I believe there should be house to house awareness or community one. I believe that people are creating awareness about SS but it is not just effective since it is not house to house.*

Aderonke: *Who are the people creating awareness? Eniola: We have NGOs now doing it.*

Aderonke: *How many times have you seen them on air or on the radio? See and I thank God that this thing is being recorded. You see, the NGOs, they are using us to enrich themselves. How will their programs be effective?*

Eniola: *A non-SS should not speak for us …*

Odekunle: *That is how we want it now Eniola: Yes, we don't want a non-SS to represent us, we don't want them to speak for us. We can do it and we will do it. [FGA2: 8] The participants thus recognized that as a group they needed to make strategic links to others who might help them. They realized that they need to canvass support from significant others, whether this was engaging with (currently non-representative) NGOs; educating significant others to be better advocates for SCD or educating other community leaders about SCD.*

This led group participants to consider themselves more akin to group members, who increasingly referred to themselves as people with shared collective interests. It also encouraged them to delineate the areas of social policy that concerned them, which included: campaigning for genotype tests; training people with SCD to be peer counsellors; accessing and using the media for campaigns; the importance of getting many stories of SCD into the public domain because not all SCD experiences are the same; instigating reporting mechanisms for those who abuse people with SCD; ensuring support mechanisms for people with SCD; identifying possible strategies to achieve reasonable adjustments in schools/employment; ensuring strategies for reasonable adjustments for SCD were undertaken in the hospitals, and considering microfinance and cooperative approaches to improve the finances of people living with SCD.

However, participants discussed how effective the indigenous language media has proven to be over time. Mundy & Lloyd-Laney, (1992), opined that the credibility attached to the forms of indigenous language media, and imbibing such in teaching or communicating values and opinions will have a long, lasting and desirable effect.

Hence, in a bid to tackle the myths and misconceptions about sickle cell disorder, the participants discussed the perceived failure of the traditional and modern media, thereby calling for the indigenous language media.

Eniola: *If with all the media stations we have in Nigeria and all the social media platforms, warriors like us are still faced with stigmatizations due to the misconceptions that exist in the society, then I don't think the media is helping us.*

Aderonke: *Well, I think the media is helping but do people really believe what they hear or see on television, radio or internet than what they hear directly from a credible source.*

Aderonke: *Exactly, that is why we need to go back to our old ways, I mean our indigenous ways of communication. If we can consider the use of folk media to spread more information about the disorder, then I think people will believe it more. Also, if our parents and other principal officers in children's life can make use of deliberate instructions to give accurate information on the disorder to their children in the language they are brought up with, then such a child will grow with a good knowledge of the disorder and also pass it on to colleagues, friends, relatives when such discussion occur.*

Eniola: *Truthfully, I don't think we can have a society null of misconceptions and myths about this disorder, however, like Aderonke said, there is a need to consider the importance of the indigenous language media in reducing the stigmatization caused by the myths and misconceptions.*

Odekunle: *If media fails us, our own words of mouth, and records we set cannot fail us. I think it is time, we consider this.*

DISCUSSION OF FINDINGS

In increasing awareness and eradicating stereotypes as regards sickle cell disorder, the discussions unearth the importance of incorporating Indigenous language and communication techniques. It is believed that the authenticity attached to indigenous communication techniques via indigenous language can be used effectively to teach the peculiarities of sickle cell disorder. The discussions also emphasized how indigenous communication can facilitate learning and understanding of the disorder majorly in rural areas and some urban areas where knowledge of the disorder is assessed low.

Many times, societies have succeeded in spreading misconceptions about the sickle cell disease or disorder especially in areas where there is paucity or lack of adequate information that will guide the overall wellness of victims (Panepinto, Pajewsk, Foerster, Sabins & Hoffman, 2009).

Some patents of sickle cell diseases who are also residents in these rural areas agree with the incorrect notion about sickle cell diseases and mostly this fallacy is disseminated via various means of communication, such as community meetings, traditional beliefs and norms about the sickle cell disease which may lead to fetish propitiations and other unhealthy cultural practices, thereby worsening the health status of patents (Platt, Thorngton, Bramblla, Milner, Rosse, Vchnsky & Kinney, 1991; Quinn, Rogers & Buchanan, 2004 and Rees, Williams & Gladwin, 2010). More so, the evaluation of the use of media in addressing the need for information regarding sickle cell disorders is important because of the enormity of the problem (Siddiqui, Schmuk, Batista, Adames, Ayala & Stix, 2012).

According to Ohaer and Shokunbi (2001), sickle cell disorder (SCD) afflicts about 100 million people worldwide. Of these, four million are in Nigeria. The magnitude of the disorder in Nigeria is best appreciated when one considers that more than one in four, or 40 million Nigerians, are careers of the sickle cell trait and that, annually, 20 per 1,000 babes are born with the disease, translating to over 150,000 babes born annually with sickle cell anemia (Omotade, 1995).

To this end, the incorporation of indigenous language in sickle cell disorder education both in rural and urban areas will be potent enough to help in tackling myths and misconceptions as regards the disorder. Furthermore, it will help reduce the rate at which children with the disorder are born in Nigeria and also avail parents and other care givers comprehensible information enough to cater and manage the disorder.

CONCLUSION

Though Nigeria happens to be the highest country with sickle cell patients, the level of information is still very low. People have little or no information about the rudiments of sickle cell. The negative attitude as regards SCD is discovered to be the result of low level of information (Smith, 2015).

In a bid to tackle this, health education about the concept of SCD should be made available to adolescences in schools and through the indigenous media platforms. Information about SCD should be given more publicity, thereby creating more awareness about the disorder and given genuine facts to the public which will help eradicate negative social attitudes about sickle cell disorder.

This information publicity should take into consideration the credibility and effectiveness of the indigenous language media to tackle the stigmatization that occurs as a result of the myths and misconceptions about the disorder.

FUTURE RESEARCH DIRECTIONS

There is a need for more study on the impact of indigenous media information, most especially home videos and documentaries should be made available as regards Sickle Cell Disorder. This can be achieved by media coverage and reportage of accurate and relevant information on sickle cell disorder crisis and management. Furthermore, Health centers should emphasize the need of genetic counselling and testing so as to help prevent the annual increase of the disorder.

CONFLICT OF INTEREST

The authors declare that there is no conflict of interest regarding the paper

ETHICAL CONSIDERATION

Ethical approval obtained from the Ethics and Research Committee of the authors' institution. Participation was voluntary and anonymous. All participant's confidentiality is maintained, although, names and state of origin were mentioned as part of the discussions, however, no means of further identification was revealed and participants are assured contentment confidentiality of their data collected.

Obtained permission from director of each research setting to conduct the study, after explaining the purpose, the consent from participants will be self-determined through their agreement to participate in the study and then the group discussion.

ACKNOWLEDGEMENT

The authors recognize and appreciate the responses from our anonymous respondents as their contributions to humanity.

REFERENCES

Adegbite, W. (2002) The promotion of reading habits in Yoruba and English through the media: Case study of some media. Activities in Southern Nigeria. *Literacy and Reading in Nigeria 9*(2).

Adegoke, S. A., & Kuteyi, E. A. (2012). Psychosocial burden of sickle cell disorder on the family, Nigeria. *African Journal of Primary Health Care & Family Medicine, 4*(1), 1–6. doi:10.4102/phcfm.v4i1.380

Akinleye, J. O. (1988) A comparative study of the cost effectiveness of instructional television and conventional classroom instruction in non-formal education. (Unpublished PhD thesis), University of Ibadan.

Aliyu, Z., Tumblin, A., & Kato, G. (2016). Current therapy of sickle cell disease. *Haematologica, 91*, 7–10. PMID:16434364

Awoniyi, A. (1995). Determining language in education policy: The dilemma in Africa. In K. Owolabi (Ed.), *Language in Nigeria, Essays in Honour of Ayo Bamgbose*. Ibadan: Group Publishers.

Ballas, S. K. (2009). The cost of health care for patients with sickle cell disease. *American Journal of Hematology, 84*(6), 320–322. doi:10.1002/ajh.21443 PMID:19415728

Barakat, P., Simon, K., Schwartz, L., & Radcliffe, J. (2016). Correlates of pain rating, Concordance for adolescents with sickle cell disease and their caregivers. *Clinical Pain Journal, 24*(5), 438–446. doi:10.1097/AJP.0b013e3181646038 PMID:18496309

Booth, C., Inusa, B., & Obaro, S. K. (2009). Infection in sickle cell disease: A review. *International Journal of Infectious Diseases, 14*(1). doi:10.1016/j.ijid.2009.03.010 PMID:19497774

Broughton, G., Brumfit, C., Flavell, R., Hill, P., & Pincas, A. (1978). *Teaching English as a Foreign Language*. London, UK: Routledge and Kegan Paul.

Bunn, H. F., & Forget, B. F. (1977). *Human hematology*. Philadelphia, PA: WB Saunders.

Cheyney, A. B. (1992). *Teaching Reading Skills through the Newspaper*. Newark, DE: International Reading Association.

Egbokhare, F. O. (2004). *Breaking Barriers: ICT, Language Policy and Development. Ibadan*. Nigeria: The Postgraduate School University of Ibadan.

Egbokhare, F. O., Oyetade, S. O., Eno-Abasi, U., & Ahmed, H. A. (2001) Language Clusters in Nigeria. CASAS Monograph Series, No. 12. Cape Town, South Africa.

Elguero, E., Délicat-Loembet, L. M., Rougeron, V., Arnathau, C., Roche, B., Becquart, P., . . . Prugnolle, F. (2015). Malaria continues to select for sickle cell trait in Central Africa. *Proceedings of the National Academy of Sciences of the United States of America, 112*(22), 1-4. 10.1073/pnas.1505665112

Elmariah, H., Garrett, M. E., De Castro, L. M., Jonassaint, J. C., Ataga, K. I., Eckman, J. R., ... Telen, M. J. (2014). Factors associated with survival in a contemporary adult sickle cell disease cohort. *American Journal of Hematology, 89*(5), 530–535. doi:10.1002/ajh.23683 PMID:24478166

Emenyonu, P. T. (1982). Promoting the reading habit in Nigeria. In *Literacy and Reading in Nigeria.*

Eyoh, H. N. (1986). Theatre of relevance: An interview with Ngugi Wa Thiong'o. *African Theatre Review, 1*(2), 110–114.

Folarin, B. (2000). *Foundation of Broadcasting*. Ibadan: Atlantis Books.

Gray, A. (2018). Observations from indigenous languages in Northern Territory, Australia. *The Lancet. Global Health, 6*(5), e496. doi:10.1016/S2214-109X(18)30075-5 PMID:29653621

Kaur, M., Dangi, C. B. S., & Singh, M. (2013). An overview on sickle cell disease profile. *Asian Journal of Pharmaceutical and Clinical Research, 6*(1), 25–37.

Lasswell, H. (1948). Mass communication, popular taste and organised social actions. In L. Bryson (Ed.), *The Communication of Ideas*. New York: Institute for Religious and Social Studies.

Lasswell, H. (1960). The structure and functions of communication in society. In W. Schramm (Ed.), *Mass Communications*. Urbana: Urbana University of Illinois Press.

Lawal, B. (1989). An analytical study of the reading habits of some secondary students in Oyo Town. In R. A. Omojuwa & ... (Eds.), *Literacy and Reading in Nigeria 4.*

Ohaeri, J. U., & Shokunbi, W. A. (2001). Attitudes and beliefs of relatives of patients with sickle cell disease. *East African Medical Journal, 78*(4), 180–186. doi:10.4314/eamj.v78i4.9058 PMID:12002066

Olakunle, O. S., Kenneth, E., Olalekan, A. W., & Adenike, O. B. (2014). Knowledge and attitude of secondary school students in Jos, Nigeria on sickle cell disorder. *The Pan African Medical Journal, 15*(1), 12–15.

Omotade, O. O. (1995). Perception of sickle cell haemoglobinopathy among would be counselors. *African Journal of Medicine and Medical Sciences*, *24*(2), 315–320. PMID:8886144

Osgood, C. E. (Ed.). (1954). *Psycholinguistics: A survey of theory and research problem. Journal of Abnormal and Social Psychology, 49 (Oct.).* Morton Prince Memorial Supplement.

Oyero, O. (2007). Dynamics of indigenous languages in environmental communication. In I. Nwosu, & O. Soola (Eds.), *Communication in global, ICTs and ecosystem perspectives- Insights from Nigeria*. Enugu: Precisions Publishers.

Oyero, O. S., Oyesomi, K. O, Abioye, T, Ajiboye E, & Kayode-Adedeji, K. T. (2018). Strategic \ communication for climate change awareness and behavioural change in Ado-Odo/Ota Local Government of Ogun State. *African Population Studies, 32*(1), (Supp.).Oyesomi, K, Okorie, N, Ahmadu, F., & Itsekor, V. (2014). Where is the African culture? Assessing the uniqueness of indigenous communication in galvanising women's political participation at the local level. *Journal of New Media and Mass Communication, 25,* USA. pp. 1-8.

Oyesomi, K. O., & Salawu, A. (2019). Assessing the Uniqueness of Indigenous Language in Advertising: Analysis of Figurative Language Used in Selected Telecommunication Yoruba Advertisement in Nigeria. *Qualitative Report*, *24*(10), 2574–2591. Retrieved from https://nsuworks.nova.edu/tqr/vol24/iss10/12

Oyesomi, K. O, Salawu, A., & Olorunyomi, B. (2017). Indigenous Communication: Socio-Economic Characteristics Influencing Contemporary Female Political Participation. *Journal of International Women Studies (JIWS), 18*(4), pp. 164-181.

Oyetunde, T. O., & Umolu, J. J. (1991). The current view of the reading process and its implications for English reading instruction in Nigeria: An afterword. *Literacy and Reading in Nigeria 5.*

Palermo, T. M., Riley, C. A., & Mitchell, B. A. (2008). Daily functioning and quality of life in children with sickle cell disease pain: Relationship with family and neighborhood socioeconomic distress. *The Journal of Pain: Official Journal of the American Pain Society*, *9*(9), 833–840. doi:10.1016/j.jpain.2008.04.002 PMID:18550443

Panepinto, J. A., Pajewski, N. M., Foerster, L. M., Sabnis, S., & Hoffmann, R. G. (2009). Impact of family income and sickle cell disease on the health-related quality of life of children. *Quality of Life Research: An International Journal of Quality of Life Aspects of Treatment, Care and Rehabilitation*, *18*(1), 5–13. doi:10.100711136-008-9412-8 PMID:18989755

Piel, F. B., Hay, S. I., Gupta, S., Weatherall, D. J., & Williams, T. N. (2013). Global Burden of Sickle Cell Anaemia in Children under Five, 2010–2050: Modelling Based on Demographics, Excess Mortality, and Interventions. *PLoS Medicine, 10*(7). doi:10.1371/journal.pmed.1001484 PMID:23874164

Platt, O. S., Thorington, B. D., Brambilla, D. J., Milner, P. F., Rosse, W. F., Vichinsky, E., & Kinney, T. R. (1991). Pain in sickle cell disease – rates and risk factors. *The New England Journal of Medicine, 325*(1), 11–16. doi:10.1056/NEJM199107043250103 PMID:1710777

Prah, K. K. (1999). Workshop Working Paper on the Harmonization and Standardization of Nigerian Languages. Lagos.

Prah, K. K. (2001). The idea of an African Renaissance, the languages of the Renaissance and the challenges of the 21st century. In E. Kurimoto (Ed.), *JCAS Symposium Series 14*. JCAS, Osaka, Japan.

Quinn, C. T., Rogers, Z. R., & Buchanan, G. R. (2004). Survival of children with sickle cell disease. *Blood, 103*(11), 4023–4027. doi:10.1182/blood-2003-11-3758 PMID:14764527

Rees, D. C., Williams, T. N., & Gladwin, M. T. (2010). Sickle-cell disease. *Lancet, 376*(9757), 2018–2031. doi:10.1016/S0140-6736(10)61029-X PMID:21131035

Salawu, A. S. (2001) An evaluation of development communication content of Yoruba newspapers. (Unpublished PhD thesis), University of Ibadan.

Salawu, A. S. (2004a). The Yoruba and their language newspapers: Origin, nature, problems, and prospects. *Studies of Tribes and Tribals, 2*(2), 97–104. doi:10.1080/0972639X.2004.11886508

Salawu, A. S. (2004b) Social status as a factor for the readership of Yoruba newspapers in Nigeria. *Nordic Journal of African Studies 13*(2), pp. 200-215.

Salawu, A. S. (2004c). Contents and styles of Alaroye news publications. In O. Ndimele (Ed.), *Language and Culture in Nigeria: A Festschrift for Okon Essien. Aba: NINLAN.*

Salawu, A. S. (2004d). A readership survey of Yoruba newspapers for development messages. *Journal of Social Sciences, 8*(3), 197–202. doi:10.1080/09718923.2004.11892414

Schramm, W. (Ed.). (1954). How communication works. In the Process and Effects of Mass Communication (Ch. I). Urbana: University of IIlinois Press.

Severin, W. J., & Tankard, J. W. Jr. (1992). *Communication Theories: Origins, Methods and Uses in the Mass Media*. London, UK: Longman.

Siddiqui, S., Schunk, K., Batista, M., Adames, F., Ayala, P., Stix, B., ... Green, N. S. (2012). Awareness of sickle cell among of reproductive age: Dominicans and African Americans in northern Manhattan. *Journal of Urban Health, 89*(1), 53–58. doi:10.100711524-011-9618-x PMID:22009200

Smith, M. T. (2015). *Factors That Contribute To the Knowledge, Health Beliefs, Attitudes, and Behaviors Regarding Sickle Cell Disorder among College Students.* Heritage Press.

The Fourth Estate. (2000). No. 9., Nov./Dec. Lagos: IJC/JODER.

Uche, L. U. (1989). *Mass Media, People, and Politics in Nigeria.* New Delhi, India: Concept Publishing.

UNESCO. (1974). *Television traffic _ a one-way street? Reports and Papers on Mass Communication, No. 70.* Paris, France: UNESCO.

Webster, P. (2018). Language barriers restricting access to health care for Indigenous populations. *Canadian Medical Association Journal, 190*(24), E754–E755. doi:10.1503/cmaj.109-5613 PMID:29914917

Westley, B. H., & MacLean, M. (1957). A conceptual model for communication research. *Journalism Quarterly, 34,* 31-38.

Chapter 7
Indigenous Language Media and Communication for Health Purposes in the Digital Age

Toyosi Olugbenga Samson Owolabi
Lagos State University, Nigeria

Nahimah Ajikanle Nurudeen
Lagos State University, Nigeria

ABSTRACT

All over the world, the issues of health and ill health have generated heightened attention among health professionals and communication experts. This is expected in view of the prevalence of increasingly life-threatening ailments. It is therefore not surprising that matters bordering on health have been elevated to the front burner of policy and decision making both at the national and multinational levels. This chapter, therefore, observes that the reason most health information doesn't get to the intended audiences and produce the desired effect is because they are not communicated in the most intelligible language to the people. Indigenous language media are potential channels through which health information could reach the grassroots where more than 70 percent of the nation's populations are resident. It also perceived that health communication could be made to produce more effect in this digital era as more citizen journalists could be raised to communicate in the indigenous language.

DOI: 10.4018/978-1-7998-2091-8.ch007

INTRODUCTION

Globally, the issues of health and ill-health have generated heightened attention among health professionals and communication experts. This is expected in view of the prevalence of increasingly life-threatening ailments. Diseases such as cancer, hepatitis, liver cirrhosis, Ebola and other infectious diseases among others have been discovered to defy curative measures. It is therefore not surprising that matters bordering on health have been elevated to the front burner of policy and decision making both at the national and multinational levels. This is based on the recognition that it is only a healthy mind that could participate in and contribute to the nation's developmental growth. Moreover, it has been observed that most of these diseases are avoidable if effective precautionary measures are taken. In spite of the dissemination of health information to the people to warn them against those risk factors that can predispose them to these diseases, many casualties are still being recorded. Recent research shows that properly designed behaviour-based health communication activities can have a significant positive impact in altering negative health-related attitudes, beliefs and behaviours if communicated through the right channel. This chapter, therefore, observes that the reason why most health information doesn't get to and produce the desired effect on the intended audiences is because they are not communicated in the most intelligible language to the people (Owolabi, Ezika, Lewitt, and Beth, 2016). Indigenous language media, including newspapers, radio and television as well as other social media platforms are potential channels through which health information could reach the grassroots where more than 70 percent of the nation's populations are resident. This is because, according to Salawu (2006, p.88), "every language reflects the culture of the people thus, it is logical that people would express themselves and their cultures better in their native language".

Language is a unique human endowment, which defines human's humanity, that is, it makes man species specific (Amuseghan, 2010). It is used as an instrument of communication in all spheres of life. The home language of an indigenous group of people is known as indigenous language, it is the language that carries a people's knowledge, culture and identity. An indigenous language is a language that is native to a region and spoken by indigenous people. This language is from a linguistically distinct community that originated in the area. It is regarded as a local means of communication between members of a community because it contains within it the essence of considerable information, knowledge and wisdom of the people. An indigenous language is the language spoken within an ethnic community where the language is part of their identity and some traits of their customs are preserved through it. An indigenous language can also be a native to a country and can serve as a mother tongue to some of its indigenes. According to Oyesomi and Salawu (2019), Indigenous language is a language that is spoken by a group of people that resides in a locality or region. It is therefore not surprising that there has been significant growth in the volume of information being disseminated through the indigenous languages across the print and broadcast spectrum as most media owners acknowledge the need to be relevant to local audiences (Olaoye, 2013).

Indigenous language media, according to Wilson and Stewart (2008) is therefore, the forms of media expression that are conceptualized, produced and/or created by indigenous people and is used as vehicles for communication, cultural preservation, cultural and artistic expression, political self-determination, and cultural sovereignty. Indigenous communication includes the transmission of entertainment, news, persuasion, announcements, and social exchanges of every type (Mundy and Lloyd-Laney, 1992). Oyesomi, Salawu and Ọlorunyomi (2017) opine that indigenous communication enjoys high credibility because it is familiar and controlled locally. Indigenous communication has value in its own right. While contributing to the indigenous language media discourse, Olukotun (2006) also adds that indigenous language media in Nigeria include the indigenous language service of the federal, state and emerging private electronic and print media.

According to Jowitt (1987) cited by Oso (2006), about 44 Nigerian languages were used by radio and television services for daily news broadcast. However, Bolarin (2013) observed that with the deregulation of broadcast media by the Federal government in 1992, the number may be more as more private investors and governments at the Federal and states have developed interest in the sub-sector; apparently because of its potential use in reaching the grassroots with their policies and programmes. Although the number of electronic media may be increasing in Nigeria however, Oso (2006) notes that this may be far from truth about the print media. The reason, according to him is because print media demand some level of literacy ability and standard orthography which are both lacking among the over 250 languages in Nigeria (Omu, 2008). It is therefore not surprising that despite that the first newspaper to be published in Nigeria was in Yoruba, an indigenous language of the south-west; English language has become the prime language of the press in the country. English language assumed this enviable position because it appeals to advertisers. The electronic media are aware of this twist and this explains why series of programmes that could attract more listeners and viewers are introduced. For example, *koko inu iwe iroyin,* (a newspaper review) and *lori papa*, (sport commentary) are two of such programmes which are believed to have wide audience going by the manner in which advertisers scramble to air their advertisements during the programme (Popoola, 2006).

Communication in general is today supported by ICTs, and the lack of terminology in African languages establishes and entrenches the digital divide, making it nearly impossible for them to compete with English language. Websites in African languages tend to be lean and most people who are literate enough to browse in

African languages may find it more economical to do so in a European language (English or French) (Olúbòdé-Sàwè, 2010).

Most African countries are multilingual societies and explicit choices have to be made among alternative language varieties about which language variety fulfills which role. This role differentiation involves language planning which can only be defined by the government and its agencies as well as language groups to influence the behaviour of users with respect to the acquisition, structure or functional allocation of their language codes (Cooper 1989, cited in UNESCO, 2005, p.5).

Indigenous language media overlap with, and are on the same spectrum with other types of minority-produced media, and quite often, they share a kinship regarding many philosophical and political motivations (Wilson et al., 2017). While the study of indigenous peoples has traditionally been in the domain of anthropology, indigenous language media are now a significant focus of interdisciplinary study (including media and communication, ethnic studies, cultural studies, art history, geography, development studies and political communication). However, there has not been much focus on the potentials of indigenous language media use for health communication.

Media campaigns in indigenous languages offer opportunities to educate and inform large populations by using traditional media, such as television, radio and newspapers.

Over time, a lot of health-related messages are being propagated but with marginal benefit to Nigerians especially the rural populace. This is because the information apart from not tailored to Nigeria, the messages are not disseminated in the languages that are intelligible to the people. According to Ransom-Kuti (2009), it is impossible to appropriately communicate health messages to largely rural communities as we have in Nigeria without engaging indigenous language media. Speaking further, he said many attempts in the media by medical experts to communicate health messages have ended as worthless efforts because they are pitched above the level of the grassroots audience. Researches have equally shown that the use of a selection of mass media channels communicating in the indigenous language is more likely to result in an effective health campaign (Corcoran, 2010).

Another dimension to the observed lopsidedness in information sharing process is that, in the digital space, available materials on the internet are only in the languages of the developed nations. The use of digital technology by the media to promote health issues is a growing field despite the obvious gaps in the rural and urban information consumption. The communication media such as radio, television, newspapers, and magazines are the most conspicuous channels of transmitting appropriate information to a large number of people. The evolution of the information superhighway offered by the internet also provides a greater access to both the senders and receivers of information in the 21st century. One of the distinct advantages of the mass media connectivity to the internet is the engagement of the audience. This is unlike the traditional mass media where the audience only acts as passive receiver of messages.

This method of accessing health information enables the receivers to be actively engaged in information seeking and processing (Corcoran 2010).Notwithstanding the potential of the digital technologies, most people especially in the rural communities are still being denied access to information. The reason is that most of the English language media are known for their urban-centred bias and their contemptuous neglect of the rural communities (Olukotun, 2006, p.132). As new technologies are evolving and the information gathering and processing are going digital, more and more information lopsidedness are created between the urban and rural areas. This, according to Korp (2006, p.82), is true to the extent that those who are well educated and well off are greater beneficiaries of digital technology. Thus, income and education are strong factors within the notion of 'digital divide'.

According to Olukotun (2006), matters are made worse by the fact that most newspapers and broadcasting organisations have no reporters covering the rural communities. Although the media have been credited to play a vital role in Nigeria's democratic journey since it gained independence on October 1, 1960, not much has been achieved in the area of health information delivery. It is important to note that there have been arguments about narrowing the rural-urban information gap, which are relevant to health improvement project. This perhaps explains why there is a call for creating alternative media where local languages will be used along with English in satisfying the information needs of the rural populace. It is against this background that this chapter will, among others place health communication and indigenous language media in perspective, look at the centrality of indigenous language in health communication process, examine the issues and trends in communicating health messages to rural populace in the digital era. Lastly, the concluding part will identify some limitations that may constitute a drag in the wheel of effective health communication using indigenous language channels and the way forward.

THEORETICAL FOUNDATION

This study is anchored on the Development Media theory. This theory is believed to possess the variables by which this study can be exhaustively discussed.

Development Media Theory: This theory was propounded by Dennis McQuail in (2010). According to Folarin (2002) cited in Anaeto et al (2008, p. 64), the theory emerged to fill the apparently existing gap between the developed and developing countries. The theory makes an assumption that "the media should accept and carry out positive development tasks in line with nationally established policy without prejudice to their traditional functions of information, education and entertainment of the public". Development media theory further states that "the freedom of the media should be opened to economic priorities and development needs of the society". These assumptions gave a clear mandate to the mass media in general and the indigenous language media in particular. In this study, the indigenous language media have a role to play in communicating health-related messages to the grassroots with the purpose of enhancing the development profile of the nation thus, bridging the gap between the developed and developing economy of the world. If the media have actually accepted to carry out positive development tasks as claimed by Olise (2008), it therefore goes to show that the media as a significant part of the society are free to imbibe the Information and Communication Technologies (ICTs) skills available in this digital era to communicate messages that can positively influence attitude and behavior change to health risks.

The relevance of this theory to the study is that it provides insight into the socio-economic implication of ill-health on the nation if not addressed through effective communication especially, to the grassroots that constitute the larger majority of national population.

Health Communication and Indigenous Language Media in Perspective

Over the years, there has been an established linkage between the domains of communication and health. Health communication represents the interface between communication and health and is recognized as an important factor for improving both personal and public health. Health communication contributes to all aspects of disease prevention and health promotion. Communication refers to the transmission or exchange of information and implies the sharing of meaning among those who are communicating. According to Healthy People (2010) guidelines, health communication encompasses the study and use of communication strategies to inform and influence individual and community decisions with the purpose of enhancing health and wellbeing.

Mass media as communication channels have become increasingly more influential in stimulating health campaigns that can effectively inform the citizens; inspires idea and feelings, stimulate discussions and assist in creating public awareness. Furthermore, it has been observed that there is rapid improvement in health message delivery in this digital era. Digital technology such as CD-ROM and the World Wide Web, which can target audiences with customized messages and engage people in interactive session have become common experience (Baran, 2004). Availability of relevant health-enhancing messages to the right people at the right time is no doubt the key to promoting healthy living and contributing to all aspect of disease prevention.

Despite the globalised characteristic and popularity of English language media in many countries, it has been observed that the mass-mediated messages in English usually do not get to the grassroots especially in a country like Nigeria where there are multiplicity of ethnic groups and languages competing alongside English (Owolabi 2014). For example, the print media is elitist in culture and content and will not make as much impact among the illiterate rural dwellers that constitute about 57% of the populations unless they are printed in the indigenous language (Owolabi, 2014). The same is what obtains in the broadcast media where more than 70% of their programmes are transmitted in English (Owolabi and O'Neil, 2014). Media scholars have therefore understood the necessity of using both national and all the minority indigenous languages to disseminate health and development messages in the media (Amuseghan, Ayenigbara and Orimogunje. 2010). English is both the national and official language of Nigeria with wider acceptance among the citizens. However, in spite of its popularity, it is still limited in its ability to carry health messages to the rural communities where a larger majority is believed to be poor and uneducated to correctly decode the information. This is the basis of Adedeji's (2015) observation that since indigenous languages fare better in the broadcast media than in the print media that give preference to English language, both can be used as the language of the media.

Communication as a mean of expressing feelings, worthwhile inter-personal relationship, and conformity to societal norms, convenience, security, innovation and change implies its pivotal role to human existence (Aristole, 1987). It is the avenue through which members of a society are informed Indigenous language media have therefore transformed itself into potential instrument for communicating social change and innovation. More importantly, communication has now become advanced and applicable in various fields of human endeavour such as environmental maintenance, public administration, civic responsibilities, social change and innovation as well as public health and hygiene.

There has been an encouraging growth in audiences for radio and television broadcast. Statistics has shown that the number of television sets in developing countries has increased from 13 million in 1955 to 707 million in 1995. Broadcast on these channels has continually provided a powerful leveler for behavioural change with a reasonable and affordable cost-benefit (Piotrow et al., 1997) cited in Amuseghan (2008b).Through communication efforts, the people can have access to information that will deepen their knowledge about new innovations and other development laden incidence around them. Apart from fostering healthy and secured quality of life it also enables the people to avoid habits that may constitute health risk in the society (Amuseghan et al (2010).

In Nigeria as in other parts of the world, health communication has now attained the position of not only steering the wheel but also the pivot on which the wheel of public health programmes rotate. This is in view of the prevalence of increasingly life-threatening ailments in the society. Diseases such as cancer, hepatitis, liver cirrhosis, Ebola and other infectious diseases among others have been discovered to defy curative measures. However, most of these diseases are avoidable if effective precautionary measures are taken. In spite of the dissemination of health information to the people to warn them against those risk factors that can predispose them to these diseases, many casualties are still being recorded. Recent researches show that properly designed behaviour-based health communication activities can have a significant positive impact in altering negative health-related attitudes, beliefs and behaviours if communicated through the right channel hence, the urgent need to develop indigenous language media.

Centrality of Indigenous Language in Communicating Health Messages

It has been established in the earlier part of this chapter that indigenous language is central to achieving health communication objectives. Communicating development messages with the people in their mother tongue brings about effective understanding of the complexity of a particular disease or health situation. For instance, the media played a crucial role in stemming Ebola Virus Disease (EVD) outbreak in Nigeria. People desperately needed information on how to prevent and treat EVD (Musa et al, 2016).

However, at the onset of the outbreak, the reportage in electronic and print media fueled a lot of fear as contracting EVD was considered a death sentence. Stigmatization and misinformation among members of the public were widespread at the start of the plague. In one instance, misinformation prompted some people to drink salty water to prevent EVD as a result of which many people died in the process. Early and intensive dissemination of appropriate messages to the public on EVD immediately the outbreak was declared, using a wide range of media would have prevented such a situation.

Subsequently, publicity was intensified through the media, providing continuous and coordinated information about the disease, including its mode of spread, preventive measures and actions being undertaken to stop the disease.

An interview was conducted with Lucy Osuizogbo-Okechukwu, a Senior Correspondent with News Agency of Nigeria in which she opines that "using indigenous languages is what many stakeholders in the health and development sectors have been advocating". While expatiating further on the role of indigenous media in disseminating health-related messages, she said, "when we look at various diseases index in the country, they are prevalent in the rural areas and this is because most rural dwellers are probably illiterates who are ignorant of the problem associated with diseases control and health communications generally". Oftentimes, the intervention programmes are done in English language, which is unintelligible to them. So, if health campaigns messages are to get to the grassroots people, it has to be communicated in the language they understand. She believed that if health promotional messages are packaged in indigenous languages, diseases such as infant and maternal mortality rate will reduce. It will be easier for them to key in properly into immunization and other intervention programmes by the time they understand well.

Also, Chioma Obinna, assistant health editor with *Vanguard* newspaper, said it will be a good development if indigenous media can have dedicated columns or programmes on health because the local people depend on these media as sources of daily information. She also emphasized the need to consider target audience of each health campaigns so as to explore best language option(s) in achieving the objectives of such programmes.

While talking about the success rate of past health intervention programmes, Obinna confirmed that some health programmes in past failed because of the adoption of top-down model of communication which pays attention to the message at the expense of the intended audience. She said, "using indigenous languages would make it bottom -up approach where the people can align with the messages and get themselves well equipped with the right and useful information to protect themselves or seek help from the right channel".

According to Salawu (2004), the indigenous media (prints and broadcast) possess an incredible power to better interpret development messages thus, placing the facts and issues in better perspective. While lending his voice to the recurring debate on the role of indigenous language in communicating health information to diverse audience, Ojebode (2004, p.90-91) identifies twelve major formats for disseminating health information to the grassroots. These include: straight news, editorials, news analysis, features, group discussion, lecture or straight talk, interviews, testimonial, entertainment, jingles, poetry and music.

Communicating Health Messages in Indigenous Language Media: Issues and Trends in the Digital age

As internet access continues to expand, it has continued to serve as a rich health information resource in the environments that lack health expertise. Regardless of location, the internet technology allows people to gain access to a wide array of health-related information globally at a mouse click. The local cyber café may even begin to serve as a health information hub. Since the internet transcends geographical barriers, there is plenty of potential for websites to provide a valuable source of health information, thus enhancing health and wellbeing of people in developing countries.

However, as the amount of information grows at an unprecedented rate, so does the amount of falsehood and potentially harmful information. Misinformation, either due to inaccuracy or misinterpretation of health information, have been found to cause terrible consequences by instigating mass panics among the ignorant citizens while it can also mislead uninformed policy-makers.

The local and international media have played a vital role as the link between health workers and the general public. Health authorities educate and entrust the media with essential health information, which is then relayed to the public in readily accessible formats through a variety of media channels. Most of the public health interventions through the media do not sufficiently engage the local people as well as translating to improved positive attitudinal and behavioral changes because they were not carried out using indigenous language media platform.

A 2002 study by Momodu which examines rural Nigerian communities' health information needs and their information seeking behavior identified radio, television, newspapers, health extension workers and health agents as Information sources in rural communities. This research further indicated that rural communities look for information to handle the incidence of epidemic outbreaks, to identify the best treatment options, to get good health facilities and to implore the government to support them in their health problems. Women in particular were found to be interested in seeking information on pre- and post-natal care and on immunization facilities for their children and themselves.

Momodu's study serves as an attestation to the importance of local languages to disseminating health messages. While a considerable number of local newspapers, television and radio stations have specialized health programmes for public education on various health matters, there is none that currently has health programmes in any of the local languages.

Findings from a study conducted in Ghana by Aryee (2014) shows a considerable use of mobile phones for disseminating and seeking health information in rural communities of Ghana. The study further shows that health-related activities performed on and with mobile phones include: (i) inquiring about health concerns from friends, family, or healthcare personnel (ii) practicing tele-consultation, and tele-health with health help lines that address specific health issues such as pregnancy and cholera outbreak; (iii) clarifying any health symptom before travelling to healthcare centres (iv) scrutinizing counterfeit medications entering the country (Aryee (2014, p.123).

However, the effectiveness of this media for disseminating and accessing health information is influenced by the interplay of a number of individual factors including a person's age, gender, level of education, individual innovativeness (National Research Council, 2011), the community's cultural practices (Van Biljon & Kotzé, 2008), and the nature of information content sought (Chetley, Davies, Trude, McConnell, Ramirez, Shields, et al. 2006) cited in (Sokey et al 2018).

These factors, in the view of Van Biljon & Kotzé (2008) are referred to as social constructs which they defined as a change in an individual's thoughts, feelings, attitudes, or behaviours that results from interaction with another individual or a group. This influence includes: cultural practices and interests of an individual, such as beliefs about using for example, mobile phones to get important information about health as a mode of promoting a healthy lifestyle (Gerber et al., 2009).

There are 100 of mobile applications available across Android, iOS and other platforms but, access to modern communication technologies and medical assistance is a problem for the majority of people living in developing countries, particularly in rural communities (Cashen et al. 2004). This, for instance is because majority of the people in need of medical assistance are not so literate enough to operate and access medical services via these technologies. Majority of the mobile health applications are programmed in English which makes them restricted to only educated elites.

Another limitation in this regard is the fact of the issues of digital divide as access to modern internet facilities of infrastructure such broadband is still very poor in most of the developing countries like Nigeria because investments in this area has been concentrated mainly in the city centres.

Additionally, the social media have proved to be a veritable tool for information dissemination to the public on health and diseases. For example, Facebook and tweeter provides platforms for giving feedback on questions and comments from the public, addressing misinformation and monitoring community alerts among others. However, the challenge in all these options provided by social media or digital platforms is still language restrictions because most feed posts from digital handles are in English.

Indigenous Language Media as Health Information Channel: Some Limitations

There has been considerable amount of documentation regarding general barriers to adoption and implementation of health information technology. Rice, Royce, and Thompson (2016) identified illiteracy and language barriers as obstacles to health information dissemination which is a pointer to the need for health communication in domestic language or local dialect.

There is also paucity of literature on the part of the limitations in the indigenous language media as health information medium. Nevertheless, there is the issue of public acceptability as general limitation to indigenous language media. One of the arguments against the use and development of African indigenous languages as languages of the media is the multiplicity of languages; African is said to have 2000 languages, 400 of which are found in Nigeria alone, (Salawu 2006).

Barriers to Effective Health Communication

Good communication is believed to be the cornerstone of an effective healthcare delivery system; the absence of which the entire process suffers serious failure. It has been observed that about 80 percent of serious medical errors are traceable to miscommunication by the healthcare providers while about 1,744 deaths were also believed to be the consequence of the same problem within the last five years (CRICO Comparative Benchmarking System, 2016).

Low Health Literacy: Because health information is normally relayed in the form of written communication, the illiterate/semi-illiterate often cannot access the information. Thus, health literature should be customised for each target audience and written in a style appropriate to their level of comprehension. At the same time, health literacy programs should train low-literacy individuals to avail themselves of these health resources.

- **Limited Internet Access:** The Internet has become the channel of choice for information delivery worldwide. However, in certain communities, even in the developed world, internet access is still too costly, and in some cases, out-rightly unavailable. Moreover, though there is abundant health information on the internet, it is still out of reach of those in resource-poor settings. Given the importance of the internet in disseminating vital health information, there should be increased effort to bring access to rural communities and the developing world. In particular, this effort should involve both the public and private sectors, namely the government agencies and technology corporations,
- **Lack of Research Activity in Developing Countries:** Research and evaluation are required in order to design, develop and implement effective health communication interventions. Unfortunately, most research is done with an eye to solving health problems in the developed world, while pressing health problems in the developing world are often neglected. Even if research is done in developing countries, it seldom comes to the attention of health professionals.

"Few reports of health research from developing countries are published in journals indexed by Western services such as Medline. Western indexing services cover some 3000 journals of which 98% are from the developed world. For instance, the whole of Latin America accounted for 0.39% of the total number of articles referenced by Medline in 1996, down from a "high" of 2.03% in 1966. Because only a small number of journals from developing countries are indexed by Medline, research from these countries is almost invisible."

- **Proliferation of Low Quality Healthcare Information on the Internet:** As the volume of Internet content increases on a daily basis, consumers need help evaluating the reliability of the information that they are bombarded with. According to the Office of Disease Prevention and Health Promotion, "people are using the internet to look up information, purchase medications, consult remotely with providers, and maintain their personal health records". Approximately 70 million persons in the United States use the internet for health-related reasons, and the potential for harm from inaccurate information, inferior quality goods, and inappropriate services is t rife. In order to protect consumers, internet health resources and health-related Web sites should be required to adhere to a strict code of conduct. Site owners should disclose their identity and essential contact information clearly and honestly. They should explicitly state the purpose of their site and provide proper citation for the content they display. They should inform their users how personal information is used, and whether the content is periodically updated to prevent misinformation.
- **Inability of Health Workers to Communicate With Patients:** Due to various communication hurdles such as language barriers, socio-cultural differences among others, health workers sometimes have difficulty in transmitting vital health information to their patients. Moreover, given the shortage of human resources, which is a common problem in developing countries, health workers often deal with multiple patients at a time, making communication even more difficult (Weller, Boyd and Cumin, 2014, p.151-152)

Strategies to Improve on Health Communication in Indigenous Language Media

Effective health communication is essential because it equips the public with the tools and knowledge to respond appropriately to health crises such as flu outbreaks, HIV/AIDS, malaria etc. High impact health communication catalyzes behavioral changes on a societal level; it galvanizes entire communities into action, prompting them to live a healthy lifestyle by taking the necessary measures to prevent disease and to protect, maintain and improve their own health, such as good nutrition, regular exercise, responsible sexual behavior, eschewing negative behaviors such as cigarette smoking, drug abuse etc.

In order for a health communication program to have an impact, it should disseminate appropriate health content that satisfies the following criteria, as prescribed by the Office of Disease Prevention and Health Promotion (2016, p.21):

- **Accuracy**: The content is valid and without errors of fact, interpretation, or judgment.
- **Availability**: The content (whether targeted message or other information) must be delivered or placed where the audience can easily access it. Placement varies according to the audience, message complexity, and purpose, ranging from interpersonal and social networks to billboards and mass transit signs to prime-time TV or radio, to public kiosks (print or electronic), to the Internet.
- **Balance**: Where appropriate, the content presents the benefits and risks of potential actions or recognizes different and valid perspectives on the issue.
- **Consistency**: The content remains internally consistent over time and also is consistent with information from other sources (the latter is a problem when other widely available content is not accurate or reliable).
- **Cultural Competence**: The design, implementation, and evaluation process that accounts must be taken into consideration especially, for special issues for select population groups (ethnic, racial, and linguistic) and also educational levels and physically challenged.
- **Evidence-Based**: Relevant scientific evidence must undergo comprehensive review and rigorous analysis to formulate practice guidelines, performance measures, review criteria, and technology assessments for tele-health applications.
- **Reach:** The content must be available to the largest possible number of people in the target population.
- **Reliability**: The source of the content is credible, and the content itself is kept current.
- **Repetition**: The delivery of/access to the content is continued or repeated over time, both to reinforce the impact with a given audience and to reach new generations.

Moreover, any effective health communication strategy must take a multi-pronged approach coupling with other interventions, such as policy changes, improvements and in health delivery systems. If a health communication initiative does not have support at the policy level, its efficacy and impact are much less predictable than if it has institutional backing.

In developing health communication initiatives, it is crucial to consider socio-cultural milieu of the target audiences with respect to their cultural characteristics, language preferences and media habits. For instance, the health communication program developer does not want to design a health education website, only to find out later that his target audience is mainly comprised of individuals who are either technologically illiterate, or simply do not have access to the digital technology.

General strategies that governmental bodies can take to enhance the quality of health communication at the macro level:

- Government agencies and technology corporations should collaborate together to bring internet access into more households.
- For the benefit of people with marginal literacy skills, pertinent health information should be written at their level of comprehension. Health literacy programs targeting their skill improvement should be organized.
- Set up training centers that equip health communication professionals and health professionals with good communication skills.

At the micro level (within organizations and communities), this study makes the following recommendations:

Workplace guides: During a disease outbreak, employers have a responsibility for employee productivity and health. The distribution of workplace guides to contain the spread of communicable disease is an important health communication strategy. These guides contain information on how to develop workplace preparedness plans, as well as prevention and support programs in a systematic manner. In addition, workplace-wide lectures, as well as providing peer educators could further enhance health communication.

Community Skits: In a community setting, it is useful to organize short dramas that portray the attitudes of the local people towards their health. By understanding local attitudes, health workers can plan interventions targeting specific behavioral changes. Theatre is also a strategic way to draw children's attention to health problems.

In addition to the above, a wide range of tools and publications have been developed by various agencies such as the Center for Global Health Communication and Marketing to provide health communication training to healthcare workers.

CONCLUSION

In this study, the traditional media of communication have been observed to be incapable of carrying health information messages to the grassroots. The print media are known to be elitist in content as most of them are usually published in English language for the English speaking audience who are fewer in number in most rural communities in Nigeria. The same reason is why the radio and television are not making much impact in the rural areas. Most of their programmes, about 70 percent are aired in English to the disadvantage of the indigenous language speakers. Most of the public health interventionist programmes through the media do not sufficiently engage the local people as well as translating to their improved positive attitudinal and behavioral changes because they were not carried out using indigenous language media platform. It has therefore been discovered that indigenous language media, including newspapers, radio and television as well as other information and communication technologies are believed to be potential channels through which the inadequacies and the information lopsidedness could be remedied.

We discovered in this study that any effective health communication strategy must take a multi-pronged approach by using different indigenous language channels of communication. These become necessary to effectively remove ignorance and influence the populace in taking informed decision that will enhance their sound health and total wellbeing.

The study also found that, apart from other factors such as low literacy level, limited internet access, lack or insignificant level of health research and low quality healthcare information on the Internet among developing countries, the inability of health workers and planners to communicate with the grassroots in indigenous language constitutes the greatest hindrance to effective transmission of vital health information especially to the rural populace.

RECOMMENDATION

On the basis of the above findings, we hereby recommend the following proven strategies for government to enhance the quality of health communication at the macro level:

- The National Broadcasting Commission should intensify efforts in its oversight functions to ensure that the broadcast media to comply with the stated rule that programmes should be aired on ratio 40:60 between indigenous languages and English

- Government agencies and technology corporations should collaborate together to make internet access into more households easier and affordable so that the grassroots people could have unlimited access to development information on the internet.
- For the benefits of people with marginal literacy skills, the health planners and workers at the various levels of government should be conscious of their peculiarity and their levels of comprehension when generating health information intended for them.
- For those without any literacy skill at all, the government should also be mindful of their distinctiveness and therefore rely heavily on indigenous language media channels to disseminate health information to them. As a matter of fact, training centers that equip health communication professionals and health professionals with good communication skills in indigenous languages could also be established for one-to-one contact with them.

FUTURE RESEARCH DIRECTIONS

Future research efforts should be geared towards the impact of indigenous language media roles in strategic communication as a step towards achieving the ongoing sustainable development goals especially among developing nations.

REFERENCES

Adedeji, O. A. (2015). Analysis of Use of English And Indigenous Languages By The Press in Selected African Countries. [OMAN Chapter]. *Arabian Journal of Business and Management Review*, *4*(8), 35–45.

Amuseghan, S. A. (2003). Prepositions in Nigerian Standard English Usage: A Study in the Domains of Science and Technology. (Doctoral Thesis), Adekunle Ajasin University, Nigeria.

Amuseghan, S. A. (2008a). 'Language, communication and information flow in entrepreneurship', in *African Journal of Business and Management*, *2*(10), 201–208.

Amuseghan, S. A. (2008b). *Language Policy Provisions and Curriculum Issues and Challenges in Nigeria.* A paper presented at the 53rd Annual Conference of International Linguistic Association held at Sunny College at Old Westbury, NY.

Amuseghan, S. A., Ayenigbara, G. O., & Orimogunje, T. (2010). Language and health Communication strategies towards effective public health communication programmes in Nigeria. *Journal Media and Communication Studies* 2(5), pp. 111-117, May 2010. Available at http://www.academicjournals.org/jmcs

Anaeto, S. G., Onabajo, S. O., & Osifeso, J. B. (2008). *Models and Theories of Communication*. Maryland: African Renaissance Books Incorporated.

Aristotle.. (1987). Poetics (S. Hal, Trans.).

Aristotle. Poetics. (1987). Translated Stephen Hallowell. Chapel Hill, NC: University of North Carolina Press.

Baran, S. (2014). *Introduction to Mass Communication: Media Literacy and Culture* (8th ed.). Boston, MA: McGraw-Hill.

Benson, O., Victor, A., Linda, I., & Ariole, I. A. (2017). "Promoting Indigenous Language in Nigeria: Issues and Challenges for the Library and Information Professionals" Library Philosophy and Practice (e-journal). 1472. Retrieved from http://digitalcommons.unl.edu/libphilprac/1472

Bolarin, O. L. (2013). Language of Communication in the Nigerian Media. *Singaporean Journal of Business Economics and Management Studies*, *1*(11).

Brieger, W. (1990). Mass media and health communication in rural Nigeria. *Health Policy and Planning*, *5*(1), 77–81. doi:10.1093/heapol/5.1.77

Cashen, M. S., Dykes, P., & Gerber, B. (2004). E-health technology and Internet Resources. Barrier for Vulnerable Population. *The Journal of Cardiovascular Nursing*, *19*(3), 209–214. doi:10.1097/00005082-200405000-00010 PMID:15191264

Collins, O. F., Banda, Z. M., & Albert, N. D. (2016). The impact of a Community driven Mass Media Campaign on the Utilization of maternal health care services in rural Malawi. Retrieved from https://www.ncbi.nlm.nih.gov/pmc/articles/PMC4730729/

Corcoran, N. (2010). Mass Media in Health Communication. In N. Corcoran (Ed.), *Communicating Health Strategies for Health Promotion* (pp. 73–93). London, UK: SAGE.

CRICO. (2016) A Report of Medical Malpractice Claims from the CRICO Comparative Benchmarking System. Retrieved from https://www.vital-learning.com › blog › barriers-healthcaren communication

Crystal, D. (1987). The Cambridge Encyclopedia of Linguistics. New York: Oxford University SPress.

Gerber, A. S., Karlan, D., & Bergan, D. (2009). Does the Media Matter? A Field Experiment Measuring the Effect of Newspapers on Voting Behavior and Political Opinions. *American Economic Journal. Applied Economics*, *1*(2), 35–52. doi:10.1257/app.1.2.35

Interview with Chioma Obinna, assistant health editor with *Vanguard* newspaper.

Interview with Lucy Osuizogbo-Okechukwu, a Senior Correspondent with News Agency of Nigeria.

John, S. (2016). The Use of Indigenous Media of Communication for Health Communication in *Olamabaro Local Government Area of Kogi State Nigeria.* Retrieved from https://www.academia.edu/33078422/The_Use_of_Indigenous_Media_of_Communication_for_Health_Commu

Korp, P. (2006). Health in the Internet: Implication for Health Promotion. *Health Education Research*, *21*(1), 78–86. doi:10.1093/her/cyh043 PMID:15994845

McQuail, D. (2010). *McQuail's Mass Communication Theory* (6th ed.). London, UK: Sage.

Momodu, M. O. (2002). Information needs and information seeking behaviour of rural dwellers in Nigeria: A case study of Ekpoma in Esan West local government area of Edo State, Nigeria. *Library Review*, *51*(8), 406–410. doi:10.1108/00242530210443145

Mundy, P., & Lloyd-Laney, M. (1992). Indigenous communication. Appropriate Technology, 19(2), IT Publications Ltd, 103-105 Southampton Row, London, UK.

Musa, E., Nasidi, A., Shuaib, F., Nguku, P. M., & Vaz, R. G. (2016). Nigeria's Ebola Outbreak Response: Lessons for Future Epidemic Preparedness. *Arch Med*, *8*(6). doi:10.21767/1989-5216.1000171

National Research Council. (2011). The US Health Disadvantage Relative to Other High-Income Countries Findings from a National Research Council/Institute of Medicine Report.

Ojebode, A. (2004). Radio as Development Communication Medium: Types, Formats, Roles and Limitation. In E. O. Soola (Ed.), *Communicating for Development Purposes* (pp. 87–99). Ibadan: Kraft Books Limited.

Olaoye, A. A. (2013).The Role of Indigenous Languages in National Development: A Case Study of Nigerian Linguistic Situation. *International Journal of Applied Linguistics and English Studies, 2*(3). Available at http://www.journals.aiac.org.au/index.php/IJALEL/article/view/847 Assessed on 20/3/2019

Olise, F. P. (2008). Communication for Development and Modern ICTs: Nigeria at Cross Roads. In E. M. Mojaye, O. O. Oyewo, R. M'Bayo, & I. A. Sobowale (Eds.), Health Communication, Gender Violence, and ICTs in Nigeria; Ibadan: Ibadan University Press, pp. 269-283.

Olúbòdé-Sàwè, F. O. (2010). Digital Communication in Indigenous Languages Federal University of Technology, Nigeria. DOI: doi:10.4018/978-1-61520-773-2.ch036

Olukotun, A. (2006). The Indigenous Language Press and Democratic Mobilisation in Nigeria: A Historical Structural Overview. In A. Salawu (Ed.), Indigenous Language Media in Africa, Lagos: Center for Black and African Arts and Civilisation (CBAAC), pp. 126-140.

Omu, F. I. A. (2008). "Ethnicity, Nationalism, and Federalism in Nigeria: An Interactive Trinity of Relationship" in F. I. A. Omu, & G. E. Oboh (Eds.), Mass Media in Nigerian Democracy. Ibadan: Stirling-Hordens Publishers (Nig) Ltd.

Oso, L. (2006). A Political Economy of Indigenous language press in Nigeria. In A. Salawu (Ed.), Indigenous Language Media in Africa. Lagos: Centre for Black and African Arts and Civilisation (CBAAC) pp. 175-195.

Owolabi, T. O. S. (2014). Media Coverage of SMEs in Nigeria: An Imperative for National Development, (Doctoral thesis), University of Strathclyde, Glasgow, UK.

Owolabi, T. O. S., Ezika, E. A., Lewitt, M., & Beth, C. (2016). Communication Media and Cardiovascular Health Promotion as Factors for Sustainable Development in Nigeria, *Journal of Sustainable Development in Africa. Clarion University of Pennsylvania*, *18*(1), 156–172.

Owolabi, T. O. S., & O'Neill, E. (2014). Communication, MSMEs, and Women Empowerment for National Development in Nigeria. *Asian Journal of Research in Social Sciences and Humanity*, *4*(3), 21–34. Retrieved from https://aijsh.com/shop/articlepdf/org/socialscience/paper686.pdf

Oyesomi, K., Salawu, A., & Olorunyomi, B. (2017). Indigenous Communication: Socio-Economic Characteristics Influencing Contemporary Female Political Participation. *Journal of International Women's Studies*, *18*(4), 164–181. Available at http://vc.bridgew.edu/jiws/vol18/iss4/12

Oyesomi, K. O., & Salawu, A. (2019). Assessing the Uniqueness of Indigenous Language in Advertising: Analysis of Figurative Language Used in Selected Telecommunication Yoruba Advertisement in Nigeria. *Qualitative Report*, *24*(10), 2574–2591. Retrieved from https://nsuworks.nova.edu/tqr/vol24/iss10/12

Healthy People. (2010). United States Department of Health and Human Services. Use Communication Strategically to Improve Health. Retrieved May 17, 2019.

Popoola, I. S. (2006). Print on the Air, an Appraisal of Koko Inu Iwe Iroyin, a Newspaper Review Programme on Metro FM, Lagos. In A. Salawu (Ed.), Indigenous Language Media in Africa. Lagos: Centre for Black and African Arts and Civilisation (CBAAC) pp. 326-346.

Ransome-Kuti, O. (2009). Health Care and the Mass media. In R. Akinfeleye (Ed.), *Health and Behavioural Change Communication for Development* (pp. 38–47). Ibadan: Spectrum Books Limited.

Rice, E. S., Haynes, E., Royce, P., & Thompson, S. C. (2016). Social media and digital t echnology use among Indigenous young people in Australia: A literature review. *International Journal for Equity in Health*, *15*(81). PMID:27225519

Rogers, E. M., & Antola, L. (1985). Telenovelas in Latin America: A Success Story. *Journal of Communication*, *35*(4), 24–35. doi:10.1111/j.1460-2466.1985.tb02970.x

Rommy, N. R. A. (2017). Researching Indigenous Ways of Knowing-and-Being, University of South Africa, South Africa. DOI: doi:10.4018/978-1-5225-0833-5.ch002

Salawu, A. (2004). Development Communication in Yoruba Newspapers. In E. O. Soola (Ed.), *Communicating for Development Purposes* (pp. 172–184). Ibadan: Kraft Books Limited.

Salawu, A. (2006). Indigenous Language Media: A Veritable Tool for African Language Learning. *Journal of Multicultural Discourses*, *1*(1), 86–95. doi:10.1080/10382040608668533

Salawu, A. (2019). Alaroye, Isoleszwe and the Adoption of Digital Technologies. In A. Salawu (Ed.), *African Language Digital Media and Communication* (pp. 33–45). London, UK: Routledge Taylor and Francis Group.

Sokey, P. P., Adjei, E., & Ankrah, E. (2018). Media use for health information dissemination to rural communities by the Ghana Health Service, 1. *Journal of Information Science Systems and Technology*, *2*(1), 13–22.

Thomas, R. K. (2006) Introduction to Health Communication. Retrieved from eknygos.lsmuni.lt/springer/189/1- 7.pdf

UNESCO. (2005). Convention on the Protection and Promotion of the Diversity of Cultural Expressions Quadrennial Periodic Report on Measures to Protect And Promote the Diversity of Cultural Expressions.

Van Biljon, J., & Kotzé, P. (2008). Cultural Factors in a Mobile Phone Adoption and Usage Model. *Journal of Universal Computer Science*, *14*(16), 2650–2679.

Weller, J., Boyd, M., & Cumin, D. (2014). Teams, tribes and patient safety: Overcoming barriers to effective teamwork in healthcare. *Postgraduate Medical Journal*, *90*(1061), 149–154. doi:10.1136/postgradmedj-2012-131168 PMID:24398594

Wilson, P., Hearne, J., Córdova, A., & Thorner, S. (2017). Indigenous Media "Native Americans" Oxford Bibliographies article DOI: doi:10.1093/OBO/9780199791286-0229

Wilson, P., & Stewart, M. (2008). "Introduction: Indigeneity and Indigenous Media on the Global Stage." In P. Wilson, & M. Stewart (Eds.), *Global Indigenous Media: Cultures, Poetics, and Politics*. Durham, NC: Duke University Press, 2008. DOI: doi:10.1215/9780822388692-001

KEY TERMS AND DEFINITIONS

Communication: This refers to the transmission or exchange of information and implies the sharing of meaning among those who are communicating.

Development Communication: This refers to the use of strategic communication to facilitate the alleviation of social problems in evolving societies. Development communication techniques include information dissemination and education, behaviour change, social marketing, social mobilization, media advocacy, communication for social change and community participation.

Digital Age: This is a period in human history where a shift process occurs from industrial based to information- based economy using computer and other technology devices as medium of communication.

Health: This is a state of complete physical, mental and social well-being and not merely the absence of disease or infirmity.

Health Communication: It encompasses the study and use of communication strategies to inform and influence individual and community decisions with the purpose of enhancing health and wellbeing.

Health Literacy: This is the degree to which an individual has the capacity to obtain, communicate, process, and understand basic health information and services in order to make appropriate health decisions.

Indigenous Language: This is a *language* that is native to a region and spoken by *indigenous* people.

Indigenous Language Media: This is the forms of media expression that are conceptualized, produced and/or created by indigenous people and is used as vehicles for communication, cultural preservation, cultural and artistic expression, political self-determination, and cultural sovereignty.

Chapter 8
Potentials of Indigenous Media Campaign Against HIV/AIDS

Olayinka Susan Ogundoyin
https://orcid.org/0000-0002-2063-6247
Bowen University Iwo, Nigeria

ABSTRACT

HIV/AIDS has become a challenge to every society all over the world. The indigenous media could serve as channels through which information dissemination about knowledge; prevention and treatment are used as weapons to curtail its devastating effect. Despite the advancement in media technologies, information about HIV/AIDS is still limited in the rural areas, as they seemed marginalized because of their socio-economic status as well as their literacy level. Therefore, this chapter examines how the grassroot media can be utilized effectively to reach the indigenous people in a way that their cultural values will reflect in all media campaign against HIV/AIDS. It was observed that health messages about HIV/AIDS could be disseminated effectively using the various indigenous media. Health message designers are therefore implored to take advantage of these indigenous media to generate local contents which could consequently be disseminated through the mediums of radio and television for wider reach.

INTRODUCTION

Information plays an important role in addressing social problems through various mass media such as radio, television, magazines, books, newspapers, billboards and internet. These media have been proven to be effective in disseminating health messages that are beneficial to the sustenance and development of every society.

DOI: 10.4018/978-1-7998-2091-8.ch008

These media are commonly relied on in the urban area for information transmission while indigenous media are common in the rural area. The indigenous media are the type of media that belong to the people. There unique feature is that they are entrenched in the culture of the people within the community where it is domiciled. Indigenous media could be described as the media that are locally owned and operated and regularly producing contents in the local language. According to Edet, Akpan & Isaac (2015) indigenous media can be used interchangeably with folk media, oramedia, traditional media, local media and informal media. Indigenous media are seen to be effective because they bring information closer to the people and messages are mostly in their local language. Before the advent of media technologies, people disseminate information using the folk media. The folk media is as old as language because it constituted part of the entertainment segment enjoyed by the people who own it. Examples of folk media utilized for information, entertainment and behaviour change are puppet shows, folk drama, storytelling, proverb, visual arts, concerts, gong beating, dirges, and songs, drumming and dancing (Edet, I., Akpan, B., & Isaac, O. (2015). However, the advancement in technology has in a way replaced some of the examples of the folk media associated with indigenous media. Radio, television, newspapers, magazines, books, billboards have taken over the functions that are hitherto performed by the folk media.

These various media are employed to perform specific functions among which are to sensitize, create awareness, inform, educate, entertain, social mobilization, persuade, dissuade, warn, and so on, in order to bring about positive change in behaviour against a social problem of which HIV/AIDS is one. This change in behaviour is important in response to the growing HIV and AIDS epidemic in Nigeria. According to The Joint United Nations Programme on HIV/AIDS (UNAIDS) (2017) report, Nigeria is the second largest country with HIV epidemic with 3.1 million living with HIV infection. The campaign against the prevention of HIV and AIDS have been on for over three decades, despite this, it is estimated that around two-thirds of new HIV infections in West and Central Africa in 2017 occurred in Nigeria (UNAIDS, 2017).

As part of the growing concern on the rate of new infections and deaths recorded annually, various bodies are involved in the campaign against this growing menace like the Government, Non-governmental organizations and the media. These bodies are saddled with the responsibility to sensitize the society about the dangers and to increase the quality of life of infected persons with the use of anti-retroviral drugs. However, since the effort to get a cure for HIV is almost impossible, one of the many ways by which the HIV and AIDS pandemic can be reduced especially in the rural areas is through the indigenous media. Therefore, this chapter is interested in the potentials of the indigenous media in the control of HIV and AIDS.

BACKGROUND

The Concept of Indigenous Media

Indigenous media can be described as forms of media expression which produces and captures the history, culture, politics, economy, religious situations, social life and identity of the indigenous people that own them.

Ansu-Kyeremeh (1998:68) defined indigenous media as,

Any form of endogenous communication system which by virtue of its origin from integration into a specific culture, serves as a channel for messages in a way and manner that requires the utilization of the values, symbols, institutions and ethos of the host culture through its unique qualities and attributes used for personal as well as group information sharing and discussion.

These media enjoy local or indigenous narratives which allow the people to construct and utilize their individual and collective identities (Wilson and Stewart, 2008). From the definition, participation of members of the indigenous group is part of the distinctive principle and in practice, the production of such media is generally multicultural in process (Font, 2014). This is what gives them a sense of belonging and control since media contents will not be imposed on them but rather, produced by them. Spitulnik (1993) cited by Font (2014) argues that the term indigenous media covers a wide area of the media, from community owned and operated, radio, television and video operations to locally produced programmes that appear on national television. Indigenous media is a powerful tool for enhancing self-expression and consolidating the overall development of the indigenous people. The concept of indigenous people is synonymous with people whose voices, points of view and vision have been ignored or repressed (Font, 2014). Though in the face of modern technology media, indigenous media is seen as outdated, archaic, backward, primitive, ancient and local (Obono, 2011) but its usefulness is as effective as modern technology media. Indigenous media is seen to have implications for promotion of knowledge and enhancement of community life (Obono, 2011) especially in this era where it has become increasingly important to get information across to the grassroot level in the face of provocative and intimidating global health challenges.

In the past, folk media was used for the dissemination of information within and across communities. This include music, dance, songs, town criers and festivals which was at that time very effective. The challenges of globalization have displaced the effectiveness of these media channels because of more challenging issues the society has to deal with as well as the acceptance of western education and technology.

Indigenous media is a veritable source of information, education, teaching and entertainment. It is a media that encourages participation especially for community and development projects. As part of the attributes that makes indigenous media an effective tool is availability, accessibility, affordability, identity creation and participation.

There is no doubt that modern technology like the internet has reduced the world to a global village through the spread of information both at the local and global levels. The internet may constitute a challenge to the rural people because it requires a measure of literacy before it could be accessed unlike the indigenous media that needs no special literacy skill before contents can be produced or utilized since this is done in the local language of the indigenous people. Communication for health purposes is an essential strategy towards curbing the spread and menace of certain communicable diseases. The modern technology which is used for mass communication is very effective for disseminating information about risk behaviour, sensitization and awareness of some diseases. On the contrary, such mass media strategy may not be effective in the rural areas where elements within the content of the information disseminated is not at par with the context or environment in which the information is disseminated. Therefore, the need for a more appropriate communication channel in order to disseminate health messages that can facilitate interaction became necessary to fit into the ideologies of the indigenous people.

In order to get the people at the grassroot more involved in the utilization of health media messages, indigenous media should be considered an option because it forms a basis of interactivity and serves as a form of social cohesion.

The electronic media (radio and television) and print media (newspaper, posters, handbills, books, magazines, and brochures) are modern techniques of disseminating information to the public. The disadvantage of these communication channels is that it excludes people at the grassroot level from participating in development programmes. This is because all the contents are not localized and culture specific and therefore may not really meet the needs of the rural people. However, these media technologies could be made to serve the indigenous people by making the content local and adaptive.

Indigenous media is a tool that brings empowerment to people in all aspects especially on health-related information. Turner (2002) explains that indigenous media goes beyond the real issue of preserving the culture (though may be part of it) but the empowerment of social players to produce their own cultural meditations.

However, as part of the efforts of the federal government to reach out to the people at the grassroot level across the federation, 101 Stations of the Nigerian Television Authority (NTA) were established in 2014 in capital cities and towns of Nigeria. Of these, there are nine network centers in Ibadan, Jos, Enugu, Kaduna, Lagos, Benin, Markurdi, Maiduguri and Sokoto (Esan, 2009). Almost every town has its own television and radio stations owned either privately or by the government. This is in a bid to cater for information deficiencies of some localities.

In addition, there are many radio stations at the grassroot level in many states across the nation. This is to enable and encourage the indigenous people to lend out their voices so that they could be heard and be able to participate in the affairs of the nation. These radio stations are government and privately owned too.

The Menace of HIV and AIDS

The Human Immunodeficiency Virus (HIV) has attracted a lot of scientific efforts as far as research is concerned. The historical development of Acquired Immune Deficiency Syndrome (AIDS) was traced to the late 1970s when some young homosexual men were dying from what was termed as rare cancer and pneumonia known to be caused by benign microbes. These conditions were found to cripple the immune system and as a result became what is known as Acquired Immunodeficiency Syndrome (AIDS) (Sanyaolu, Okorie, Kumar, LaMoure, Rabadi, Hernandez and Omiloli, 2018). AIDS is caused by HIV and was discovered in 1983. After its discovery, HIV has killed men, women and children in their millions irrespective of their economic and social status, race or country of the world they belong to.

One of the major areas of concern about the virus is its incredible mutation rate. The rate at which the virus proliferate encourages resistance of drugs by infected person's system which has made it resistant to treatment thereby reducing life expectancy of infected persons. Educating people about its impact, causes, prevention and treatment of the disease became imperative in order to curb its spread. To stem the tide, massive education programmes were put in place by both government and non-governmental organizations. The essentiality of education as a veritable tool was identified as a strategy to fight against HIV and AIDS. It is believed that through literacy, HIV prevention and people's vulnerability to the disease could be subdued, as part of the educative measures taken, television, radio, newspapers, billboards, posters, handbills and so on were the medium used to reach out to vast number of people in order to create and increase awareness and knowledge about the dreadful disease. However, despite the aggressive measures taken against its spread, the effect of the infectious disease is still devastating as families have suffered due to the loss of their loved ones and its effect on the society is enormous as it cripples the economic and social state of the nation since huge amount of financial resources would be committed towards the care of affected persons. Though HIV and AIDS affect all the countries of the world, the hard-hit areas are the poorest parts of the world especially areas with low literacy level.

Globally, HIV is transmitted mainly through exposure to body fluids. These fluids include blood, semen, pre-seminal fluids, rectal fluids, vaginal and cervical fluids with mucous membranes (Kapila, 2006) and breast milk, all carrying the virus and are sources of transmission. It also spreads through any form of sexual contact with any type of partner: male-male, male-female, female-female relations. The sexual relation that poses the highest risk is the anal sex (Sanyaolu, et al 2017) and homosexual relations especially in the United States and Japan (Kapila, 2006; Sanyaolu, et al 2017) but recently, heterogeneous sexual relations constitute the highest mode of transmission in the world today (Kapila, 2006). The mode of transmission of this virus includes transfusion of contaminated blood, sharing of hypodermic needles, accidents in health care settings or certain health care products, mother-to-child transmission – through spontaneous virginal delivery (SVD) and breast milk (Kapila, 2006; Adedokun and Adedokun, 2016).

HIV/AIDS is an infection that has spread over the last three decades which has devastatingly affected all areas of the nation including but not limited to: social, health, economic and political sectors. The spread of the disease is multifaceted as inequality in socio-economic status, poverty, political instability, armed conflicts (Irwin, Millen and Fallows, 2003) war and migration are contributing factors.

In an epidemiological survey conducted by the World Health Organization (2004), it was reported that HIV has claimed more than 25 million lives over the last 30 years with an estimated number of people living with HIV (PLWHIV) approximately 36.9 (34.3-41.4) million globally. In Sub-Saharan Africa, PLWHIV are 25.8 (24.0-28.7) million out of the 36.9 million people affected in 2014 (WHO, 2004; Awofala and Ogundele, 2018), 66% of all people with HIV were living in the same region (Joint United Nations Global Fact Sheet, 2015; Awofala and Ogundele, 2018).

In 2016, Nigeria had 220, 000 (150, 000-310, 000) new HIV infections and 160, 000 (110, 000-230, 000) AIDS related deaths. Of the 3,200,000 infected population in 2016, 30% (19%-42%) were accessing anti-retroviral therapy, 32% (22%-44%) were pregnant women accessing treatment to prevent mother-to-child transmission of HIV. Also, an estimated 37, 000 (22,000-56,000) children were newly infected with HIV as a result of mothers' transmission of HIV to their children (the Joint United Nations Programmes on HIV and AIDS (UNAIDS) 2017).

Globally, 9% of PLWHIV live in Nigeria (UNAIDS 2014). Of these, the key population mostly affected are the sex workers with a prevalence rate of 14.4%; gay men and other men who have sex with men with a prevalent rate of 23% and people who inject drugs with a prevalence of 34%. These statistics reveals that the incidence of HIV is still on the rise despite the awareness created at various levels against its transmission in the country.

Nigeria is seen to be the largest HIV epidemic in the world as 3.1 people were living with HIV in 2017 (NACA 2017). In view of a survey conducted and reported by UNAIDS (2017), it is estimated that around two-thirds of new HIV infections in West and Central Africa in 2017 occurred in Nigeria.

There has been a progression in the public campaign of HIV infections. The shift was from causes, prevention and impact to the abuse of stigmatization. This measure enabled government, health message designers and policy makers encourage infected individuals on the need to promptly use anti-retroviral drugs for successful treatment (Ogundoyin, 2016a). The reason stigmatization in form of rejection and discrimination towards people with HIV was actively spoken against was because such action will likely lead to the progression and spread of the infection of HIV (Putri, Malini, Basmanelly, 2019) which will be inimical to their health and the society at large.

The symptoms of the infection according to Kapila (2006) include:

1. Large lymph nodes or swollen glands that may be enlarged for more than three months
2. Frequent fever and sweat, skin rashes or flaky skin that appears permanently
3. Short term memory loss
4. Slow growth or frequent illness in children
5. Cough and shortness of breath
6. Seizures and lack of coordination
7. Difficult or painful swallowing
8. Confusion and forgetfulness
9. Nausea, cramps, diarrhea or permanent vomiting
10. Vision loss and unexplained weight loss

In the light of this, attempt to reach mass audience especially those in the rural area can be accomplished by public communication campaign through indigenous content using the medium of radio and television in order to educate, sensitize and enlighten people about the scourge of the disease, since they are more effective than newspapers, books, posters, handbills, billboards and magazines in rural development. Also, radio and television influence our understanding of the world around us because media content can spread basic messages about the nature of reality.

Indigenous Media and Public Health Campaign

Public health campaign is a way of getting messages across to a target audience. It involves the use of media and messaging. It also organizes sets of communication activities to generate well-defined outcome in a target audience within a time frame (Dungan-Seaver, 1999; Ogundoyin, 2016b). It is used to shape and modify undesirable behaviour to a more desired one. There are two types of campaigns, they are individual behaviour change campaign and public will campaign (Dungan-Seaver, 1999; Henry and Rivera, 1998).

Individual behaviour change campaigns are also referred to as public information or public education campaigns. It attempts to change an individual behaviour from a social problem and further reinforces approved behaviour for the well-being of the society. Many of such campaigns include smoking, drug use, recycling, designated driving, seat belt usage, or fire and crime prevention (Henry and Rivera, 1998). Similarly, this type of campaign may be used in the case of HIV and AIDS using the indigenous media to project messages that can modify undesirable behaviour, acquire and strengthen knowledge through awareness.

Public will campaign is geared towards creating public will that will inspire public officials to take policy actions. It could also be referred to as a public engagement campaign. This type of campaign helps to raise the importance of a social problem in the public eye which serves as a drive for action (Henry and Rivera, 1998). It focuses less on the individual who performs the behaviour (like drug addicts and smokers) or engages in risk behaviour that can make him vulnerable to HIV and AIDS, but rather on the public's responsibility to do something that will create a conducive environment needed to support that behaviour change. This type of campaign is used for HIV and AIDS campaign which sometimes focuses on the need for members of the public to care and support people living with HIV and AIDS (PLWHA) and the need for them to adopt measures that will prevent them from contracting HIV/AIDS by not engaging in high risk behaviour that will predispose them to the disease.

Currently, almost every country in the world has been affected by HIV and AIDS according to the Joint United Nations Programmes on HIV and AIDS (UNAIDS, 1997). In response to this scourge, many countries have established a national AIDS programme and have conducted mass media HIV and AIDS campaign (WHO, 1994). Although the impact of mass media campaign on reducing AIDS risk behaviours is debated, knowledge about AIDS is obtained most often from mass media which indirectly makes it a veritable tool for reducing the spread and effect of the disease.

Since the advent of internet technologies, governmental public health authorities have shifted their attention from the indigenous media to social media facilities (Kass-Hout and Alhinawi, 2013) because of its ubiquitous nature (internet). Indigenous media also have a way of reaching the mass audience but not as much as the internet. The indigenous media have a potential to meaningfully enhance public health services by creating and establishing knowledge about HIV and AIDS to the target audience. This will assist the assimilation and retention of media messages which will later translate to behaviour change. Using the radio and television for HIV and AIDS campaign may be a good approach to tackling the disease headlong. This is because people living in the rural areas have limited access to the internet aside from the literacy skill it requires, but the medium of radio and television to create awareness and using the local language to pass the information across will go a long way to determining the efficacy of the effort. The added advantage of the television is its visual effect which adds to the retention rate of the target audience. Mass media generally and the indigenous media in particular, have a fundamental impact on collective and individual health because they have a potential of shaping human beliefs and behaviour. The basic role of the mass media is to provide information that would be beneficial to the general well-being of the public.

One of the possible barriers to the effectiveness of the internet and the print media (Books, magazine, poster, newspaper, and handbill) is language use. Most information that is common is written in English language which may pose a barrier to understanding the content of the messages presented. Therefore, for public campaign to be successful among indigenous people, indigenous media should be used as well as the indigenous language if message are to be well-understood and subsequently, followed by a change in behaviour (Ansu-Kyeremeh, Richter, Villianatos, and Aniteye, 2016).

In a survey reported by Ansu-Kyeremeh, et al (2016) congruence and simplicity in message are critical. They observed that rural women were not learned and therefore are unable to comprehend messages written in English language, though English language was the dominant means of communication in the country. In the same survey, some printed materials such as posters, flyers, stickers were analysed. It was discovered that those materials were solely written in English language and out of 24 printed materials, only one was written in both English and Hausa languages. Hausa language being the indigenous language of the respondents sampled. Also, it was observed that the most popular radio stations were found to broadcast in the Akan language which the indigenous people understood and could relate with. Their findings show that all flyers expressed in English language was of no commercial value and such information could be better expressed in the local language because illiterate women may be unable to use messages expressed in English language to understand the message presented. This clearly shows that for a successful public campaign on HIV and AIDS to take place, the various indigenous media channels should be considered using the indigenous language or dialect of the people and broadcast the messages through radio and television. Likewise, Smith and Abel (2008) claim that television is a powerful tool for adopting and stimulating any indigenous culture. This assertion directly or indirectly confers on the indigenous people the sense of responsibility and duty to identify with any public campaign that bothers on their health thereby, operating within the culture of their environment.

In communicating HIV and AIDS campaign messages, critics of the modernization paradigm are of the view that new media technologies suggest the top-down flow of communication which has failed in the areas of development in order to stand to its actual potential because it lacked the knowledge of the challenges facing the indigenous people in developing countries (Govender, 2010). Therefore, the need to explore the indigenous media channels to start off development programmes especially in the area of HIV and AIDS campaign seems expedient.

THEORETICAL FRAMEWORK

Uses and Gratifications Theory

Uses and gratifications theory was first introduced in the 1940s as interest of scholars began to shift to study the reason people use media and what they use them for. As part of the assumptions of the uses and gratification theory, media use is goal-directed, and people are motivated to consume the media (Vnney, 2001). This could be related to the careful selection of media by health message designers in order to achieve the desired goal of educating and sensitizing rural people about HIV/AIDS using the indigenous media. Another assumption states that media is selected on the expectation that it will satisfy specific needs and desires. The choice of indigenous media to disseminate health messages has implications for development programmes. This is because the indigenous people share a cultural link with these media, this in turn, will aid their cooperation to ensure the success of mounted health programmes. This sense of identity would also encourage rural people to become major actors to make any development effort a success.

Potentials of Indigenous Media Campaign Against HIV/AIDS

The use of indigenous media in dealing with health-related issues such as HIV/AIDS could be enhanced with the active use of mass media such as radio and television. Television and radio seem more appropriate to disseminate indigenous content since they reach large number of people around the world and have profound influence on society too. In addition to this, both media are essential because they cater for the need of the rural people who are unlearned. They do this by delivering indigenous contents and messages in a way the indigenous people can comprehend. These indigenous communication channels depict the values and lifestyles of people and are entrenched in their social, cultural and psychological thinking (Panford, Nyaney, Amoah, & Aidoo, 2001). Indigenous media are known to be credible sources of information. They promote local knowledge and are at the center of the socio-cultural, religious and political views of communities (Nigussie, 2015). Irrespective of which media is available either technology based or locally produced media, both have implications for campaign against HIV and AIDS. For example, folk songs as part of the traditional media could have some of its themes dominated by social, cultural and political events. These folk songs are usually composed based on the needs of the society and the richness of the culture of the people. Once a song is composed and performed in a locality, it spreads quickly to every part of the community, in that way, information gets disseminated among rural people. In this regard, the radio and television could serve as veritable tools for broadcasting these folk songs within a short period of time. These folk songs could be loaded with information on how dangerous HIV and AIDS infection is and the different modes of transmission would go a long way to equip them with the necessary knowledge that would keep them away from contracting the disease. Today, pop culture can help to transmit HIV and AIDS messages and update rural people on what is socially and morally acceptable. The songwriter would have to compose the lyrics of the song in a way that the narratives would be easier to commit to memory and becomes handy when they are faced with unacceptable situations. This method has a potential to attract the target audience to listen, watch and retain information in order to change risk behaviour. Dramas and puppet shows are also a very good means of passing messages through the electronic media. Puppet shows can be used for informing and entertaining the target audience. There are four types of puppets, the glove, string, rods and shadow puppets (Ritu, 2010). All these types are mostly used to tell a story. This story could be developed or built around sensitizing rural people about the dangers of HIV/AIDS especially when it is broadcast on the television. Dramas could be shown on television focusing on the different aspects of the disease, it will help to inform, educate and sensitize rural people who may be unaware of facts regarding HIV and AIDS.

In addition to radio dramas, radio soap operas are useful in creating awareness on HIV and AIDS. Radio opera is a serial drama that runs for a relatively long period of time. It is made up of plots that teaches different aspects of a subject in which HIV and AIDS is one. One of the advantages of soap operas is that they are entertaining and do appeal to the emotions of the target audience over a long period of time thus, encouraging the required behaviour change. People who watch or listen to soap operas tend to learn to identify with the characters in the drama, by this, the target audience retains and recapitulate more of the messages that are broadcast.

Radio

Radio is one of the main sources of health information in Nigeria. Despite the advent of new media technologies, radio failed to lose its relevance among people within the society. It is so regarded because it has the capacity to reach mass audience including those in the rural areas who receive low or no attention at all as far as information is concerned. It is a communication tool that is very cheap to operate and does not have the problem of network failure at any point. Based on the viability of the medium, health message designers have used this medium to transmit HIV and AIDS campaign messages especially in the hinterlands where limited information is made available. As part of the advantages of the medium is affordability, availability, cost effectiveness and accessibility. It is not limited by power failure as it is also battery operated.

During the peak of the campaign against HIV and AIDS in Nigeria, government and non-governmental organizations sponsored HIV campaign dramas such as One thing at a time by the Society for family health (SFH) - a pidgin drama that was aired in 1998, Garin muna fata was in Hausa (meaning 'Town of Hope') broadcast in January 2000, and the Igbo drama Odenjiji aired in 2001 and the Yoruba adaptation was Abule Oloke Merin which was produced and broadcast in 2001. All these drama programmes were aired in 42 radio stations across the country (Meekers, Rossem, Zellner & Berg, 2004 p. 16; Obono, 2011). These dramas were presented using English language, pidgin and the indigenous language for easy assimilation and comprehension. Radio dramas are aimed at increasing awareness of causes, consequences, prevention and counter to stigmatization. This clearly shows that radio is a good campaign tool for campaigning against HIV and AIDS. Radio is significant because it has the prospect of reaching those who do not have access or do not want to visit healthcare facilities because of different reasons (nonchalant attitude, distance, cost, humiliation of contracting HIV and AIDS).

In rural communities, community radios seem very appropriate in disseminating HIV and AIDS information. Community radio is one that is run by a community for its benefit. It helps to inform the indigenous people and raise awareness about ideas on HIV and AIDS and promote safe sex among adults and abstinence among youths. It is a type of radio service that offers a model of radio broadcasting beyond commercial and public service orientation.

Community radio is one that is closer to the people and is culturally sensitive. This ensures an integrated approach towards inculcating health messages on HIV that is relevant to the lives of the community and do not violate the beliefs of the people. It serves as a means of behaviour change as radio listening is an activity that encourages discussions and debates on health issues for adequate understanding.

Community radio is a good medium for HIV and AIDS awareness as PLWAs can make use of it to give mutual support to people within the locality who have the infection on how to care for themselves. It could also be used to sensitize people to integrate them into the society as normal citizens. It could be used as an avenue to encourage PLWAs to adhere to their treatment regimen in order not to suffer a relapse of the disease. This act of support given by the PLWAs to others in their category will prevent them from being marginalized within the community and would also make listeners who are HIV negative to learn more about their concern and therefore motivate them.

In order to make radio campaign (through storytelling, poetry, dramas, folk songs,) work effectively or capture public interest, significant days of the year should be targeted for HIV and AIDS campaign like Valentine's Day. In countries where Valentine's day is celebrated, youths may be prone to act carelessly due to the euphoria of the day. Condom use and abstinence from sex could be the subject of campaign few weeks to the celebration. This may provoke a form of consciousness in the youths to be careful in the face of any emotional explosion from their side. Indigenous programmes could be developed along this area in order to reinforce desirable behaviour. International AIDS Day is also an important day when awareness is created all over the world. The campaign can go on air prior to the celebration in order to have a lasting effect on the target audience. During these times, messages people hear repeatedly have the tendency to be retained in the long-term memory of their brain. Efforts could be made to develop indigenous programmes to commemorate that day. This will put a caution on any action that may contravene the content of the media message once they feel they are vulnerable to the disease. The indigenous content of drama, storytelling, folk songs, etc. would produce a better result in target audience.

Television

The television is also a medium that could transmit indigenous content. It is useful to effectively engage the public in communicating public health messages on HIV and AIDS. The difference between the radio and television is that television combines the feature of sight and sound. This feature makes it attractive and appealing to watch. Health message designers can make use of this medium to generate indigenous contents through the various indigenous channels of storytelling, drama, proverbs, puppet shows to get HIV and AIDS campaign messages across to the indigenous people. It is a medium that has the capacity to reach diverse people within a short period of time irrespective of their educational, social, economic, religious and political status. Soap operas are common as part of television programmes as well. Soap operas have their origin in folk drama. In Nigeria and in some other countries like Ghana and Philippines this method has been used to discourage sexual behaviour in the campaign against HIV and AIDS. Soap operas can repeat the same messages designed on HIV and keep it fresh by changing the storylines and characters. The concept of folk media has successfully been used in behaviour change. Folk media deals with learning from the environment by observing role models in everyday life and not excluding characters in television programmes and movies (Edet, et al, 2015). This is in a bid to ensure retention of messages and subsequently, a change in risk behaviour. As mentioned earlier, the infusion of culture into the storyline of the show would encourage the illiterate, less literate and poorer audience the opportunity to make a significant contribution in closing the gap in the socio-economic status of the target audience.

Television stations have taken over the responsibility to campaign against HIV and AIDS. One of such station is MTV which broadcast an HIV campaign drama by the MTV Staying Alive Foundation who produced the edutainment programme MTV Shuga in November 2009. It is a television drama that targets African youths. Another prominent television drama series that made the waves in the HIV prevention effort was Wetin Dey between 2007-2008. It was a Television drama series about HIV and AIDS awareness programme and the realities of living with HIV and AIDS. It is part of a larger campaign called 'STOP HIV' it was also used to address HIV and AIDS and sexual and reproductive health among Nigerian youths, it was one of the programmes that encouraged youths to know the importance of knowing their HIV status. The project was in partnership with the Society for Family Health (SFH) in Nigeria.

One of the ways the television can create awareness about HIV and AIDS is to mount up educational programmes on HIV and give rooms for debate. In the rural areas renowned health workers could be invited to educate the target audience about practicing safe sex and the devastating effect of contracting the disease. In a drama series on television, if the effect of AIDS is depicted as it is in real life especially at the final stage is shown, this will leave a lasting impression on the minds of the target audience, and this will also encourage them to avoid risk behaviour. Pictures leave a lasting impression on the mind hence; health message designers make use of pictures and scare tactics in composing messages in order to create fear in the target audience. For all these measures to work, attention should be paid to language use and appropriate indigenous channels. Drama series, advertisements against HIV and AIDS should not be presented only in English language. Attention should be paid to the different languages and dialect spoken in the various communities the health message is meant to cover. The various people that would be involved in the dialogue exchange in the drama series must be from the locality the message is designed for. The advert and the show must be presented in the context of everyday village life to help make the recall of messages very easy. Indigenous communication media such as music, poems, puppet shows and theatrical performance are not universal, (that is they are limited or restricted to the locality they belong to unlike the radio and television that have a wider coverage area) but they have been proven to be a formidable force in opinion molding which is enough for behaviour change. These indigenous media help to shape the society by correcting the ills within the community. For effectiveness of HIV messages within the indigenous locality, poems, puppet shows, music, storytelling, dramas, folklore, and theatrical performances could be made use of by the television, using the local and traditional presenters. This will help to preserve the cultural values of the locality without undermining the potency of the HIV and AIDS campaign message.

Television campaign is successful in increasing knowledge and improving risk perception about HIV and AIDS because it exerts a lot of influence on youths and adults alike. This is as a result of its extent of reach together with its visual attribute that describes real life situations. Television campaign helps to alert the populace on risks of HIV and AIDS and promote healthier behaviour through sensitization, education and community outreach especially among the youths in the rural community.

CONCLUSION

The scourge of HIV and AIDS is still an issue of concern all over the world. It is one of the most deadly and infectious diseases that has received a lot of attention globally. Various bodies which include government and non-governmental organizations have spent millions of dollars in the campaign against the disease. Different mass media channels have been utilized to reach out to diverse people for creation of awareness and sensitization about HIV, but this campaign may likely to be less effective in the rural areas because of so many reasons such as poverty, illiteracy and social status. These factors militate against the overall success of the whole effort. Hence, the need to integrate the local media into the propagation of HIV and AIDS campaign messages at the grassroot level, with proper attention paid to their cultural value as well as other intricacies that might ensure message retention and recall. This will greatly improve and enhance intelligibility and message comprehension which will consequently translate to a change in behaviour.

Entertainment constitutes an important part of any society. Folk songs, dramas, poetry, puppetry, theatrical shows are different sources of entertainment and channels for education as well. Health message designers are therefore implored to take advantage of these indifferent indigenous media to generate indigenous contents and targeting important days to disseminate HIV/AIDS message to the indigenous people through the mediums of radio and television.

FURTHER RESEARCH DIRECTIONS

As indigenous media have been seen to have potentials in educating the rural people on HIV/AIDS related messages, researchers should try to measure the effect these indigenous media have on the rural people after they might have been exposed to HIV/AIDS campaign messages.

REFERENCES

Adedokun, S., & Adedokun, A. (2016). Evaluation of the knowledge about attitude to HIV/AIDS and sexual practice among senior secondary school students in Ota Ogun State. *International Journal of Management Sciences*, *9*(1), 161–174.

Al-hassan, S., Andani, A., & Abdul-Malik, A. (2011). The role of community Radio in livelihood improvement: the case of Simli Radio. *The Journal of Field Action Report*, 5. Retrieved 7th June 2019 from https://journal.openedition.org/factsreports/docannexe/image/869

Ansu-Kyeremeh, K. (1998). Perspectives on indigenous communication in Africa: Theory and applications. School of communication studies, University of Ghana, Legion.

Ansu-Kyeremeh, K., Richter, M., Villianatos, H., & Aniteye, P. (2016). Rural women's exposure to health messages and understandings of health. *Journal of Health Care Communications*, *1*(3), 18.

Awofata, A., & Ogundele, O. (2018). HIV epidemiology in Nigeria. *Saudi Journal of Biological Sciences*, *25*(4), 697–703. doi:10.1016/j.sjbs.2016.03.006 PMID:29740232

Dungan-Seaver, D. (1999). Mass media initiatives and children's issues: An analysis of research and recent experiences relevant to potential philanthropic funders [Electronic version]. Paper prepared for the McKnight Foundation.

Edet, I., Akpan, B., & Isaac, O. (2015). Indigenous communication media and utilization of development information in rural communities of South-South Nigeria. *International Journal of English and Literature*, *5*(1), 85–96.

Esan, O. (2009). Nigerian Television: Fifty years of television in Africa. Retrieved 7th June 2019 from http://amvpublishingservices.com/pd-nigerian-televisionbrfifty.cfm

Font, L. (2014). Indigenous media: From transference to appropriation. Retrieved 25th May 2019 from http://anthrovision.revues.org/668

Govinder, E. (2010). How effective is HIV and AIDS Communication in Africa? *African Communication Research*, *3*(2), 205–234.

Henry, G., & Rivera, M. (1998). Public information campaigns and changing behaviours. Paper presented at the meeting of the association for Public Policy Analysis and Management, New York.

Irwin, A., Millen, J., & Fallows, D. (2003). *Global AIDS: Myths and facts tools for fighting the AIDS pandemic*. Massachusetts: Southend Press.

Kapila, M. (2006). HIV/AIDS, conflict and displacement. Retrieved June 6, 2019 from https://data.unaids.org>pub>report>2006.

Kass-Hout, T., & Alhinawi, H. (2013). Social media in public health. *British Medical Bulletin*, *108*(1), 5–24. doi:10.1093/bmb/ldt028 PMID:24103335

Meekers, D., Rossem, R., Zellner, S., & Berg, R. (2004). Using behaviour change Communications to overcome social marketing sales plateaus. Case study of Nigeria and India. Retrieved from https://www.shopsplusproject.org/sites/default/files/resource/910_file_07_Nigeria_and_India

NACA. (2017). National strategic framework on HIV and AIDS: 2017-2021. Retrieved from https://naca.gov.ng>2013-national-hiv-Nigeria National Agency for the control of AIDS (2021). National HIV/AIDS strategic plan 2010-2015. Abuja Nigeria. Retrieved April 26 2019 from http://nigeria.unfpa.org/pdf/nsp

Nigussie, H. (2015). Folk media and their use in HIV/AIDS prevention campaign. Retrieved May 10, 2019 from www.waccglobal.org>articles>folk-media.

Obono, K. (2011). Indigenous media preferences for reproductive health diffusion among the Yakur of Southern Nigeria. *Journal of Environment and Culture*, *8*(1), 62–77.

Obono, K. (2011). Media Strategies of HIV/AIDS Communication for behaviour change in South West Nigeria. *Africana*, *5*(2), 148–170.

Ogundoyin, O. (2016). Information and communication strategies for improving adherence to anti-retroviral drugs among patients with Human Immunodeficiency Virus infection. *International Journal of Management Sciences*, *9*(1), 1–10.

Ogundoyin, O. (2016). Perception and attitudes of respondents in Ibadan to fear appeal-based messages on HIV/AIDS. *Journal of Communication and Media Research, 8*(1) Sp. 1: 66-81.

Panford, S., Nyaney, M., Amoah, S., & Aidoo, N. (2001). Using folk media in HIV/AIDS prevention in rural Ghana. *American Journal of Public Health*, *9*(10), 1559–1562. doi:10.2105/AJPH.91.10.1559 PMID:11574305

Putri, D., Malini, H., & Basmanelly, B. (2019). Living with HIV/AIDS: Stigma and social discrimination. *Journal The Messenger*, *11*(1), 10–17. doi:10.26623/themessenger.v11i1.875

Ritu, A. (2010). Know your folks: Traditional folk media in India. Retrieved October 13, 2019 from https;//www.youthkiawaaz.com/2010/11/know-your-folks-traditional-folk-media-in-india

Sanyaolu, A., Okorie, C., Kumar, A., LaMoure, D., Rabadi, M., Hermandez, J., & Omoli, G. (2017). Current trends of HIV/AIDS in Asia. *South East Asia Journal of Public Health*, *7*(2), 3–11. doi:10.3329eajph.v7i2.38850 PMID:28857056

Smith, J., & Abel, S. (2008). Ka Whawhai Tonu Matou: Indigenous television in Aotearoa/New Zealand. *New Zealand Journal of Media Studies*, *11*(1), 1–14. doi:10.11157/medianz-vol11iss1id58

Turner, T. (2002). Indigenous media and political imaginaries in contemporary Bolivia. Retrieved May 21, 2019 from https://bools.google.com.ng/books

UNAIDS. (1997). Report on the global HIV/AIDS epidemic. Geneva. Switzerland: UNAIDS/WHO Working Group on Global HIV/AIDS. Retrieved May 16, 2019 https://www.data.unaids.org>report>2000gren.

UNAIDS. (2017). HIV and AIDS in Nigeria. Retrieved March 8, 2019 from https://www.avert.org/professionals/hiv-around-world/sub-saharan-africa/nigeria

United States Agency International Development. (2014). Orphans and Vulnerable Children Affected by HIV and AIDS. Retrieved April 9, 2019 from https://www.usaid.gov>technical-areas.

Wilson, P., & Stewart, M. (2008). *Global indigenous media. cultures, poetics and politics*. Durham, NC: Duke University Press. doi:10.1215/9780822388692

World Health Organization. (1994). AIDS: Images of the epidermic, Geneva, Switzerland. Retrieved April 2, 2019 from https://apps.who.int>iris>handle

World Health Organization Fact Sheet. (2014). *Global update on the health sector response to HIV*. Geneva.

ADDITIONAL READING

Irwin, A., Millen, J., & Fallows, D. (2003). *Global AIDS: myths and facts tools for fighting the AIDS pandemic*. Massachusetts: Southend Press.

Wilson, P., & Stewart, M. (2008). *Global indigenous media. cultures, poetics and politics*. Durham, London: Duke University Press. doi:10.1215/9780822388692

KEY TERMS AND DEFINITIONS

Campaign: It is the creation of awareness on HIV/AIDS through media messages.

Health: Is a state in which a person enjoys complete physical, mental and social wellbeing through the absence of infection and diseases.

Health Message Designers: Authorized people who decide and write contents that are used to create awareness, educate and sensitize the target audience on health-related issue.

HIV/AIDS: A communicable disease that is transmitted through infected body fluid.

Indigenous Media: The media of communication owned and operated by the indigenous people which transmit information about rural development. It includes drama, storytelling, songs, folklore, poets, proverb, and puppetry theatre performers.

Indigenous People: Are those who are resident in rural areas or less developed communities in terms of infrastructural development.

Mass Media: They are electronic media that transmit information through sound and sight to disseminate development information. They include radio and television which help to project and convey information from the indigenous media to the local people.

Potential: Is the ability or possibility of an entity to perform tasks leading to positive results.

Section 3

Indigenous Language Media/Communication and Radio/Television Programming

Chapter 9
Handling of Sexually Offensive Expressions on Zimbabwe's Selected Radio Stations

Phillip Mpofu
North-West University, South Africa & Midlands State University, Zimbabwe

Abiodun Salawu
https://orcid.org/0000-0002-1687-4621
North-West University, South Africa

ABSTRACT

Sexual and reproductive health-related communication in Africa is culturally regulated. This chapter analyses the handling of sexually offensive expressions on Zimbabwe's African language radio stations. The conceptual lens for this study is grounded in the indigenous knowledge systems perspective, which underscores indigenous communication systems as indispensable assets for African cultural communities. The chapter shows that African language radio stations are expedient channels for sexual and reproductive health-related communication in the contemporary society. However, this study shows the widespread use of inconceivable sexually explicit language and ineffective euphemisms in a manner that diminishes the relevance of the radio programmes. Therefore, the chapter maintains that it is imperative to remodel African language radio's language use conventions in programmes that relate to sexual and reproductive health issues in ways that match the cultural traditions of the respective audience.

DOI: 10.4018/978-1-7998-2091-8.ch009

INTRODUCTION

Present studies underscore sexual and reproductive health related communication as a human right and an enormously important public health issue (see Iliyasu et al., 2012; De Jesus, 2013; Melaku et al, 2014; Ngwenya, 2016; Rodrigues da Silva, 2018). For that reason, it is vital for members of any given community to be availed with sexual and reproductive health information at all stages of social progression. De Jesus (2013) maintains that mass media are vital channels of health communication in a polity.

Indigenous language print or broadcast media are expedient channels for disseminating development communication to African communities (Mpofu and Salawu, 2018). However, before considering the modern forms of communication, it is worth noting that traditional African communities have organised and dynamic social structures that comprise channels and institutions that disseminate developmental information (Ansu-Kyeremeh, 2005; Salawu, 2004). In particular there are specific settings and timing were specific sexual and reproductive health related communication is disseminated by designated individuals to community members of all age groups (see Ndlovu & Hove, 2015; Mumvana, 2018).

With specific reference to the Shona people of Zimbabwe, sexual and reproductive health training was characteristically a private, gendered and compartmentalised activity (Mano, 2004). This indicates that sexual and reproductive communication was not a public pursuit, rather it occurred in private settings of women, or of men, or people of the same social category using appropriate language. In these restricted settings, perspicuous language that is viewed as obscene, indecent, X-rated or simply sexually offensive in the public domain is admissible. This form of communication equips members of the Shona cultural community with important and necessary sexual and reproductive health knowledge and abilities (Gwandure & Mayekiso, 2012; Ndlovu & Hove, 2015). This also shows that though sexual and reproductive health related communication looks like a contemporary concept which is a creation or preserve of modern institutions, this study demystifies that perspective, and shows that it is not a novel practice in the Shona tradition.

In spite of the facts stated in the preceding paragraph, the modern world exposes members of the Shona cultural community, and other African cultural communities with a plethora of channels and spaces through which sexual and reproductive information is disseminated and can be accessed. Such channels of sexual and reproductive health-related communication include among others, fliers, workshops, peer education, the Internet, social media, as well as print and broadcast media. Generally, due to factors such as urbanisation, education, globalisation and other technological advancements, the modern society is also epitomised by the demise and diminished importance of the traditional social structures and institutions that were key in delivering sexual and reproductive health related communication. Thus, in the absence of the Shona fundamental such social infrastructure, the media in general, and broadcast media in particular have become veritable, alternative and expedient spaces for cultural information such as sexual and reproductive health related communication (see Mano, 2004). Zimbabwe's African radio broadcast media in particular is now awash with programmes which sexual and reproductive related issues such as sex and sexual rights, family planning, sexually transmitted diseases, mensuration, sex and marriage, and maternal health.

It is also worth noting that explicit public discussions on sex and reproductive health related issues that may include descriptions of human sexual reproductive organs and processes are ordinarily despicable and indecorous utterances among the Shona people of Zimbabwe (Mpofu, 2003; Mabaso, 2009; Museka & Kaguda, 2013; Mubonderi & Mpofu-Hamadziripi, 2018). In modern-day Shona society, particularly among the educated people intimates, articulating sexual and reproductive health related issues in the exotic language- English is to some extent stomached. However, explicit sexual and reproductive health related discourse in the native language- Shona is deemed uncouth, insolent, disgraceful, and totally unacceptable in the public domain. In fact, such utterances are categorised as vulgar or obscenities, and therefore constitute taboo language in public spaces.

However, over the years, there has been proliferation of diverse programmes that have been, and are still aired on Zimbabwe's African language national and regional radio stations. Such programmes, are popular and are a major attraction to the audience (Mpofu and Salawu, forthcoming). These radio programmes include among others, *Zvavakuru* (for the mature) on National FM radio in Harare, *Pamubheda* (on the bed), and *Chakafukidza Dzimba Matenga* (what covers people's homes are just but roofs)- both on Radio Zimbabwe in Harare, as well as *Couples Quality Time* on Star FM radio in Harare, and *Dandaro Revakuru* (popularly known as *Moto Mubhurugwa*) on Ya FM radio in Zvishavane.

Therefore, against the above discussed background it is critical to find out how producers/presenters of radio programmes that treat sexual and reproductive related issues handle taboo linguistic terms on a public platform like a radio. The terms include reproductive organs such as penis, vagina, testes, labia minora, and reproductive processes such as sexual intercourse, ejaculation, and mensuration. Against this background, this chapter analyses the handling of sexually offensive terms on selected African language national and regional radio stations using examples of three programmes which are *Chakafukidza Dzimba Matenga* (Radio Zimbabwe); *Couples Quality Time* (Star FM), and *Moto Mubhurugwa* (Ya FM).

The chapter shows the conundrums of performing sexual and reproductive health related communication on Zimbabwe's African language radio given that the practice itself is originally and routinely culturally regulated. As this chapter reveals, one of the major challenges is the handling of sexually offensive terms. As a result, the studied radio programmes- *Couples Quality Time* and *Moto Muburugwa* show widespread and ludicrous use of explicit language and inconsequential euphemisms which devalues the relevance of the African language radio programmes to the targeted cultural community. This chapter provides sociolinguistic and cultural insights towards understanding the problems of sexual and reproductive health related communication on African language radio in particular, and African language media in general.

BACKGROUND

This section contextualises the treatment of sexually offensive language in sexual and reproductive health related communication on Zimbabwe's African language radio by way of reviewing existing studies on sexual and reproductive health related issues in Shona tradition, and Africa in general. The section also shows the important roles and function of mass media in health communication in general, and sexual and reproductive health-related communication in particular. In view of the conceptual grounding that is set in this section, the section that follows critiques the handling of sexually offensive terms in the selected radio programmes.

Globally, existing scholarship show that communication on sexual and reproductive health related issues such as relationships, menstruation, and maternity care among others is an important subject and practice (Iliyasu et al, 2012; De Jesus, 2013; Melaku, et al. 2014). With specific to young generation, Rodrigues da Silva (2018) maintains that sexual and reproductive health information is a priority, especially on issues that include HIV and AIDS, sexually transmitted infections, negotiation for safe sex, and methods of contraception. Melaku et al (2014) illuminates that sexual and reproductive health-related issues include sexually transmitted infections, unwanted pregnancy and abortion, sexual organs and sexual intercourse, contraceptive methods and menstruation. Ngwenya (2016) emphasises sexual and reproductive health rights that include seeking, receiving and imparting information related to sexuality; receiving sexual education, choosing partners, bodily integrity, decisions on being sexually active or not, having consensual sexual relations and marriages, as well as pursuance of safe, satisfying, and pleasurable sexual life. In view of this understanding, it is imperative to establish how these sexual and reproductive health related issues are captured in an African language, in this case, Shona on radio given most of these concepts constitute what is termed linguistic taboos (Mbaya, 2002; Mubonderi & Mpofu-Hamadziripi, 2018).

Sexual and reproductive health related communication equips individuals of both gender with awareness of their sexual and reproductive health needs, and solutions to challenges they can face in that regard at any given stage of social development. The other important point that emerges in existing scholarship on sexual and reproductive health related communication in Africa is that it is a cultural event, which is therefore culturally determined (Salawu, 2011; Gwandure & Mayekiso, 2012; Ndlovu & Hove, 2015; Mumvana, 2018; Rodrigues da Silva, L.B.V. 2018). This observation implies that the understanding of sexual and reproductive health related issues, and how information is conveyed should be understood from the perspectives of members of a given cultural community since they are culture specific. Consequently, announcers of sexual and reproductive related issues on African language radio must be sensitive to the accepted moral language use practices of their audience.

Among the Shona people of Zimbabwe, sexual and reproductive health knowledge and skills are passed and acquired through the use of various methods and agents of socialisation (Gwandure & Mayekiso, 2012; Ndlovu & Hove, 2015; Mumvana, 2012). Shona refers to the largest ethnic group in Zimbabwe, whose members speak Shona, a language that comprises four mutually intelligible dialects (Mpofu and Salawu, 2019). In this cultural grouping the perspectives and actions about sexual and reproductive health are systematically and culturally acquired, and the related problems are generally solved through cultural means. This indicates that sexual and reproductive health related issues of the Shona people are grounded in their culture and philosophy.

As mentioned in the introductory section of the chapter, there are vital social structures in Shona tradition that are instrumental in disseminating sexual and reproductive health related communication to adolescents and adults (Chiwome, 1996; Gwandure & Mayekiso, 2012; Ndlovu & Hove, 2015; Mumvana, 2019). It is also important to note that sexual and reproductive knowledge is also dependent on gender, age and level of social development. To augment this observation, Mano (2004) argues that the instruction is a gendered process which occurs within split camps and same-sex contexts. Thus, communication on sexual and reproductive health related issues is contingent to people's social category. Also it is privately propagated to specific social groups at a given moment. In Shona tradition, it is in these private spaces where the use of explicit language on sexual and reproductive health related issues is permissible. In Mano's (2004: 332) words, the invented old tradition on radio "has to self-censor itself when it extends the old symbolic vocabulary from previously distinct and gendered spaces to new national limit." Hence, it is important to find out how the producers/presenters of African language radio on sexual and reproductive health related handle sexually offensive terms to the audiences of different gender, age and social classes.

The Shona social infrastructure that disseminates sexual and reproductive-related issues involves members and institutions of the extended family. The members of the extended family specifically include the aunts, uncles, grandmothers and grandfathers who are perceived to have the experience, information and license to provide sexual and reproductive health instruction. The aunts and the grandmothers are responsible for the female relatives, while the uncles and grandfathers serve the male relatives of the family (Chiwome, 1996). Using their knowledge and experience, they wittingly employ the appropriate language to the relevant members of the family, and at the appropriate time.

Rodrigues da Silva (2018) maintains that culture plays an important role in the improvement of efficient communication strategies for public health campaigns. This scholar reasons that the culture of a community may lead to their recognition or rejection of the health related communication. This implies that if sexual and reproductive health related programmes that are on African language radio neglect or contradict the culture and philosophy of the target audiences, especially by using unfitting of terminology of taboo terms; the efforts of the producers/presenters of broadcasts will be in vain, as audience may shun the programmes and eventually the radio station.

Existing studies also show that explicit sexual and reproductive health discourses in public spaces are taboo among the Shona and in most African cultural communities (see Salawu, 2011; Museka & Kaguda, 2013; Melaku et al, 2014; Rodrigues da Silva, 2018). Public utterances of words that refer to reproductive body parts such as penis, vagina, testes, labia minora, sexual intercourse, and other reproductive process such as mensuration is an offensive and disgraceful act in Shona tradition, and in most African cultures. Rodrigues da Silva (2018) show that even in Mozambique show that talking openly about sex and sexuality is unrefined and not accepted in the Changana community. This confirms the argument that sex and sexuality issues, which are part of sexual and reproductive communication are sensitive topics that should not be openly discussed. In a study by Rodrigues da Silva (2018), language and health terminologies were identified by the participants as a cultural challenge since open discussion on sexuality and sexual issues are considered bad-mannered and disrespectful in the Changana community. Similarly, in the Nigerian context, it is abominable for Yoruba women to openly talk about sex (Salawu, 2011). The submissions by these scholars show that public inter-generational deliberations on sex-related matters are taboo in much of Africa (Melaku et al, 2014).

The above discussed issues are perhaps the reasons why Iliyasu et al (2012) are against the introduction of sexuality education in school curriculum. Therefore, this validates the contention that contemporary communication on sexual and reproductive health related issues must be done with understanding that it is a culturally determined practice. People from different cultural communities have diverse views regarding what is deemed acceptable and unacceptable sexual and reproductive health related communication, and of course language use. Therefore, radio producers/presenters of African language radio programmes that treat sexuality and other sexual and reproductive health related issues should show respect of the audiences' culture and philosophy by avoiding explicit sexually offensive language.

In modern-day Zimbabwe, the Shona people are now exposed to multiple and different sources of sexual and reproductive health related information that contrast with the traditional ones in a number of ways. This kind of information can be accessed in music, films, Internet, and magazines as well as print, broadcast and social media. Existing scholarship show that mass media health related communication has enormous potential to change how health-related information is disseminated and obtained by different populations (De Jesus, 2013). In these spheres, different forms of sexual and reproductive health related information are presented. In the process, members of the Shona community are exposed to foreign and often contrasting forms of sexual and reproductive health related communication. Therefore, it is crucial to check the handling of sexually offensive language on African language radio programmes that deal with sexual and reproductive health related issues. Globally, the inclusion of sexualised content in the media has been contested and despised in existing literature (Attwood, 2007; Ybarra, Strasburger & Mitchell, 2014).

Mpofu (2003) and Mabaso (2009) show that words that relate to sexual and reproductive health related issues such as sexual intercourse, reproductive sex organs, sexually transmitted diseases are tabooed subjects among the Shona, and therefore must not be uttered in public. Linguistic taboo, cultural taboo or tabooed language refers to the prohibition of mentioning certain words and expressions in public spaces (Mbaya, 2002; Ndlovu & Botha, 2017; Mubonderi & Mpofu-Hamadziripi, 2018). In inescapable situation where they are mentioned, they are captured with veiled language or euphemisms. Euphemisms are courteous words or expressions that are used to replace expressions to do with sexual activity and other bodily functions that are deemed obscene and embarrassing. This is contrary to what Ndlovu and Botha (2017) term explicitness which is a form of communication where ideas are put across plainly and openly without hesitation or fear of condemnation. Therefore, it is important to find out if presenters on African language radio manage to employ well-thought-of euphemisms in programmes that deal with sexuality and reproductive health related issues, or they resort to explicitness.

This chapter is not the first study to appraise programmes dealing with sexual and reproductive related-issues on African language radio. Mano's (2004) study of the *Chakafukidza Dzimba Matenga* (what covers people's homes are just but roofs) analyses the invention of Shona traditional practice dare in the radio programme on Radio Zimbabwe. *Chakafukidza Dzimba Matenga* is a conversational programme that has a long history that dates back to 1981, which broadcast every Tuesdays at

2100hrs. Mano's focus was on the adaptability of a Shona cultural institution on national radio. The scholar argues that, the programme retains the essential elements of the Shona tradition *dare*, and shows continuity of traditional authorities as shown by elderly woman who acts as the *tete* (aunt), *sekuru* (grandfather/uncle) and the producer/presenter of the programme. The programme customarily treats issues that are related to sexual and reproductive health which revolves around relationships and marriages. Though Mano's gaze into this radio programme was from a broadcasting point of view, he noted courteousness of presenter and his participants in handling linguistic taboos since they adhere to the use "toned down language" (Mano, 2004: 327). Therefore, it is imperative to compare the rookie radio stations -Star FM and Ya FM's handling of sexually offensive terms in *Couples Quality Time* and *Moto Mubhurugwa,* with the language use conventions in the established *Chakafukidza Dzimba Matenga* on Radio Zimbabwe.

This chapter exposes the inaptness of uncensored use of sexually explicit language on Star FM and Ya FM radios to the Shona audience. The chapter shows the need for African language radio producers/presenters of sexual and reproductive health related issues to be sensitive to the culture of their audience in a bid to appropriate tradition in their broadcast content in an acceptable manner. It is esoteric and important to disseminate sexual and reproductive related communication through African language radio; however language use conventions in such programmes should be responsive to Shona moral standards and the culturally acceptable ways of treating sexuality and reproductive health related terminology.

CONCEPTUAL FRAMEWORK

The conceptual gaze for this chapter is grounded in the indigenous knowledge systems perspective. Indigenous knowledge is a body of knowledge that embodies specific norms, values and mental constructs that guide, organise and control a particular people's lives and how they view the world (Dei, Hall & Rosenburg, 2000). Shizha (2007) argues that indigenous knowledge is situational, culture and context-specific, dynamic and adaptive; holistic in nature; and is intimately related to the survival of indigenous people. It is shared knowledge, skills, and attitudes that belong to a community that arose from personal and community experiences (Ocholla & Onyancha, 2005). Existing literature underscores indigenous knowledge systems as indispensable assets for African cultural communities (Maunganidze, 2016).

According to Shizha (2007), indigenous knowledge exists in many forms that include among others music, spirituality, dance, song, ceremonies, ecological knowledge, symbols, scientific and agricultural knowledge, designs and languages. This indigenous knowledge is implanted in the rituals, customs, habits, and social institutions of a cultural community. It is interesting to note that language is also included in the list of aspects of indigenous knowledge. Language does not only function as a means for communication, but expresses the culture and identity of a people (wa Thiong'o, 1986). Therefore, understanding of language use in sexual and reproductive health related African language radio programmes is enhanced by the indigenous knowledge perspective.

In indigenous communication studies, aspects of indigenous communication systems are also grounded on indigenous knowledge, and they are termed indigenous media, folk media, informal media, communal media, traditional media or oramedia in different studies (Ugboajah, 1985; Ansu-Kyeremeh, 2005; Salawu, 2004; 2015, Oyesomi, Salawu & Olorunyomi, 2017). Oramedia are channels of communication that are grounded on indigenous culture and produced by members of a group (Ugboajah, 1986). Salawu (2004) shows that broadcast media are indispensable in the use of oramedia for development purposes. Therefore, it is imperative for broadcasters to appropriate oramedia on African language radio in programmes that treat sexual and reproductive health related issues in ways that are rooted in the culture of the audience.

Against the above stated erudition, this study is predicated on the contention that; the Shona people have their own indigenous knowledge systems, and indigenous communication systems in particular that reflect their value systems and their perception about appropriate or offensive language. As demonstrated in existent scholarship, the Shona people have fundamental social infrastructure that help in disseminating sexual and reproductive health-related issues to adolescents and adults in appropriate settings (Chiwome, 1996; Ndlovu & Hove, 2015; Mumvana, 2018).

Since language is an aspect of indigenous knowledge, and is fundamental to understanding the cultural reality of a people (Shizha, 2005), it is imperative for producers/presenters of African language radio programmes that cover issues related to sexual and reproductive health to package their messages in courteous language that adhere to the cultural conventions and philosophies of the Shona people, who are their audience. This is because the culture of a group may lead to the acceptance or rejection of sex and sexuality messages (see Rodrigues da Silva, 2018).

Hence, against this conceptual foundation, the chapter disapproves what Ndlovu and Botha (2017) terms explicitness, which is a form of communication where concepts on sex and sexuality are put across bluntly without hesitancy or fear of disapproval. Among the Shona people of Zimbabwe, terminology that relate to sexual and reproductive health related issues that include sexual intercourse, reproductive sex organs, sexually transmitted diseases are tabooed subjects which must not be uttered at all in public spaces (Mpofu, 2003; Mabaso, 2009). These are linguistic taboos or tabooed language which is the prohibition of mentioning certain words and expressions in public spaces (Mbaya, 2002; Mubonderi & Mpofu-Hamadziripi, 2018).

Therefore, this study subscribes to the use of veiled language or reputable euphemisms and avoidance of explicitness on African language radio programmes that discuss issues related to sexual and reproductive health. Thus, the producers/ presenters of sex and sexuality issues on Radio Zimbabwe, Star FM and Ya FM must ruminate on the language use conventions of the Shona people, particularly the treatment of sexually offensive terminology. This indicates that the maintenance of the Shona tradition on African language radio can only be efficient if the actors involved (producers/presenters and audience) are equipped with the rightful cultural knowledge (see Mano, 2004).

METHODOLOGY

This qualitative study was designed to analyse the handling of sexually offensive terminology on selected national and regional radio stations. The study focused on three purposively selected African language radio programmes that deal with sexual and reproductive related-issues that are *Chakafukidza Dzimba Matenga* on Radio Zimbabwe, *Couples Quality Time* on Star FM, and *Moto Mubhurugwa* on Ya FM. The primary focus for this study was on *Moto Mubhurugwa* and *Couples Quality Time*, while *Chakafukidza Dzimba Matenga* was used as for cross-referencing purposes. Primary data were collected for Star FM and Ya FM programmes, while secondary data were used for the Radio Zimbabwe programme, *Chakafukidza Dzimba Matenga*. Secondary data was collected from published work on, particularly Mano's (2004) publication.

This qualitative study adopted the interpretive paradigm. Interpretivists submit to socially construct multiple realities, where truth and reality are created not discovered (Guba & Lincoln, 2005:204). Therefore, the study sought to understand the handling of sexually sensitive terminology in selected radio broadcasts from the subjective view point of the producers/presenters and audiences. Data were collected from forty-two purposively and conveniently selected respondents consisting of two radio presenters, and forty radio audiences. Precisely, we interviewed the producer/ presenter of *Moto Mubhurugwa* on Ya FM, and made use Mumvana's (2018) interview with the Tilder Moyo, the producer/presenter of *Couples Quality Time* on Star FM. These two respondents provided data on the original purposes of the respective programmes and how they handle sexually offensive language. Data from the audiences were collected using focus group discussions that were administered by the first of author of this chapter in four settings.

The data from the audiences of the programmes being investigated showed audiences' perceptions on the handling of sexually offensive words on the selected programmes and radio stations. The collected data were augmented by content analysis of ten recordings of *Moto Mubhurugwa* and *Couples Quality Time*. In analysing data, the study employed thematic analysis. The objective of thematic analysis is to identify themes, that is, patterns of data that emerge from the data and are important in addressing the research question (Maguire & Delahunt, 2017).

FINDINGS

Handling of Sexually Offensive Lingo on Radio

The previous section exhibited interesting facts with regards to sexual and reproductive health-related communication, and the expected language use conventions in Shona tradition. Firstly, the preceding section shows that sexual and reproductive health communication on issues such as sexual relationships, reproductive body parts, menstruation, and maternity care among others is esoteric to the Shona community in particular, and African cultural communities in general. Secondly, sexual and reproductive health-related communication in Africa is a culturally determined phenomenon. Therefore, it is important to recognise the existing Shona social infrastructure which is made up of strategically positioned members of the extended family; which are involved in disseminating sexual and reproductive health-related communication to adolescents and adults. Thirdly, sexual and reproductive communication is a gendered and private process that is also social class specific. The fourth point is that aspects that relate to sex and sexuality are tabooed expressions that cannot be easily uttered in public spaces, particularly in the Shona language.

However, these authors note that there is growing interest in sexual and reproductive health-related content in broadcast media, as shown by the increasing number of programmes on African language radio stations in modern-day Zimbabwe. Over and above the classical *Chakafukidza Dzimba Matenga* which has been on Radio Zimbabwe (formerly known as Radio 2) since 1981 (Mano, 2004), *Couples Quality Time* and *Moto Mubhurugwa* on Star FM and Ya FM respectively are to a greater extend analogous broadcasts that have significantly attracted audiences' interest. Therefore, this section presents the findings of the study that highlight the treatment of sex and sexuality terminology which can be sexually offensive if uttered in a public space like radio, and in an African language like Shona.

Couples Quality Time is a popular broadcast on Star FM, a radio station that is situated in Zimbabwe's capital, Harare. Though, the title is English language, *Couples Quality Time* is broadcast in an African language- Shona between 2300hrs-0000hrs every Tuesday of the week. It is produced and presented by Tilder Moyo, also referred to as *tete* (aunt) by her audience during the programme. The programme focuses on sex and sexuality issues in relationships, especially those that concern married couples. Some of the topics that are covered in this programme include sex positions, male and female orgasm, and erectile dysfunctional problems among many other sexually related subjects. The programme is highly interactive; it is characterised by active participation of audience through WhatsApp or telephone. Therefore, it is imperative to analyse how the producer/presenter and her audience handle sexually suggestive terms in their discussion on air.

Moto Mubhurugwa, a Shona phrase which literary means 'fire in pants' is a programme that is broadcast on Ya FM radio, a regional station that is based in Zvishavane, in the Midlands province. At its inception, the programme was known *Dandaro Revakuru* (the adults' forum), but was popularised as *Moto Mubhurugwa*, a sexually suggested description of sexual arousal. The programme is presented by Israel Mundawarara who is affectionately known as *Sekuru* Munda (Uncle Munda) by his admirers. This is a weekly programme that is broadcast between 2300hrs and 0000hrs every Wednesday. Just like *Couples' Quality Time*, *Moto Mubhurugwa* is basically interactive as it involves audience participation through WhatsApp and telephone. The programme also covers wide ranging problems bedevilling marriages and relationship, and the issues discussed to a larger extend are related to sexual and reproductive health. The two programmes are mould in the frame of the established *Chakafukidza Dzimba Matenga* (What covers roofs are roofs), a programme which has been broadcast on Radio Zimbabwe (formerly Radio 2) for many years now.

Content analysis of the selected recordings of *Couples Quality Time* which we retrieved from YouTube showed that the programme surprisingly is awash with sexually explicit terminologies that are considered taboo language among the Shona. In one of the studied recordings, the presenter deliberately inspires callers to mention the actual terms that refer to sex and sexuality issues, and discourages them from using veiled language during phone-in conversations with the audience. The study established that even in instances where callers find it difficult to utter sex and sexuality terms, she probes them to say it out as it is in the indigenous language. As a result sexually explicit terms which are linguistically tabooed among the Shona are surprisingly uttered on a number of occasions in the studied recordings. For instance, excerpts of a phone in conversation below is laden with indescribable words which cannot be uttered in public, but were uttered on air:

Presenter: *Munoita sei kana mava kuda zvinhu zvenyu.*

Caller 1: *Ndinoti baba huyai timbotamba.*

Presenter: *Aiwa kumbotamba kudiiko, ndopandakambobvunza umwe waiti ndaiti. amai huyai timborara ah ah hakuna zvinhu zvakambodaro.*

Caller 1: *Baba huyai timbokwirarana chaiko.*

Presenter: *Ehe ka, taurai sezvazviri handisi kuda kunzwa language iyoyo.*

Caller 2: *... ndave kunzwa kuda* ***kuiswa****.*

Caller 3: Manje ini **masviriro** *andinoita, ndinoita kudambura.*

Caller 4: *ini ndinoti huyai tipinde pabonde.*

Presenter: *mmm language dzanamai vedu idzo.*

Caller 5: *Isu tava masenior* ***pakusvira****... kana newe* ***ndikakukwira unotunda****...*

Caller 6*: ...ndipewo* ***mboro****..*

Caller 7: *kana tava kuda* ***kusvira*** *ndinoti ndiri kuda* ***beche****...chero newe* ***unotunda****.*

Translation

Presenter: *What do you say when you want to make love?*

Caller 1: *I say dad, come let us play.*

Presenter: *No! playing, what does that mean? I once rebuked someone who said let us sleep, there is nothing like that.*

Caller 1*: Dad, let us make love (using colloquial language).*

Presenter*: Yes, that good. Let us say things as they are, we do not want that language (referring to the use of euphemisms).*

Caller 2: *...I want to make love (using colloquial language).*

Caller 3: *Myself I can hammer seriously (referring to sexual intercourse).*

Caller 4: *I say come let us make love (using a culturally accepted euphemism).*

Presenter: *That language belongs our mothers.*

Caller 5: *I am now a senior in making love… even if in do it with you, you squirt.*

Caller 6: *…May I have my penis*

Caller 7: *When I horny, I say give me my vagina.*

The above excerpt is a transcript of the conversation with seven listeners who phoned in to participate in the discussion where the question was: *Munoti kudii kana mava kunwa kuda*? (What do you say when you want to make love?). The first key talking point in this dialogue is that sexually offensive language, or tabooed language is audaciously uttered on a public space, in this case radio. The unspeakable terms include *mboro* (penis), *kusvira* (sexual intercourse), beche (vagina), and *kutunda* (ejaculation). Secondly, where callers for example like Caller 1 find it difficult to utter sexually explicit terminology, the presenter implores them to say it as it is, and discourages them from using euphemisms. The presenter refers to a culturally accepted euphemism for sexual intercourse (*bonde*) as outmoded language that does not belong to this generation. And thirdly, instances where callers, for instance Callers 5, 6 and 7 excessively use sexually explicit language, the presenter does not rebuke them. While there is an attempt to use what might not appear as explicit language at face value, like *kukwira/kudambura* (sexual intercourse), it is colloquial language which is too direct and obvious and not euphemisms. There are many other sexually offensive terms that were observed in other recordings that were studied and these include *matinji (*labia), *machende* (testes), *kupurojusa* (ejaculation), *kukoira* (sexual intercourse), *gambi* (vagina), *punani* (vagina) and *chikapa* (a particular sex position).

The above highlighted of lexical items are obscene and must not be uttered in public spaces. However, an excuse was given that the programme is done towards midnight, therefore supposedly children should be in bed; this is inconsequential in the digital era where radio stations can be accessed on the Internet and mobile devices. More so, different recordings of *Couples Quality Time* are available and can be retrieved from on You Tube at any time. In an interview with Mumvana on 17 April 2018, the presenter defended the use of sexually explicit language an African language radio as part of her role as an aunt as in the Shona tradition. This study notes that she is oblivious of the fact that in Shona tradition, it is only permissible in private and gendered settings, and among people of the same social category (see Chiwome, 1996; Mano, 2004; Gwandure & Mayekiso, 2012), not on a public platform like a radio.

The foregoing occurrence contradicts Shona moral standards which enshrine that words that relate to sexual and reproductive health such as sex, genitals, sexually transmitted diseases are tabooed and must not be uttered in public (Mpofu, 2003; Mabaso, 2009). If ever they are to be mentioned, courteous words or expressions called euphemisms must be employed. The use of euphemisms is corroborated by the producer/presenter of *Moto Mubhurugwa* on Ya FM who argued that "*tinonzvenga nematauriro atinoita, hatitauri mazita sezvazviri*" (we use euphemisms, we do not use explicit Shona terms) (Personal interview, 23 May 2018). For that reason, the findings of this study show that sexually offensive terms were comparably handled in a decent manner on Ya FM radio's *Moto Mubhurugwa* as shown by the use of euphemisms like *chivakashure* (buttocks), and *kudzikisa gejo* (sexual intercourse). However, some of the terminologies they consider to be euphemisms are common colloquial terms which equally explicit and sexually offensive.

This is contrary to the seminal *Chakapfukidza Dzimba Matenga* on Radio Zimbabwe which have consistently employed euphemistic language. In Mano's (2004), on *Chakafukidza Dzimba Matenga* the presenter/producer and other participants adhere to the use "toned down language" (Mano, 2004: 327) which is respectable. This exposé shows that while sexual and reproductive health communication through African language radio remains essential in modern-day world, it is the handling of sexually offensive terms on African language radio proves to be a challenge, since some presenters prefer and condone what Ndlovu and Botha (2017) call explicitness, a form of communication where sex and sexuality issues are put across plainly and openly without hesitation or shame.

Research findings show that while the audiences applauded Star FM radio's *Couples Quality Time* and Ya FM radio's *Moto mubhurugwa* as important broadcasts which deal with important issues; they all disapproved the use of sexually explicit language which is obscene and embarrassing in the Shona society. In a focus group discussion, one respondent argued "*zvekutauravo zvinyadzi paredhiyo, kuya kwava kumbairashika kuya...* (uttering obscenities on radio is losing the plot) (Group interview, 18 October 2018). This suggests that the use of sexually explicit language contravenes the Shona people's culture and philosophy on the language use conventions in public spaces.

Therefore, this chapter argues that language use in African language radio programmes on sexual and reproductive health must reflect the language conventions of the Shona value systems. While the chapter appreciates the role played by African language radio in sexual and reproductive health-related communication, it calls for increased caution and sensitivity in in the treatment of sexually offensive words. The chapter shows that African language radio are expedient channels for sexual and reproductive health-related education in the contemporary society. However, it queries the capturing of sex and sexuality issues where the presenters condone explicitness and uncivil way of handling sexually offensive terms on radio.

SOLUTIONS AND RECOMMENDATIONS

The preceding section showed the conundrums of sexual and reproductive health related communication which is conveyed through African language radio to cultural communities which traditionally have their own frames of acceptable and unacceptable language use conventions in public spaces. This has been exemplified by the excessive and obnoxious use of sexually explicit terms on Star FM radio's *Couples Quality Time*, and revealing euphemisms on Ya FM radio's *Moto Mubhurugwa.* The main challenge of sexual and reproductive health related communication on these two Zimbabwean radio stations is the predominant use of sexually explicit terms which is an unacceptable practice in the Shona tradition, therefore inappropriate to the audiences. Such that, on one end sexual and reproductive health related communication on African language radio is perceived as an expedient re-establishment of Shona tradition in broadcast media the context of modernisation; while on the other end the use of sexually explicit language in discussions relating to sexuality and reproductive health related issues in public spaces, radio included is a disgraceful development which inadvertently diminishes the morality of the African language radio programmes.

Hence, there is need to transfigure the language use conventions in African language radio's broadcast programmes that relate to sexual and reproduction issues, especially the unrelenting use of sexually revealing language, and flimsy euphemisms. Firstly, this chapter advocates the spreading out of themes discussed on the selected African language radio programmes beyond sex focused subjects to also include other sexual and reproductive related-subjects as outlined by Melaku et al (2014) and Ngwenya (2016). Secondly, the authors implore the producer/presenters of the sexual and reproductive health-related radio programmes to be sensitive to the cultures of the audiences they serve by avoiding the use of sexually explicit language, as presenters/producers of *Chakafukidza Dzimba Matenga* on Radio Zimbabwe have strived to achieve over many years. Though there could be other commercial imperatives pushing them to do so, broadcasters of African language radio programmes related to sexuality and reproductive health related issues should abide by the cultural value systems of the audiences' language use conventions if the programmes could remain relevant and respectable.

FUTURE RESEARCH DIRECTIONS

This chapter has shown the perils of Star FM and Ya FM radio producers/presenters' fascination with sexually explicit language in ways that are at odds with the Shona cultural conventions which regard words or expressions which describe sexual reproductive organs, sexual intercourse or other sexual and reproductive related-issues as obscene and forbidden in public spaces. This chapter shows that this is an emerging and perturbing feature in Zimbabwe's African language radio that appears to be instigated partly by the commercial necessity for new radio stations to gain competitive advantage in a highly competitive broadcasting market with already established radio stations (Mpofu & Salawu, forthcoming).

This chapter provides critical sociolinguistic and cultural insights to the understanding of the challenges of sexual and reproductive health-related communication on African language radio stations in the modern society. Given that this chapter focused on the handling of sexually offensive language on Zimbabwean radio stations, it is imperative for researchers from other parts of the African continent who are interested in health communication and African language media to join the discourse community of sexual and reproductive health-related communication in African language media for comparative purposes. More so, since this study has looked the handling of sexually offensive language on African language radio stations from sociolinguistic and indigenous knowledge perspectives, future researchers can also consider employing other theoretical paradigms to understand the use of sexually implicit language on African language radio, and African language media in general.

CONCLUSION

This chapter makes a sociolinguistic and cultural contribution to understanding the conundrums of sexual and reproductive health related communication on African language radio in particular, and African language media in general. The chapter analysed the handling of sexually offensive terms in two Zimbabwean radio stations, Ya FM and Star FM. Given that health communication is esoteric and imperative, sexual and reproductive health related communication in Africa is rooted in culture, and therefore uttering terms that relate to sexual and reproductive health related issues in public is culturally unacceptable; language use on African language radio programmes that discuss sexual and reproductive health related issues must be sensitive to the culture of the audience. However, this chapter show that in the studied radio programmes there is prevalent use of unthinkable sexually offensive language and weak euphemisms in a manner that diminishes the expediency of the African language broadcasts to the target audience. Hence, the chapter argues for the fashioning and modifying of language use traditions of sexually offensive terminology on African language radio in ways that are commensurate to the cultural traditions of the audiences.

CONFLICT OF INTEREST

The authors declare that they have no competing interests.

ETHICAL CONSIDERATIONS

Consent was sought from and granted by the producer/presenter of *Moto Mubhurugwa* at Ya FM, and he voluntarily participated in the study. Consent was also sought from and given by Otilia Mumvana to use her interview recording with the presenter of *Couples Quality Time*, Tilder Moyo. The authors ensured that the anonymity and privacy rights of the audiences who participated in this study were respected.

ACKNOWLEDGEMENT

We would like to thank Otilia Mumvana who granted us permission to use her interview recording with the presenter of *Couples Quality Time* on Star FM, Tilder Moyo for the purposes of this study. We would also like to extend our sincere appreciation to the interviewees who participated in this study. Special mention to Sekuru Munda (Israel Mundawarara).

REFERENCES

Ansu-Kyeremeh, K. (Ed.). (2005). *Indigenous Communication in Africa: Concept, Application, and Prospects*. Accra: Ghana Universities Press.

Attwood, F. (2007). 'Other' or 'one of us'? The porn user in public and academic discourse. *Participations*, *4*, 1.

Chiwome, E. (1996) Communicating with children on sexual Issues. In S. Mutsvairo, E. Chiwome, N. E. Mberi, A. Masasire, & M. Furusa (Eds.), Introduction to Shona Culture. pp. 51-64. Kwekwe: Juta Zimbabwe (Pvt) Limited.

De Jesus, M. (2013). The impact of mass media health communication on health decision-making and medical advice-seeking behaviour of U.S. Hispanic Population. *Health Communication*, *28*(5), 525–529. doi:10.1080/10410236.2012.701584 PMID:22888787

Guba, E. G., & Lincoln, Y. S. (2005). Paradigmatic controversies, contradictions, and emerging confluences. In N. K. Denzin, & Y. S. Lincoln (Eds.), *The Sage handbook of qualitative research* (pp. 191–215). Thousand Oaks, CA: Sage.

Gwandure, C., & Mayekiso, T. (2012). Sexual desire and expression among girls in a traditional Shona context. *Anthropologist, 14*(5), 415–423. doi:10.1080/0972 0073.2012.11891264

Iliyasu, Z., Aliyu, M. H., Abubakar, I. S., & Galadanci, H. S. (2012). Sexual and reproductive health related communication between mothers and their adolescent daughters in northern Nigeria. *Health Care for Women International, 33*(2), 138–152. doi:10.1080/07399332.2011.562996 PMID:22242654

Dei, G. J., Hall, B. L., & Rosenberg, D. G. (2000). Indigenous Knowledges in Global Contexts: Multiple Readings in our World (pp. 3–18). Toronto, Canada: University of Toronto Press.

Mabaso, P. (2009). The compilation of a Shona children's dictionary: Challenges and solutions. *Lexikos,* 19, *Supplement* (*AFRILEX-reeks/series*), 19, 112-119.

Maguire, M., & Delahunt, B. (2017). Doing thematic analysis: A practical, step by step guide for learning and teaching scholars. *AISHE-J, 8*(3), 3351–3369.

Mano, W. (2004). Renegotiating tradition on Radio Zimbabwe. *Media Culture & Society, 26*(3), 315–336. doi:10.1177/0163443704041176

Maunganidze, L. (2016). A moral compass that slipped: Indigenous knowledge systems and rural development in Zimbabwe. *Cogent Social Sciences, 2*(1), 1–12. doi:10.1080/23311886.2016.1266749

Mbaya, M. (2002). Linguistic taboo in African marriage context: A study of the Oromo Laguu. *Nordic Journal of African Studies, 11*(2), 224–235.

Melaku, Y. M., Berhane, Y., Kinsman, J., & Reda, H. L. (2014). Sexual and reproductive health related communication and awareness of contraceptive methods among secondary school female students, northern Ethiopia: A cross-sectional study. *BMC Public Health, 14*(252), 1–11. PMID:24628909

Mpofu, N. (2003). Cultural aspects in the Shona monolingual dictionary Duramazwi Guru reChiShona. *Lexikos,* 13, (*AFRILEX-reeks/series),* 13, 232-239.

Mpofu, P., & Salawu, A. (2019). Interrogating the autonomy of previously marginalised languages in Zimbabwe's indigenous language press. *Language Matters: Studies in the Languages of Africa, 50*(1), 25–44. doi:10.1080/10228195.2018.1541925

Mpofu, P., & Salawu, A. (forthcoming). Sex and sexual fantasies on Zimbabwe's Ya FM and Star FM radio stations. *African Identities*.

Mubonderi, B., & Mpofu-Hamadziripi, N. (2018). Speaking the unspeakable: A socio-cultural analysis of tabooed language in Shona society. *The Fountain Journal of Interdisciplinary Studies*, *2*(1), 104–118.

Mumvana, O. V. (2018). *Transformations and challenges of sex education in selected radio programmes*, (Honours Dissertation), Midlands State University, Zvishavane.

Museka, J., & Kaguda, D. (2013). The school and the 'second sex': A feminist response to verbal and non-verbal sexual harassment of girls by boys in Zimbabwe's secondary schools. *Journal of Emerging Trends in Educational Research and Policy Studies*, *4*(2), 308–314.

Ndhlovu, K., & Botha, R. (2017). Euphemism vs explicitness: A corpus- based analysis of translated taboo words from English to Zimbabwean Ndebele. *South African Journal of African Languages*, *37*(2), 235–243. doi:10.1080/02572117.2017.1378278

Ndlovu, S., & Hove, E. F. (2015). Old wine in new skins: Revisiting counselling in Traditional Ndebele & Shona societies. *Journal of the Humanities and Social Sciences*, *20*, 101–105.

Ngwenya, S. (2016). Communication of reproductive health information to the rural girl child in Filabusi, Zimbabwe. *African Health Sciences*, *16*(2), 451–461. doi:10.4314/ahs.v16i2.13 PMID:27605960

Ocholla, D. N., & Onyancha, O. B. (2005). The marginalized knowledge: An informetric analysis of indigenous knowledge publications (1990-2004). *South African Journal of Library and Information Science*, *71*, 247–248.

Oyesomi, K., Salawu, A., & Olorunyomi, B. (2017). Indigenous Communication: Socio-Economic Characteristics Influencing Contemporary Female Political Participation. *Journal of International Women's Studies*, *18*(4), 164–181. Available at http://vc.bridgew.edu/jiws/vol18/iss4/12

Rodrigues da Silva, L. B. V. (2018). Communication strategies of adolescent sexual and reproductive health programmes in Mozambique: Cultural challenges. *Open Access Journal of Public Health*, *2*(3), 1–11.

Salawu, A. (2004). The intrinsic value of oramedia for development. *Humanities Review Journal*, 4, 18-30.

Salawu, A. (2011). Breaking the culture of mute sensation: Female expression of power in Sexual contest with men in Yoruba newspapers. *Soc Sci*, *27*(1), 39–51.

Salawu, A. (2015). Oramedia as a vehicle for development in Africa: The imperative for the ethical paradigm of development. *Journal of Sociology and Social Anthropology*, *6*(2), 209–216. doi:10.1080/09766634.2015.11885660

Shizha, E. (2005). Reclaiming our memories: The education dilemma in postcolonial African school curricula. In A. Abdi, & A. Cleghorn (Eds.), *Issues in African education: Sociological perspectives* (pp. 65–83). New York: Palgrave Macmillan. doi:10.1057/9781403977199_4

Shizha, E. (2007). Critical analysis of problems encountered in incorporating indigenous knowledge in science teaching by primary school teachers in Zimbabwe. *The Alberta Journal of Educational Research*, *53*(3), 302–319.

Ugboajah, F. O. (1985). Oramedia in Africa. In F. O. Ugboajah (Ed.), *Mass Communication, Culture, and Society in West Africa* (pp. 165–176). New York: K. G. Saur.

wa Thiong'o, N. (1986). Decolonizing the mind: The politics of language in African literature. Portsmouth: Heinemann.

Ybarra, M. L., Strasburger, V. C., & Mitchell, K. J. (2014). Sexual media exposure, sexual behaviour, and sexual violence victimization in adolescence. *Clinical Paediatrics*, 1-9.

KEY TERMS AND DEFINITIONS

African Language Media: refers to print, broadcast, or digital media that disseminate content in an African language.

African Language Radio: refers to a radio station that broadcasts content in an African language.

Euphemisms: these are courteous words or expressions that are used to replace explicit expressions for reproductive organs, sexual activity or other bodily functions that are deemed culturally obscene and embarrassing.

Explicitness: refers to a form of communication which puts across sexual and reproductive health related issues plainly, openly and clearly without hesitation or fear of condemnation (Ndlovu & Botha, 2017).

Indigenous Knowledge System: is a situational, culture and context-specific, dynamic and adaptive body of knowledge which embodies specific norms, values and mental constructs that guide, organise and control a particular people's lives and how they view the world. It is shared knowledge, skills, and attitudes that belong to a community that arose from personal and community experiences (Dei, Hall & Rosenburg, 2000; Ocholla & Onyancha, 2005; Shizha, 2007).

Linguistic Taboo/Tabooed Language: refers to the prohibition of mentioning certain words and expressions in public spaces (Mbaya, 2002; Mubonderi & Mpofu-Hamadziripi, 2018).

Oramedia: refers to small group oriented, orally based, and two way dialogical channels of communication such as games, folktales, drama, that are grounded on indigenous culture and produced by members of a group (Ugboajah, 1986; Ansu Kyeremeh, 2005).

Radio Zimbabwe: formerly Radio 2, is Zimbabwe Broadcasting Corporation (ZBC) owned radio station that broadcasts in two widely spoken African languages in Zimbabwe- Shona and Ndebele, and is based in Harare.

Sexual and Reproductive Health-related Issues: these include sexually transmitted infections, unwanted pregnancy and abortion, sexual organs and sexual intercourse, contraceptive methods and menstruation (Melaku et al, 2014).

Sexual and Reproductive Health Rights: refers to issues such seeking, receiving and imparting information related to sexuality, receiving sexual education, respect for bodily integrity, deciding on being sexually active or not, having consensual sexual relations, getting into consensual marriages, and practicing satisfying, safe and pleasurable sexual life (Ngwenya, 2016).

Shona: refers to the largest ethnic group in Zimbabwe, whose members speak Shona, a language that comprises four mutually intelligible dialects (Mpofu and Salawu, 2019).

Star FM: is a Zimbabwe Newspapers owned radio station which broadcasts from Harare.

Ya FM: is a regional radio station which is located in Zvishavane, in the Midlands province of Zimbabwe.

Chapter 10
A SWOT Analysis of Indigenous Language Use in Agricultural Radio Programming in Nigeria

Babatunde Adeyeye
Covenant University, Nigeria

Lanre Amodu
Covenant University, Nigeria

Odiboh Oscar
https://orcid.org/0000-0001-5870-6223
Covenant University, Nigeria

Oladokun Omojola
https://orcid.org/0000-0001-8362-4588
Covenant University, Nigeria

Evaristus Adesina
Covenant University, Nigeria

Charity Amaka Ben-Enukora
Covenant University, Nigeria

ABSTRACT

This chapter investigates the strengths, weaknesses, opportunities, and threats of indigenous language use in agricultural radio programming in Nigeria within the theoretical frame of diffusion of innovations as well as the theory of planned behaviour. This discourse affirms existing assertions that using indigenous languages in agricultural radio programming can guarantee farmers' access to information on issues of agro materials, utility applications, support accessories, funding, technology, conservation, marketing, and pedagogy. The study concludes that indigenous language use in agricultural radio programming engages agricultural programme producers and farmers through their opinion leaders. It recommends that the use of indigenous languages in agricultural radio programming in Nigeria should continue. However, the country's agro policy should protect all farmers irrespective of cultural or ethnic divides; and specifically cater to the needs of minority ethnic groups of farmers.

DOI: 10.4018/978-1-7998-2091-8.ch010

INTRODUCTION

Access to agricultural information around the world allows farmers to make sensitive decisions leading to increased productivity in agriculture (Stefano, Hendriks, Stilwell, & Morris, 2005; Wang *et al.*, 2017; Khan, Aziz, & Ahmed, 2018). In spite of this significance, Ozowa (1995) considers that the vital role that information plays in developing countries for agricultural and modern development is ignored and given a reduced status than other sectors of the economy. Alam and Haque (2014) support this perspective just as Wojcik, Jeziorska, Biel and Czapiewski (2019) who argue that a big part of rural regions still needs information and agricultural expertise to assist in modernizing their farming methods. Padre, Sundarshana and Tripp (2003) note that food production is reaching a point where unhindered information flow is becoming germane to stakeholders' achievements. Additionally, the adoption of Information Technology can significantly boost agricultural output (Waqas, Khan, Akhter, Noor, & Ashraf, 2017; Ahmad *et al.*, 2016).

Consequently, access to information has turned into an essential asset for agricultural development. In this unique situation, information is required to maximize openings and bring to limelight issues of present-day cultivation innovations. The Food and Agricultural Organization, FAO, (2006) states that sustained agricultural growth depends, at all phases of the agricultural production chain, on material input, human resources, farmers' comprehension and communication of data. Adeyeye *et al.*, (2019) provide insight into the relationship between the use of new media for farmers ‘ training by extension workers and the rate of innovation by farmers. Agricultural expansion has been imagined with imparting research discoveries and enhanced agricultural practices, and the effectiveness with which this information and practices are passed on would decide the level of farmers' efficiency (Ani, 2001; Donye, 2018; Moyo & Salawu, 2018). The most potent channel of this impartation are the media of mass communication (Odiboh, Salawu & Doghudje, 2019; Odiboh & Ekanem, 2019).

Among members of communication media, radio and its aired content are adduced the most ideal tool for achieving improved development of rural small-scale farmers in Africa (Ozowa, 2005). Additionally, advancements in information and communication technologies (ICTs) have made it fundamentally simpler and more reasonable to connect through and collaborate among audience members over the radio (Adeyeye *et al.*, 2018). By utilizing new media technologies, it is conceivable to upgrade the potential of radio as a proficient circulation channel beyond mere expression. Radio programmes urge rural dwellers to take interest in development by embracing new innovations. Radio programmes empower groups to explain their encounters and basically look at issues and arrangements influencing their lives.

Communication in indigenous languages has been observed to enhance social harmony thereby encouraging African cultures to be preserved (Salawu, 2006). . According to Oyesomi and Salawu (2019), Indigenous language is a language that is spoken by a group of people that resides in a locality or region. Sonderling (2009, p. 85) points out that language plays a main role in all fields of human endeavour because it is a conduit through which people interact. Such communication varies from circumstances of face to face to tactical mass mediation. Through the media, the use of indigenous languages to communicate with agrarian groups, particularly radio, provides the listener a feeling of belonging. Studies have shown that the use of native language in radio broadcasting is the best conduit of mass interaction as it achieves more easily than other media and is understood by the audience group (Mufwene, 2002; Manyozo, 2009). This constantly increases agricultural productivity in general terms.

This chapter therefore seeks to fill the lacuna that characterizes agriculture in many of the world's emerging economies exemplified by Nigeria. Approximately 924,000 square kilometres of arable land and 133.4 million farmers' constituting 70% of the country's population has been disconnected by inadequate farming information. Mass mediated communication and inappropriate linguistic drivers explain the disconnection and lacuna in question. Bridging this gap calls for intense collaboration between agro-focused mass mediators and the farmers' themselves; thus, bringing about a need for synergy between the two key sectorial stakeholders. In this regard, farmers' craving for productivity-enhancing information, mass mediation outputs of agricultural radio programmes and the desire of programme producers to meet such needs must synchronize. Scholars agree that communicating in indigenous languages would give farmers a sense of belonging in Nigeria's agro-refocusing economy. However, the cultural diversity and multi-ethnicity of the country pose as challenges to radio programme producers. This narrative draws the need to examine the strengths and weaknesses of using indigenous languages in radio agricultural programming in today's Nigeria. It also analyses the threats and opportunities of using indigenous languages in disseminating agricultural information to 21st century farmers' in the country.

METHODOLOGY

Qualitative research method is applied in this study. According to Reinard (2001), by using general opinions of social action, qualitative studies attempt to define the human condition. Also, the chapter is approached from the descriptive and analytical perspectives. As Okoro (2001) illustrates, the purpose of descriptive research is to designate a specific phenomenon as its name indicates. Robson (2011) observed that the distinction between descriptive and analytical methods is that while descriptive studies define what is, analytical studies determine its existentiality. This is in line with Wimmer and Dominick's (2013) statement that while descriptive study compares and explains what phenomena are, analytical study is generally concerned with causal-effect interactions; and generally, the outcome allows researchers to examine and create explanatory inferences on the interrelationship between factors. Using this inquiry method, we analyse the power and weakness of indigenous language use in agricultural radio programming using a technique of SWOT analysis as it relates to agricultural productivity.

LITERATURE REVIEW AND THEORETICAL FRAMEWORK

Radio

Radio is a medium used by electronic waves to send and receive messages through the atmosphere. According to Idebi, (2008). Radio involves broadcasting programmes for listening to the public using the mechanism of electrical signals transmission over a distance (BBC English Dictionary, 1992). Radio acts as an audio medium that offers data, it is very important for individuals everywhere to be mobilized by mass. Okunna (1999) recognized radio as having the ability to break down the obstacles of analphabetism and infrastructural deficiencies that are significant constraints on the print media.

The primary alternative methods of communication have traditionally been television and newspapers (Onabajo, 1999). However, IT development has considerably changed the landscape as social media and associated types of communication have emerged to play a key role in communication. McKenzie (2006) claims that radio is one of the most common communication instruments in rural residences. Affordable and available it disseminates significant information to rural audiences through entertainment, information and education. Sakwa (2012) observes that, compared to other communication media, radio has a broad coverage with greater persuasion and impact. These studies assist to demonstrate that radio can be used to educate society on significant problems such as health, growth, agriculture, and family.

Indigenous Languages

Language is a means of transmitting the culture, standards, thoughts and beliefs of people. The repository of the identity and manner of life of people are encapsulated in and transmitted through their language to newer generations (Emeka-Nwobia, 2015). Eyisi (2000) states that language is the subject of every conceivable human activity;

used to convey love, hate, rage, happiness, praise, satisfaction, and unhappiness. It is also used for commenting on political, social, educational and financial circumstances of a nation; confirming or expressing religious views, commenting on the weather and even filling a void when there is nothing else to do particularly in pleasantry communion. Therefore, human beings are naturally endowed with the tendency to always use language for mutual social relations with their fellow people and achieve their daily goals for their individual and collective well-being. When their communication flows, people get on well; when the contrary occurs, people experience dissonance.

Language is essential to supporting groups of individuals; it is the vehicle that acquires, shares and transmits other constituents of society. Without language, thoughts, ideas, data, and society would be redundant and useless. Hanafi (2013) sees language as the foundation of every culture. Language is a non-specific system of words, meanings and symbols for all cultural components, including speech, written characters, numerals, symbols, and non-verbal expressions of communication.

Language remains inseparable from culture to indigenise communication. Cultural context and intimacy with a culture offers a greater significance to the comprehension of language and the circumstances under which it happens determines the credibility and truism of communication (Wallace, 1996). Language aids comprehension, assists assimilation and complement the recall of such messages when transmitted to individuals in their indigenous languages (Oyero, 2003). By decreasing knotty extraneous terms in indigenous language development texts, the audience will understand the profound meanings of such texts. Bamgbose (1991) believes that literacy enables a farmer for instance, to gain knowledge in fertilizer utilization, pricing and other processes.

The implication of the farmers' analogy above is that the use of indigenous languages in the education of farmers can go a long way in securing a stream of data on fertilizers, pesticides, high yield crop range, suitable seasons of planting, irrigation and conservation as well as marketing outlets (Odiboh, 2011; 2002; Odiboh & Oladunjoye, 2019; Odiboh & Ajayi, 2019; Odiboh, Ezenagu & Okuobeya, 2019). According to (Lawal, 2015), the formal and informal education scheme, that is, the stage of enculturation, plays a very important role in indigenous languages. The use of local languages in farming education and expansion centres would be made easier, thereby transforming rural farmers' new agro-technologies to increase returns, incomes and living standards. That is why Geekie (1995) affirms that helping rural people to read, write, and converse in their native languages helps them and stakeholders in countryside living in dealing with everyday problems.

Agricultural Radio Programmes

Rural agrarian communities are most of the time, the focus of agricultural radio programmes. On-air conversations are components of the communication element that is critical to sharing pluses in agriculture among stakeholders. From its founding in Africa in the 1920s, when mass media were regarded as powerful tools with which authoritarian governments mobilized groups and rallied them around the growth agenda, the potential of radio in socioeconomic development became evident. Radio is the medium of global understanding for farming groups (African Farm Radio Research Initiative, 2008). Maputseni (2006) believes that its perceived strengths were what motivated the use of radio programmes as a pedagogical and educational instrument. Other academics have enumerated the strengths of radio programmes as realized by the consumers. It is based on oral tradition, it appeals to and depends on the viewers imagination, it can cross time and space without limits, it can go through locations and evoke true life imaginations; and it is a private medium (being a companion) that can reach millions of listeners at once with the power to talk separately to each of them (Fossard, 1996).

Moemeka (1980) exemplified Tanzania and Colombia as nations that used radio to raise rural communities' intellectual and living standards, Tanzania's instructional project has been regularly broadcast to countless listening groups across the nation on domestic radio stations. On the other side, Columbia removed physical distance by setting up rural radio stations. According to Bell, Payne and Bohn (2011) the tasks of agricultural radio programmes are to connect farmers to markets, increase overall awareness of productivity possibilities, provide technical data in training and application, and diagnose issues and suggest alternatives (Odiboh, Adeyeye & Ekanem, 2018). Other tasks are: to answer client-related follow-up questions, provide mass advice, promote access to credit and inputs, help with business planning, and perform surveys.

Indigenous Languages, Agricultural Information And Farmers In Nigeria

Many problems arise when knowledge is disseminated to farmers in indigenous languages. The Opubor reference by Lawal (2015) points to Nigeria's elite-oriented media content, the triple equivalent of radio and television media coverage, and the near non-existence of media coverage in minority languages. This is illustrated in agricultural programmes on TV and radio broadcast for peasants. The dominance of English over local dialects is still felt through newscasts, documentaries on agricultural news, among others. Bamgbose (1991) supports this statement by noting that almost all Nigerian radio stations are owned by the government, and the majority of programmes that will help local farmers to increase returns, and other innovations are not incorporated in their understanding of languages.

Nigeria has more than four hundred languages and is a multilingual nation. Only a few farmers in the nation use modern farming techniques. Therefore, in the face of this multi-ethnic structure, a question emerges about the real role of language. The reality is that language has no part to play if the country is really aiming at achieving the required agricultural development. It is said that linguistically heterogeneous states are generally underdeveloped economically while homogeneous states are extremely advanced (Bamgbose, 1991).

Ndaghu and Taru (2012) provide available information showing that compared to other developing nations, Nigeria has a virile broadcasting structure. However, the enormous chance of these media is yet to be fully utilized for farmers in agriculture. The reasons for this range from staggering transmission expenditure to the non-attendance of lawful framework to integrate the media into the rural advancement drive as well as the use of indigenous languages in bringing the farmers along. In addition, Nigeria's media framework is centralized in urban regions without resorting to rural farmers ' needs and plight. Therefore, the necessary data aimed at farmers for productive farming does not reach this group of individuals. Even if it does; these programmes are not packaged in such a manner that farmers appreciate them. Similarly, on the other side of the divide, there is the issue of illiterate farmers who cannot read and understand the data accessible to them. Similarly, publishers and program managers are more enthusiastic about generating programmes of high company esteem, hosting data intended for farmers.

THEORETICAL FRAMEWORK

The study is anchored on the theories of Diffusion of Innovations and Planned Behaviour.

Diffusion of Innovations Theory

Diffusion of Innovations provides three insights into the process of social change, highlighting:

- The things that influence the spread of innovation
- The significance of peer to peer discussions and peer to peer networks
- The requirements of distinct customer understanding

These insights have been tested in over 6000 study surveys and field trials, making them some of the most socially reliable. Innovation diffusion requires a radically distinct strategy to most other change theories. Rather than concentrating on persuading people to change, it considers change as mainly about the evolution or reinvention of products and behaviours so that they become better suited to individual and group requirements.

The theory describes how innovations in a population are taken up. An innovation is an idea, behaviour or object that its audience perceives as fresh. Accordingly, Rogers (2003) further argued that the innovation-decision method is an information-seeking and information-processing activity where an individual is motivated to decrease uncertainty about its benefits and disadvantages. This method of innovation-motivation includes understanding, persuasion, decision-making, execution and confirmation. Typically, these five phases follow one another in a timely way.

Rogers (2003) defined the process of innovation-diffusion as a method of reduction of uncertainty, proposing innovation fundamentals that assist to reduce uncertainty about innovation. Innovation attributes include five innovation features, including: relative advantage, compatibility, complexity, trialability, and observability. He further stated that the views of these features by people predict the rate of innovation acceptance. Nevertheless, diffusion researchers think that a population can be divided into five distinct sections based on their propensity to embrace a particular innovation. These include: innovators, early adopters, early majority, late majority and late majority (Rogers, 2003).

Diffusion of innovation theory is important to this chapter because indigenous-language agricultural radio programmes provide a range of new agricultural technologies that require farmers to adopt if they wish to improve their general production. By adopting these technological developments in agriculture, farmers' yields are enhanced as a consequence of which availability of enhanced, tested and trusted food security techniques is fully assured.

Theory of Planned Behaviour

Icek Ajzen created the concept of planned behaviour in 1991 as a derivation of Ajzen and Fishbein's suggested concept of reasoned action (1980). A key factor in planned behaviour theory is the individual's intention to execute certain behaviours. The intention to act is the instant determinant of the behaviour, according to Ajzen (2005). The planned behaviour theory assumes that the greater the intention to behave, the more probable their performance will be (Ajzen, 1991). Ajzen (1991) asserts that an intention results in behaviour only if the individual can willingly decide whether or not to participate in the behaviour. Most behaviours however, rely, to some extent, on the accessibility of no motivational variables, such as possibilities and resources (economic abilities and others' collaboration). Considering that an individual has the possibilities and resources and intends to behave, he or she must do it (Ajzen, 1991).

The theory of planned behaviour is derived from three concepts: attitude, subjective norm and perceived behavioural regulation. Attitude refers to the degree of a favourable or unfavourable behavioural perception by a person (Ajzen 1991). The attitudes of individuals are defined by their understanding of what can be true about a particular subject, often influenced by beliefs and values (Willock *et al.*, 1999). Subjective norm is a social factor which suits or does not interpret the social pressure to act. Perceived behavioural regulation refers to the person's ease or difficulty in carrying out his actions (Ajzen 1991). Perceived behaviour management refers to individual behavioural ease and complexity (Ajzen 1991). The more beneficial these three mechanisms are, the more an individual wants to act (Ajzen, 1991). There is therefore projected to differentiate between behaviour and circumstances in the relative importance of attitude, subjective normality and perceived conduct control in predicting intent (Ajzen 1991)

The concept of planned behaviour is important to this chapter because it reveals that the greater the intention to participate in behaviour, the more probably their performance is that an intention leads to behaviour only if the individual can willingly choose to participate in the behaviour or not. Farmers therefore decide whether or not to embrace new farming methods in accordance with their intention to participate. This intention to participate invariably relies on the nature of the indigenous languages to which agricultural radio programmes are subjected.

A SWOT ANALYSIS OF INDIGENOUS LANGUAGE USE IN AGRICULTURAL RADIO PROGRAMMING IN NIGERIA

Indigenous language use in agricultural radio programming in Nigeria is characterised by certain strengths, weaknesses, opportunities and threats. These are analysed as follows:

Strengths

Indigenous languages as established in literature gives farmers a sense of belonging thereby fostering a deep desire to apply whatever is disseminated on radio. To achieve meaningful development, indigenous languages are sacrosanct (Ndhlovu, 2008), and radio is viewed as the far-reaching medium that can encourage the use of these languages, particularly in supporting the growth of agriculture.

Agricultural radio programs in indigenous languages have potential for growth as the added benefits of being able to deliver warmth and humanity to all messages transmitted in local dialects. Salawu (2006) indicates that the ability to interact with the target audience on air in indigenous languages is better and the outcome can produce more than other media. Literature suggests less than one would like to learn, because even in schools with restricted media both print and electronics, mother languages are now compelled to break up. Salawu (2004) agrees that a conscious and honest effort must be made to learn and teach the language in its original form both officially and informally as it ensures the survival of indigenous languages and culture.

In human society, the function of language is essential. It offers social, management and organizational resources. Development, however, offers a means of conveying a social, social, political, socio-cultural and technological change through enhanced agricultural production. Consequently, language is used in domestic growth as a catalyst. In agricultural radio, the use of indigenous languages is essential to any nation's overall growth. In order to guarantee complete involvement of all citizens (including farmers) in the development process, the linguistic characteristics are important for efficient communication in indigenous languages. This is because the use of foreign languages will subvert citizens' involvement at the grassroots in particular.

To ensure full and equal participation of all citizens in all sectors of the country, there is need for understanding of concepts conveyed. The use of indigenous languages is pivotal for agricultural, technological, social, political, economic and scientific advancement. It is not just enough to formulate policies and programmes, it is of more importance to be able to transfer and interpret such policies to the end users; and also, to ensure that they understand what is being transmitted. Unfortunately, not all the population is educated. If this must be done, then there is need to use the indigenous languages for transfer and transmission of such.

Weaknesses

The fundamental problem presented by the diversity of indigenous languages is how the mass participation and grassroots involvement can be effectively accomplished with a view to ensuring complete and genuine farm growth. There is not much that has been done in this area of mass communication, i.es. there is no flow of information, because communication experts think indigenous languages are not enough to be experienced by the audience. Nigerian farmers are most likely to continue farmers who can only receive information in local languages about fertilizers, pesticides, high-yield crop varieties, suitable seasons of planting, irrigation and survival, and marketing outlets.

In the face of multiplicity of indigenous languages especially within the same environment, it becomes difficult for radio programme producers to come up with programmes the suits all residents which invariably make information dissemination difficult. Hence, Bamgbose (1991) opined that some type of 'semi-communication' across languages is feasible even where languages are not the same. However, only a few of these languages are so similar to supporting this statement. In addition to the primary languages (Hausa, Yoruba and Igbo), the remaining hundreds of linguistic groups did not do much in the language they could understand to convey foreign ideas, ideas and technology in spite of being agricultural powerhouses in the country. One point of observation is that agricultural development and technology attained by nations such as Japan, China and Germany was not based on the extensive dissemination of English, popularly known as the global language, but on the indigenization of technology in those nations and the translation of procedures into terms that are commonplace. The situation of Nigeria should not be an exception.

The challenge, then, is how far can the capacity of Nigerian languages be built so that they can be relevant in the ongoing dialogue for Nigeria's sustainable Agricultural development agenda? Technology and sustainable development have always been implicitly central to an understanding of what language is or can be. It is difficult to achieve technology in an imported language. Unfortunately, during the twentieth century, however, as is widely known and recognized, English language colonized indigenous languages, which in turn, became subject languages, just as the people who speak them became subject citizens. Indeed, by dint of historical accident, past and present empires, and lately, through a virtual monopoly of Microsoft, English language has increasing expanded in the global communication network. The implication includes a steeply subordinated position of indigenous languages. The ultimate challenge is to develop the indigenous languages to the extent that they become economically empowering. According to Rob Pope (2002), English language is the major invisible exports of Britain, the USA and Australia. In contrast, there is no indigenous Nigerian language that is in any great demand. Nigeria's position as a major stake holder in the oil market and as the most populous black nation in the world should confer a major economic and political status on, at least, one of the major languages of Hausa, Yoruba and Igbo.

Most Nigerian languages lack adequate lexicon for certain etymological words, especially international technology and science issues. With these, the use of metal vocabulary appears to revert. This cannot however solve the problem because the abstract and mental sense of the foreign word can be substantially separated from it semantically. In certain cases, the meaning of words in the source language (maybe English) and the recipient language (mostly indigenous languages not being standardized) cannot always be one - to-one. Uno (1987) noted that the lack of a systematically developed metal language and specialized vocabulary to effectively disseminate information in the various fields of human activity can hamper efforts to achieve sustainable development objectives aimed at improving agricultural productivity in the language of the Nigerian language.

Other problems include misrepresentation and erroneous understanding of ideas and cultural inhibition when the mother-speakers cannot even cooperate in developing their language.

Opportunities

Chinese language has acquired more global status because Europe and America want to tap from the achievement of the Chinese civilization, culture and technology. Every human civilization starts with language, which has the power of constructing possible models of human experience. Therefore, the empowerment of indigenous languages in agricultural radio programming will enhance the achievement of literacy and an interactive positive attitude towards people from other ethnic groups thus leading to improved agricultural productivity. Agricultural radio programming provides the opportunity of the Chinese experience for Nigerian languages.

Brumfit (1995) argues that although knowledge is not merely power, language use, and knowledge about language have a specifiable relationship to power; hence the debate about the future of Nigerian languages, in part, about the potential for power of their use in official communication through agricultural programmes. If other foreign languages are becoming immensely important international languages today, Igbo, Yoruba or Hausa can also become West African lingua franca.

It became evident that national goals and philosophies in the native languages were better communicated. Nigerian can both be an inclusive language and can promote positive attitudes and identification for groups. Accommodation in indigenous languages will therefore encourage multiculturalism and pave the way for sustainable national development in relation to agricultural productivity. Afolayan (1995) observes that English was introduced into Nigeria in order to groom Nigerian citizens for service in the British colonial administration. The time has come to mould an indigenous language into an instrument capable of maximally developing the capacity of Nigerians to utilize the vast development opportunities in the twenty-first century. This means that while an indigenous language becomes a second language, English can serve as a foreign language. Incorporating it into agricultural radio programming will also go a long way in improving the desire of farmers to embrace technologies in agricultural production since they are engaged in a language they can relate with.

Of so many indigenous languages, only too few in Nigeria have been recorded and represented in a significant way apart from Hausa, Igbo and Yoruba. The underuse of indigenous languages is regarded as one region that slows down the rate of linguistic and agricultural growth in all its implications. Skutnabb-Kangas (2000) states that if this message is transmitted, people appreciate information better. The rural areas are home to a bigger percentage of Nigerians. Almost everyone is monolingual with only very few of them being bilingual. They do not therefore understand English as the language of print and electronic media. Due to this challenge, they cannot reach SDG's purpose and expectations, as the information is not conveyed through the language they understand, to communicate it using English medium. In other words, it is imperative that rural communities should be reached within a context to which they can respond and contribute to the efforts of facilitators to achieve the desired outcome and its effect as anticipated. The above therefore calls for the creation and effective use of our agricultural radio programs in indigenous languages.

Cyber knowledge diffusion can be useful through the development of Nigerian languages, Urua (2005). Hence, it is possible to mobilize individuals and distribute agricultural data to individuals in their local languages by using modern Information Technology (IT) resources and IT centres. This concept was utilized by a "simputer project" in India which offers individuals in rural environments data in an accessible level, using their local languages. A cheap and handy alternative to PCs,' simputer' offers opportunities for the ordinary person. Crystal (2003) captures most of what simpler a language does to make it concrete by providing a public profile. Through this simpler technique, information is therefore distributed in their indigenous languages on government and other development agencies such as SDG programs, targets, principles, farm developments, ideas and ideals as well as on any other cruise with human and community well-being.

Threats

There are fears that indigenous language agricultural programmes will not do enough to safeguard the different indigenous languages that are slowly disappearing. Some scientists agree that most indigenous languages face imminent fatalities. (Salawu, 2006; Manyozo, 2009; Mabika, 2011).

Mavesera (2009) argues that young people do not see the need to learn the indigenous languages because, as with English and other foreign languages, they do not have an academic or economic advantage. Indigenous languages are important for speakers because they enable people to have free faith and speech. Radio broadcasting in indigenous languages, particularly among social groups such as young people who no longer recognize the importance of their own languages, is important since it can add value to moving languages. The revitalisation of indigenous language includes the use of languages that are moribund or threatened with incremental restitution (O'Laoire, 2008). If fully exploited, radio is a mass media that offers almost limitless resources to minority languages and groups (Ndamba, 2008).

CONCLUSION AND RECOMMENDATIONS

The chapter attempted to analyse the strengths and weaknesses of indigenous language utilization in agricultural radio programmes. Discussions verify the viability of Nigeria's agricultural radio programmes in indigenous languages. Radio broadcasting is currently more competitive and varied than it has been historically in terms of program and channel spread. The argument is not that broadcasting programmes have become ways of corroding their languages and cultures, as some communications academics insist, but that radio programmes in indigenous languages efficiently transmit messages of rural development and edify native languages and cultural skills. Radio programmes in indigenous languages, for example, have the capacity to integrate farmers into the public agenda's mainstream. It follows that media policymakers cannot ignore the potential of indigenous languages as cultural expressions and identity-building means. In this age of people-centred development, it is noteworthy that farmers prefer to listen to the programmes they receive in an embraced language.

This discourse affirms current assertions that using indigenous languages in agricultural radio programming can ensure that farmers have access to data on agro-material problems, utility apps, supporting accessories, financing, technology, preservation, marketing and pedagogy. The research concludes that, through their opinion leaders, indigenous language use in agricultural radio programming involves manufacturers and farmers of agricultural programmes. It is suggested that indigenous languages continue to be used in Nigeria's agricultural radio programming. The agro-politics of the country should, however, safeguard all farmers regardless of cultural or ethnic divisions; and specifically address the requirements of minority ethnic farmers' organizations. The amount of radio programmes in native languages on Nigerian radio needs to be increased. This is because rural development programmes are efficiently communicated to the target audience. Broadcasting should strictly adhere to the Nigeria Broadcasting Code regulations. For example, the code indicates that there should be 70% local content of a station's entire programming. Including indigenous language as a content requirement and such programmes incorporating agriculture should be harnessed.

FUTURE RESEARCH DIRECTIONS

There is a need for more study using the quantitative method to feel the impulse of farmers' first-hand so as to know how indigenous language use in agricultural radio programming have impacted on the practice of agriculture. Furthermore, media establishments should emphasize the need of coming up with other programmes in indigenous languages beyond agricultural programmes.

CONFLICT OF INTEREST

The authors declare that there is no conflict of interest regarding the paper

ETHICAL CONSIDERATION

Ethical consent was acquired for the study from Covenant Health Research Ethics Committee (CHREC).

ACKNOWLEDGEMENT

We appreciate the Covenant University Centre for Research, Innovation and Discovery (CUCRID) for the moral support and enabling environment for this publication.

REFERENCES

Adeyeye, B., Amodu, L., Odiboh, O., Okorie, N., Adesina, E., Yartey, D., & Ekanem, T. (2019). Data on new media use for agricultural training and research at Agricultural Services and Training Centre (ASTC). *Data in Brief*, *22*, 181–184. doi:10.1016/j.dib.2018.11.031 PMID:30581923

Adeyeye, B., Odiboh, O., Adesina, E., Yartey, D., Ekanem, T., & Ben-Enukora, C. (2018). An examination of Information Communication Technology for Agriculture-Focused Teaching, Learning and Communication Research in the 21st Century. *Proceedings of the 31st International Business Information Management Association Conference (IBIMA)*, pp. 6384- 6390. Milan, Italy.

Afolayan, A. (1995). In A. Bamgbose, A. Banjo, & A. Thomas (Eds.), *Ineffectiveness in the Presentation of English in Nigeria: Sources and Remedies. New Englishes: A West African Perspective* (pp. 113–129). Ibadan: Mosuro.

AFRRI. (2008). *Communicating with radio: what do we know? Findings from selected rural radio effectiveness evaluations, African Farm Radio Research Initiative (AFRRI).* Ottawa, Canada: Farm Radio International.

Ahmad, W., Noor, M. A., Afzal, I., Bakhtavar, M. A., Nawaz, M. M., Sun, X., ... Zhao, M. (2016). Improvement of Sorghum Crop through Exogenous Application of Natural Growth-Promoting Substances under a Changing Climate. *Sustainability*, *8*(12), 1330. doi:10.3390u8121330

Ajzen, I. (1991). The theory of planned behaviour. *Organizational Behavior and Human Decision Processes*, *50*(2), 179–211. doi:10.1016/0749-5978(91)90020-T

Ajzen, I. (2005). *Attitude, personality, and behaviour* (2nd ed.). Maidenhead: Open University Press.

Alam, M. K., & Haque, A. M. (2014). *Contribution of television channels in disseminating agricultural information for the agricultural development of Bangladesh*. Retrieved from http://digitalcommons.unl.edu/libphilprac

Ani, A. O. (2001). *The essence of monitoring and evaluation in extension delivery*. A paper presented at a training Workshop on Extension Communication for ADPs.

Bamgbose, A. (1991). *Language and the nation: The language question in sub-Saharan Africa*. Great Britain: Edinburgh University Press.

Bell, M., Payne, J., & Bohn, A. (2011). *ICT Options in Relation to Extension Functions*. MEAS. Available at www.meas-extension.org/resources/ict

Brumfit, C. (1995). English as a Second Language and English Language Teaching: Retrospect and Prospect. In A. Bamgbose, A. Banjo, & A. Thomas (Eds.), *New Englishes: A West African Perspective* (pp. 99–112). Ibadan: Mosuro.

Crystal, D. (2000). *Language Death*. Cambridge: Cambridge University Press. doi:10.1017/CBO9781139106856

Donye, A. O. (2018). Assessment of mass media performance in agricultural information dissemination to rural farmers in Girei Local Government Area of Adamawa State, Nigeria. *International Journal of Agricultural Extension and Rural Development*, *6*(5), 639–647.

Emeka-Nwobia, N. U. (2015). The Place of Indigenous Nigerian Languages in National Development. *Research on Humanities and Social Sciences*, *5*(12), 112–117.

English Dictionary, B. B. C. (1992). *A dictionary for the world*. London, UK: Harper-Collins Publisher.

Eyisi, J. (2000). Language and education: The raison d'être for political socialization. *African Journal of Research in Education*, *1*(2).

FAO. (2006). *Framework on effective rural communication for development*. Rome, Italy: FAO.

Fossard, E. (1996). *Writing and producing radio dramas*. India: Sage.

Geekie, R. (1995). Mali: Championing women's literacy programme' in African farmer. *The Hunger Project*, *15*, 34–50.

Hanafi, A. (2013). *Indigenous Languages as Developmentals* (pp. 1–37). University of Leeds.

Head, S. W., Sterling, C. H., Schofield, L. S., Spann, T., & McGregor, M. (1998). *Broadcasting in America: A survey of electronic media*. Boston, MA: Houghton Mifflin.

Idebi, S. K. (2008). *Fundamentals of radio production*. Ibadan: Impact Motion Pictures and Media Koncept Nig.

Khan, R., Aziz, Z., & Ahmed, V. (2018). Building integrated agriculture information modelling (BIAIM): An integrated approach towards urban agriculture. *Sustainable cities and society, 37*, 594-607.

Lawal, O. A. (2015). Indigenous languages as tools for effective communication of science and technology for food production in Nigeria. *Theory and Practice in Language Studies*, *5*(3), 463–468. doi:10.17507/tpls.0503.02

Manyozo, L. (2009). Mobilizing rural and community radio in Africa. *Ecquid Novi: African Journal Studies*, *30*(1), 1–23. doi:10.1080/02560054.2009.9653389

Maputseni, C. (2006). *Using radio for advocacy and communication of issues affecting farm communities in Zimbabwe*. (Thesis), Malmo University, Sweden.

Mavesera, M. (2009). *Empowerment through language: exploring possibilities of using African languages and literature to promote socio-cultural and economic development in Zimbabwe* (Doctoral dissertation).

McKenzie, R. (2006). *Comparing media from around the world*. Boston, MA: Pearson.

Moemeka, A. (1980). *Mass media in a mass literacy campaign: guidelines for action in Africa*. Discussion paper. Federal ministry of education.

Moyo, R., & Salawu, A. (2018). A survey of communication effectiveness by agricultural extension in the Gweru district of Zimbabwe. *Journal of Rural Studies*, *60*, 32–42. doi:10.1016/j.jrurstud.2018.03.002

Mufwene, S. S. (2002). Colonisation, Globalisation and the Future of Languages in the Twenty first Century. *MOST Journal on Multicultural Societies*, 19-48.

Ndaghu, A. A., & Taru, V. B. (2012). Role of mass media in agricultural productivity in Adamawa State, Nigeria. *Global Journal of Agricultural Sciences*, *11*(2), 111–116.

Ndamba, G. T. (2008). Mother Tongue Usage in Learning: An Examination of Language Preferences in Zimbabwe. *The Journal of Pan African Studies*, *2*(4).

Odiboh, O., Adeyeye, B., & Ekanem, T. (2018). Awareness of e-Transaction among Consumers of Indigenous Herbal Remedies in Ota, Nigeria: A Case for e-Herbals. In *Proceedings of the 4th IEEE International Conference on Information Management, (ICIM 2018),* Oxford, UK, pp. 179-183. 10.1109/INFOMAN.2018.8392831

Odiboh, O., & Ajayi, F. (2019). Integrated Marketing Communication And Carbonated Drinks Consumers in Nigeria: A Consumerist Analysis. In *Proceedings of the 33rd International Business Information Management Association (IBIMA)*, April 10-11, 2019, Granada, Spain. Academic Press.

Odiboh, O., & Ekanem, T. (2019). *Mass Communication Book of Book Reviews* (Vol. 1). Germany: Academy Publishers.

Odiboh, O., Ezenagu, A., & Okuobeya, V. (2019). Integrated Marketing Communication Tools and Facials Consumers in Nigeria: Applications and Connexions. In *Proceedings of the 33rd International Business Information Management Association (IBIMA)*, April 10-11, 2019, Granada, Spain. Academic Press.

Odiboh, O., & Oladunjoye, A. (2019). Application of Integrated Marketing Communication Tools for Promoting Computers in Nigeria. In *Proceedings of the 33rd International Business Information Management Association (IBIMA)*, April 10-11, 2019, Granada, Spain. Academic Press.

Odiboh, O., Salawu, A., & Doghudje, C. (Eds.). (2019). *Introduction to Philosophy of Mass Communication for Higher Institutions*. Ibadan: Stirling Horden.

Odiboh, O. O. (2002). *Integrated Marketing Communication*. Lagos: APCON.

Odiboh, O. O. (2011). *A Philosophy of Marketing Communication: Through Gabriel Marcel's Theory of Intersubjectivity*. Germany: VDM.

Okoro, N. (2001). Mass communication research: Issues and methodologies. Nsukka: AP Express publishers.

Okunna, C. S. (1999). *Introduction to Mass Communication* (2nd ed.). Enugu: New Generation Books.

Onabajo, S. (1999). *Essentials of Broadcast Writing and Production.* Lagos: Gabi Concept Ltd.

Oyero, O. S. (2003). Indigenous language radio for development purposes. In E. O. Soola, (Ed.), Communicating for Development Purposes. Ibadan: Krafts Books.

Oyesomi, K. O., & Salawu, A. (2019). Assessing the Uniqueness of Indigenous Language in Advertising: Analysis of Figurative Language Used in Selected Telecommunication Yoruba Advertisement in Nigeria. *Qualitative Report, 24*(10), 2574–2591. Retrieved from https://nsuworks.nova.edu/tqr/vol24/iss10/12

Ozowa, V. N. (1995). Information needs of small-scale farmers' in Africa: The Nigerian example. Quarterly *Bulletin of the International Association of Agricultural Information Specialists, 40*(1).

Ozowa, V. N. (2005). Information needs of small-scale farmers' in Africa: The Nigerian example. Quarterly Bulletin of the International Association of Agricultural Information Specialists, IAALD/CABI, 40(1).

Padre, S., Sundarshana, N., & Tripp, R. (2003) Performing farm journalism: the experience of Adike Parttirike. Agricultural research and extension Network (AGREEN) Network paper No. 128, London, UK.

Pope, R. (2002). *The English Studies Book: An Introduction to Language, Literature and Culture* (2nd ed.). London, UK: Routledge.

Porter, J. R., Xie, L., Challinor, A. J., Cochrane, K., Howden, S. M., Iqbal, M. M., ... Travasso, M. I. (2014). Food security and food production systems. Cambridge University Press. *Climatic Change, 2014*, 485–533.

Reinard, J. C. (2001). *Introduction to communication research.* McGraw-Hill Humanities, Social Sciences & World Languages.

Robson, C. (2011). *Real world research* (Vol. 3). Chichester: Wiley.

Rogers, E. M. (2003). *The diffusion of innovation* (5th ed.). New York: Free Press.

Sakwa, C. P. (2012). *Gender stereotyping in radio programming: the case of Kenya Broadcasting Corporation* (Master's Thesis), University of Nairobi, Kenya.

Salawu, A. (2006). Paradox of a milieu: communicating in African indigenous languages in the age of globalization. In A. Salawu (Ed.), Indigenous Language Media in Africa (pp. 1-20). Lagos, Nigeria: Centre for Black and African Arts and Civilization (CBAAC).

Skutnabb-Kangas, T. (2000). *Linguistic Genocide in Education or Worldwide Diversity and Human Rights?* London, UK: Erlbaum.

Sonderling, S. (2009). Media, language and discourse. In P. J. Fourie (Ed.), *Media Studies: Media Content and Media Audiences* (pp. 83–115). Cape Town, South Africa: Juta & Co. Ltd.

Stefano, L. A., Hendriks, S. L., Stilwell, C., & Morris, C. (2005). *Printed information needs of small-scale organic farmers in Kwazulu-Natal.* Availablc at www.librijournal.org/pdf/005 1pp56-66.pdf

Uno, S. O. (1987). Information Dissemination: How effective through local (Nigerian) languages. In S. O. Uno (Ed.), *Tropical Issues in Communication Arts. Uyo.* Modern Business Press Ltd.

Urua, E. E. (2005). Exploiting Information Technology Resources in the Human Development of Nigerian Languages. In O. M. Ndimele (Ed.), *Globalization and the Study of languages in Africa. Port-Harcourt: Grand Orbit Communications.*

Wallace, L. (1996). Media, writers, arts session summary. In G. Cantoni (Ed.), *Stabilizing Indigenous Languages.* Flagstaff: Northern Arizona University.

Wang, T., Wu, G., Chen, J., Cui, P., Chen, Z., Yan, Y., ... Chen, H. (2017). Integration of solar technology to modern greenhouse in China: Current status, challenges and prospect. *Renewable & Sustainable Energy Reviews, 70*, 1178–1188. doi:10.1016/j.rser.2016.12.020

Waqas, M. A., Khan, I., Akhter, M. J., Noor, M. A., & Ashraf, U. (2017). Exogenous application of plant growth regulators (PGRs) induces chilling tolerance in short-duration hybrid maize. *Environmental Science and Pollution Research International, 24*(12), 11459–11471. doi:10.100711356-017-8768-0 PMID:28316047

Willock, J., Deary, I. J., Edwards-Jones, G., Gibson, G. J., McGregor, M. J., Sutherland, A., ... Grieve, R. (1999). The role of attitude and objectives in farmer decision making: Business and environmentally-oriented behaviour in Scotland. *Journal of Agricultural Economics, 50*(2), 286–303. doi:10.1111/j.1477-9552.1999.tb00814.x

Wimmer, R. D., & Dominick, J. R. (2013). *Mass media research.* London, UK: Cengage Learning.

Wójcik, M., Jeziorska-Biel, P., & Czapiewski, K. (2019). Between words: A generational discussion about farming knowledge sources. *Journal of Rural Studies*, *67*, 130–141. doi:10.1016/j.jrurstud.2019.02.024

KEY TERMS AND DEFINITIONS

Agricultural Communication: This includes all types of human communication related to farming, food, natural resources and rural concerns.

Agricultural Radio Programmes: This is used in this study to refer to the use of radio as a medium to exchange views from various sources by allowing Members of a specific group in order to obtain access to their data.

Agriculture: This refers to the method by which certain crops are grown to produce food, feed, fiber and many other required products. There are two ways to see agriculture; traditional and modern. Traditional agriculture uses techniques developed over decades or centuries to ensure good, sustainable yield over time in a particular area or geopolitical area based on mixed crops complementing each other. On tiny family farms and in developing nations, traditional agricultural methods are most commonly practiced. Crops are mixed, often using the same crop's various varieties, and are sometimes planted in related communities. Modern agriculture, on the other hand, is an emerging approach to agricultural innovation and farming methods that helps farmers boost effectiveness and decrease the quantity of natural resources such as water, soil and power needed to satisfy the requirements of the world in terms of food, fuel and fiber.

Broadcasting: Head, Sterling, Schefield, Spinn and McGregor (1998, p. 16) see broadcasting as the act of transmitting sound and images through radio waves to the general public through room for reception. This is the way to go in which broadcasting is used in this study.

Farmers: This refers to individuals engaged in agriculture and raising food crops in North-Central Nigeria.

Farming: It is the act or method of soil cultivation, seed planting, and growing edible plants. It is also called, among other things, the process of raising cattle for milk or meat.

Food security: it is the situation in which all individuals have physical, social and financial access to adequate, secure and nutritious food at all times that meets their nutritional requirements and food preferences for active and healthy living. (Porter *et al.*, 2014).

Indigenous Languages: These are languages native to a country and spoken as a mother tongue by some of its indigenes. It also signifies people's knowledge culture and identity.

Innovation: refers an idea, exercise or object perceived as fresh in a social system by a person or group of individuals. Regardless of when the concept or exercise was initially created, it is an innovation for the individual when a individual first becomes conscious of it. An innovation may also be an improvement over the existing practice. Once such an improvement is new, it is regarded as an innovation.

Radio: The medium for transmitting electromagnetic signals through the atmosphere aimed at informing farmers about agricultural innovations.

Radio Broadcasting: Radio broadcasting is the radio wave transmission aimed at reaching a broad audience. Therefore, stations are connected to broadcast a popular radio format in radio networks, either in broadcast syndication or simulcasting or both.

Chapter 11
Global Media, Television, and the Americanization of Young Africans

Nelson Okorie
Covenant University, Nigeria

ABSTRACT

This chapter examined the perception of young Africans on American values as portrayed in popular entertainment programs. This chapter examined use DSTV as a study example because it is the most popular digital-pay TV with the highest subscription in Africa. Furthermore, the objectives are: (1) To ascertain the major type of western programmes preferred on DSTV among young Africans, (2) To examine the perception of young Africans on whether these TV channels influence the adoption of western values. This research adopted the use of the survey method to achieve the objectives of the study. A value contribution of this chapter is that global television has created multiple media products that have unique elements of American culture, which will distort African values. Also, the influence of American values will have a snowball effect on African youths in different spheres of life.

INTRODUCTION

Media experts suggest that the influence of the media on our social realities correlates with the extent of our dependence on the media for information (Okorie & Bwala, 2016; Lee, 2017; Okorie & Salawu, 2017; Okorie &Bwala, 2017; Oduaran & Okorie, 2018). Lippmann (1934) as cited in Odukomaiya (1992) explained how we form "the pictures in our heads". Since people cannot possibly experience most events

DOI: 10.4018/978-1-7998-2091-8.ch011

of the real world first-hand, they derive their knowledge of the world through a "window" provided by the media, even though what people see through this media window is not the actual reality of life but a pseudo-reality.

In the same vein, media viewing have been ascertained to be largely inculcated into our systems, that we do not even realize how much effect it has on an individual's life; from a young schoolboy who is eager to skip school, just to watch cartoons, to a young teenager who craves after the latest musical videos, movies, and idolizes celebrities and other larger-than-life images exposed to on the television. Television has been observed to be one major way of driving information into our systems, whether good or bad, because of the sound coupled with sight advantage it possesses over other media, hence the saying; "Seeing is believing."

Interestingly, the proliferation of cable and digital television stations in Africa have further increased media viewing among young people. Importantly, Western-American content dominates most of the cable and digital television stations. Okorie (2010) citing Bagdikan (2000) observed that "By 1984, 50 corporations had established a controlling interest of diverse media in the United States. By 1987, the number of firms having the controlling interest was reduced to twenty-six. By 1990, it fell to twenty-three and by 1996; the number was closer to ten. This acceleration pace of global media system is now dominated by nine giant firms. The five largest are Time Warner ($24 billion), Disney ($22 billion), Bertelsmann ($15 billion), Viacom ($13 billion), and Rupert Murdoch's News Corporation ($11 billion). While, Viacom, Disney and AOL Time Warner are U.S owned, many non-U.S. owned companies dominate the roster of the largest media groups: News Corporation (Australia), Bertelsmann (Germany), Reed-Elsavier (Britain/Netherlands), Vivendi and Lagadere-Hachette(France) and Sony Corporation (Japan)". Besides needing global scope to compete, the rules of thumb for global media giants are twofold: First, to get bigger so as to dominate markets and your competition can't buy such firms out. Firms like Disney and Time Warner have almost tripled in size this decade. Secondly, they have interests in numerous media industries, such as film production, book publishing, music, TV channels and networks, retail stores, amusement parks, magazines, newspapers and the likes.

Scholars, Amosu, 2016; Okorie & Salawu, 2016; Usaini & Ekeanyanwu, 2017; Lee, (2017) agree that these TV products have cultural values that have been embedded in their programmes; a teenager would gladly tune to MTV to catch-up with the latest hit songs; Fox and BET channels to see the recent blockbuster movies and E! TV to watch celebrities shows..

Against this background, this chapter examined the perception of young Africans on American values as portrayed in popular entertainment programs from the United States. This chapter examined the use of DSTV as a study example because it is the most popular digital-pay TV with the highest subscription in Africa, using Nigeria as a study example. Furthermore, the objectives are: (1) To ascertain the major type of western programmes preferred on DSTV among young Africans, (2) To examine the perception of young Africans on whether these TV channels influence the adoption of western values

Conceptual Definition of Terms

1. **Digital Satellite Television (DSTV)**: DSTV is Multi Choice's multi-channel digital satellite TV service established in South Africa in 1995. It broadcasts on Ku band via the Intelsat 7 and 10 satellites (PAS7 and PAS10). Some of the channels available on DSTV include; M-Net, MTV Base, African Magic Movie Magic, E! TV, Channel O, Cartoon Network, BBC World, CNN International, etc.
2. **Values:** Values in this context refers to socio-cultural beliefs of a people in a particular society. For the purpose of this study, values and culture was used interchangeably. Western values, therefore can be referred to as those values from the United States of America, which is also known as American values
3. **Western Programs:** This refers to any programme that has its origin from the United States. In essence, these programmes were created and produced in the United States. In this chapter, Western programmes also refer to American programmes aired on DSTV. Some of these programmes include: *Glee*, *Ugly Betty*, *30 Rock*, *How I met your mother*, *the Wendy Show*, *The Real*, *Cheaters*, *Judge Judy*, etc.

Global Media and Americanisation

In the discussion about the global media and the Americanisation of the world, one cannot but mention the concept of the global village and the interconnection of all societies around thc world, in the era of globalization. It is important to therefore define the concepts-global media and Americanization. Americanization can be defined as European media forms that bear a resemblance to American media forms and have been directly influenced by American (Miller, 2010). According to Hallin and Mancini, Americanization as a concept has been popular since the 1960s. Americanization means that European media forms are exhibiting direct influence by and a strong resemblance to American media. This argument is closely linked to the idea of cultural imperialism and the United States as a global cultural power. The chapter states that while American influence is great in European media, its influence must not be exaggerated and that the key driving force behind media change in Europe is still changes within the countries themselves and not outside influences (Miller, 2010).

As observed by Olausson(2011), there have been doubts around the concept of the global media. The media has long been described and argued, as a being western or American, in the well standing field of global communication. Most scholars have argued that, there has been western or American bias, in terms of ownership and in dissemination of media products.

According to Hjarvard (n.d.), in terms of the history of programming, the influence of American television on European television has been substantial (p. 74). The presence of media giants in America and in the west in general, who introduce and immerse people with American or western lifestyles, should not be taken for granted. This is a sign of cultural imperialism, which means that these western culture portrayed on the media, are subliminally produced in a way that matches the target audience, to make them a potential market for their western products (Sparks, 2007b as cited in Olausson, 2011). According to Hjarvard (n.d.), global media cultures represent a cultural otherness, at times a threat to cultural tradition and autonomy (p. 72).

As stated by an article titled "Impacts of Americanization" (n.d.), ''Americanization has had many impacts on the world - some of them good, some of them bad''. The positive impacts of Americanization, is the fact that the American way of life is spread globally and also, their constant innovation are disseminated globally in a way that the rest of the world wants to be like America. The negative impacts include the fact that ''Americanization removes and strips ethnic areas of their cultural uniqueness, leaving the once beautiful ethnic areas as Americanized and bland'' and also the fact that, ''It also means that everything exhumed by the media, whether it be from the film industry, the music industry, the news industry -it'd be to meet America's standards, which also means that everything will be left from America's point of view''("Impacts of Americanization," n.d.).Miller (2010) & Hafez (2009); Thussu (2003), as cited in Olausson (2011) agreed that, another negative part of Americanization is the dissemination of propaganda, because it causes homogenization in the media. It was reported that, ''National propaganda is often present in transnational media as well, not least in CNN, as are stereotypical and negative depictions of the 'others.'''

Another article titled "Examples of Americanization" (n.d.)cited examples of Americanization. It was stated that, the two most popular brands in the entire world, McDonald's and Starbucks, are the most iconic companies of America. Their spread around the world is an example of Americanization, since the American products have made their way into other countries, influencing them accordingly. It also shows the sales of the fast food industries that originate from America, which is another good example of Americanization.

We cannot mention the Americanization of the world, without referring to the role that Hollywood has played since its inception till date. According to Nye (2018), the Hollywood industry rely on an extremely important domestic market and American cinema is an instrument for the Americanization of migrants. It is a patchwork of myths from a variety of countries that are myths arranged according to the American vision.

Global Television, Americanization and African Audiences

Society has metamorphosed from one era to the other starting with the local through to the modern and the technologically advanced. This trend is hinged on the need for communication between individuals and a group of people as well as the society at large. The arrival of mass communication on the scene changed everything as it penetrated communication limitations between societies. Television in particular has transformed the way humans relate and interact with one another to the point that the world has not remained the same as a result of the impact of Television. This advancement has led to transnational communication between people from different parts of the world converging together and relating with each other seamlessly. Hence this relationship is referred to as global Television

Over the years, the need to communicate has become germane to the success between different countries of the world. Studies have shown that television have impacted on the cultural values of audiences scattered across the globe (Chalaby, 2016; Morales & Simelio, 2015). Allen (1992) observers that close to 3.5 billion hours are spent on watching television across the globe (p. 110).

It has been argued that the United States is leading the world in the entertainment stage. This is evident in the communication flow globally as information flows in a disproportionate way from the United States to the rest of the world. This has led critics to describe this pattern of communication to be one sided (Padovani, 2008). The outcome of this dominance of the media landscape by the United States results in unbalanced flow of information from the US to other countries of the world especially Africa. This leads to the promotion of American culture, ideas and perception to the world without concomitant flow of information from Africa and other developing countries. Hence the image of Africa is seen by the world in bad light. The portrayal of Africa in bad light has negative implications on the audiences which invariably showcase make them feel that everything emanating from such countries is terrible. This thus leads to the Americanization of African audiences.

Countries of the world run international broadcasting for certain reasons. These reasons include: enhancement of national prestige, promotion of national interest, religious, ideological or political indoctrination, fostering of cultural ties, trade in international markets and promotion of access to pay-television broadcasts (Entman,

2004). Additionally, Kamalipour (2007) observes that E-commerce in terms of trans-border trade, selling of culture and information across borders, entertainment in terms of music, video, drama, personal and group expression of identity, ideology and religion, promoting access to global traditional media organisations are some other reasons why global television encouraged among nations.

Locally produced television content has not triumphed over foreign media content in many parts of Africa (Tindi & Ayiku, 2018). In Europe and Latin-America, studies have revealed that audiences have strong affinity to local and regional productions (Ksiazek & Webster 2008). The situation in Africa is different as audiences in this part of the world prefer foreign content as against local content. Against this backdrop, local producers are shaping media output according to audience preference (Haynes, 2011; Endong, 2014). The reverse scenario is also possible as audience preference for foreign content can possibly be the result of media producers' priming of such content. With this scenario, it can now be said of the existence of a global television industry which is a mosaic of international production and distribution networks with the content value chain at its core (Chalaby, 2016).

Audience experiences with global television are occurring simultaneously across the world but with different consequences. Accordingly, studies have shown audiences experience with global television and the Americanization of the world. An analysis of the consumption pattern of global television content shows that these global television texts facilitate identity construction (Morales & Simelio, 2015; Adia, 2014). Global television changes local identities in dynamic ways by altering the symbolic environment subtly (D'Silva, 2000).

As ideological re-presentations, television texts are borne of audience. Hence, the broadcast of foreign television texts in local areas may conceal local experiences, knowledge and tradition. Whilst this is true, Tomlinson, (2012) and Magu (2015) aver that local audiences are not necessarily victims of global television because audiences can also adopt and integrate the attraction of globalization. However, there is much more to be desired in the resilience of local audiences as global television intensifies.

Dstv as a Vector of Americanization in Africa: The Nigerian Perspective

The conveyance and the appropriateness of American values and identity across the Atlantic to the African continent has a long been a subject of controversy among scholars. While some proponents recognize it as a welcome and authentic phenomenon engendering value-added trade, facilitating networking and cooperation among peoples irrespective of their geographical inclinations, opponents of Americanization have however see it as a new form of neo - colonialism with an ulterior motive of further enriching the developed Nations (Adedimeji, 2009).

Socio-cultural dependence on westernization has been largely being influenced by global media. The global media are therefore seen as agents of neo-colonialism (Iyorza & Ekwok, 2014). The electronic and print Global media such as the Digital Satellite Television (DSTV) with a number of bundles and bouquets, together with channels stemming from foreign nations such as: news and information programs on BBC, CNN, and Al Jezeera, FOX news; showbiz programs (including sports, drama and music) on channels like Channel O, Super sports, Mnet series, E Entertainment and African Magic; adverts (commonly found in almost every program); international religious evangelism channels; and foreign educational channels including radio stations.

With approximately 12 million subscribers, Digital Satellite Television (DSTV) is a sub-Saharan broadcast satellite serviced owned by media conglomerate Multichoice. The subscribers of the broadcast satellite service are dispersed around Africa with majority being in Nigeria.

The programs offered by DSTV for viewing by the subscribers are sourced from International content providers with notable mention of news channels and entertainment channels which a large number of Nigerian. Price has not been a deterrent for the Nigerian consumer. DSTV has different packages —— DSTV Premium NGN15800; DSTV Compact Plus NGN10650; DSTV Compact NGN6800; DSTV Family NGN4000; DSTVAccess NGN2000; and DSTV FTA Plus NGN1600. The prices are averagely.

There is a huge correlation between media content and culture in every given society. There's a symbiotic relationship between the two elements as the media content is created within the codes, context, and expectation of the culture. Also, media content is a vehicle of culture. It is a touch point where members of a society deepen their knowledge of a culture and it is with media content that members of a society can clearly delineate between what ideas, behaviours are associated with a culture or not.

Americanization is a term that gained prominence in the light of the collapse of the Soviet Union can be viewed from various two perspectives—— one, Internal Americanization which refers to the process of identification with and the adoption of the American customs and values among immigrants. Second, it may be viewed as the influence of the American culture or practices on other countries. Third, it may be viewed loosely as globalization (Roudometof & Robertson, 1998; Jaja, 2010; Obeidat, 2010).Recognizing globalization as the buzzword of the moment, Mooney & Evans, 2007 views it as "a field of inquiry defined more by the questions it asks and its object of study: the world as a whole and parts of it in relation to this whole."

The media has been used chiefly as a tool to promote certain ideals over the other. The mass distribution and reception of these contents by international audiences have led to paradigm shift. A perfect example would be the promotion of democracy as opposed to communism and capitalism as the ideal economic system has influenced Nations that are receptive of media content from America (Anderman, Bamodu, Dine, Blecher, Brennan, & Freeman, 2006).

"The sociological view that the loss of support from objective religion and the disintegration of the last precapitalist residues, in conjunction with technical and social differentiation and specialization, have given rise to cultural chaos is refuted by daily experience. Culture today is infecting everything with sameness. Film, radio, and magazines form a system." (Horkheimer & Adorno, 2006)

The kind of content being disseminated on the DSTV platform promotes the American beliefs, values and consumption culture. This is viewed with the evident behavioural change and attitudinal dispositions among African audience. While studies (Ekwuazi, 2014) have investigated the impact, perception and reception of indigenous channels on African audience, it is important attention is giving to this phenomenon of the weaponisation of foreign content on satellite television services for the purpose of cultural preservation and the rising risks of ethnocentrism

METHOD

This research adopted the use of the survey method to achieve the objectives of the study. Tejumade (2003, p.56) sees survey as the most frequently used research method by behavioural scientists. He further explained that the method involves drawing up a set of questions on various subjects to which selected members of a population are expected to reach. For this study, the population of study was 60,000 undergraduate students of University of Lagos (UNILAG). This is due to the fact that these people are a fraction of the Nigerian youths. More so, these students are in a Nigerian institution which is believed to be the citadel of immorality. Universities are believed to imply "freedom days" of members of the youth.

Taking into consideration the fact that the entire population of the University cannot be studied a total of 300 students using the calculation for getting the population size. The total of institution of UNILAG is over 60,000 and so it would be absurd to try to even think of using the whole population (Unilag.ng, 2017). UNILAG students' campuses are dispersed around Lagos but the campus on the social ground can be used to represent most of its students.

Hence, 1% of the universities' student population will be researched due to the difficulty of researching on all students from the university; therefore, 300 students were selected from University of Lagos campus in Yaba, Lagos. The instrument

Table 1. Bio-data of the respondents

	M	F	15-25yrs	>45yrs	Single	Married	Christians	Muslims
Sex	32.5%	68.5%						
Age			74.5%	26.5%				
Marital status					90.5%	9.5%		
Religion							85.7%	14.3%

used in this work or research is the questionnaire. The questionnaire items consisted of 20 questions comprising of three sections which contain questions on level of influence of global media on youths, the first section of the questionnaire consists of the demographical information of the respondents, while the second is related to those raised in the study. Importantly, this study examined Western TV programs on Digital Satellite Television Network (DSTV). This study selected DSTV as a study example because it is the most popular and most watched digital paid television in Africa

RESULT AND DISCUSSION

The findings indicate that more than 65% of the respondents were females, while 32.5% of the respondents were males. \

Table 1 also shows that more than 90% of the respondents were Single. Also, the table shows that almost 86% of the respondents were Christians, while 14.3% of the respondents were Muslims.

Table 2 shows three most preferred Western types of programmes were Reality TV programmes, Music and Movies. Most of the respondents were favourably disposed to Reality TV programmes such as 'X-Factor', and 'Amazing Race'. Importantly, only less than 3% preferred documentary channels such 'History Channel, and 'National Geographic'. From the table, a significant number of the respondents preferred Western Entertainment channels compared to Western information channels

Table 3 shows that 80% of the respondents believed that global TV is a channel of transferring western culture to Africans, only 12% disbelieved that global TV is a channel of transferring western culture to Africans. Also, almost 81% of the respondents indicated that they learnt western values from global TV on DSTV. Interestingly, more than 65% of the African youths are respondents indicated that they loved 'American' cultural values compared to other culture.

Table 2. Respondents preference for Western TV programmes

Programme Types	
Music	15.5%
Movies	10.0%
Reality TV	20.5%
Series	7.5%
News	3.0%
Sports	7.0
Documentary	2.5
Cartoons	9.0
Total	100% n=191

Table 3. Attitude towards Western TV

Responses	Global TV is a means of cultural Transfer	I learn western values from global TV on DSTV	I love the 'American' cultural values compared to other culture
Strongly Agree	40.0%	40.8%	45.0%
Agree	40.0%	40.0%	20.3%
Disagree	7.5%	8.2%	20.6%
Strongly Disagree	4.5%	1.0%	9.1%
Undecided	8.0%	0%	5.0%
Total	100% n=300	100% n=300	100% n=300

The implication of this result is global TV networks will influence the adoption of western culture among Africans. Furthermore, African youths will prefer the American identities compared to African identities. It is this type of thinking that made Ekeanyanwru (2005) to assert that there have been the massive flows of American culture into non-western societies of the developing world leading to cultural domination. To this end, African culture has been distorted and displaced, and also the increase in the adaptation of foreign values, life style. A value contribution of this chapter is that Global television has created multiple media products that have unique elements of American culture, which will distort African values. Also, the influence of American values will have a snowball effect on African youths in different spheres of life,

FUTURE RESEARCH DIRECTIONS

For future directions, this study re commends that there is a need to investigate global media coverage of American culture in Asia and Europe. Such type of study will explore the dynamics of media culture influence on Asians and Europeans

CONCLUSION

Television is an agent of societal change in both developed and developing countries. More so, television has the influence to reshape the cultures of individuals in any modern society. The advent of global TV networks has redefined the media landscape by creating multiple media products that have a unique effect on individuals in African countries. Importantly, the domination of global media will continue to erode indigenous African culture as well as promote American culture to the world.

RECOMMENDATION

It is recommended that more digital media products should be created to reflect hybrid cultures of America and African cultures. It is essential media and film producers consider elements of subcultures to promote social inclusion and global citizenship

REFERENCES

Adedimeji, M. A. (2009). Globalization and the survival of the Nigerian cultural and linguistic heritage: The American paradigm. *The Sociolinguistics of English and Nigerian Languages*, 69-87.

Adia, E. A. (2014). Programme element importance: An analysis of telenovela in the Ghanaian media. *International Journal of ICT and Management*, *2*(1), 96–101.

Allen, D. (Ed.). (1992). *Women transforming communications: Global interactions*. Thousand Oaks, CA: Sage.

Anderman, S., Bamodu, G., Dine, J., Blecher, M., Brennan, F., & Freeman, M. (2006). *Human rights and capitalism: a multidisciplinary perspective on globalisation.* Edward Elgar.

Bagdikian, H. (2000). *The media monopoly*. New York: Beacon Press.

Chalaby, J. (2016). Television and globalization: The TV content global value chain. *Journal of Communication*, *66*(1), 1–41. doi:10.1111/jcom.12203

Chioma, P. E. (2013). News Commercialization in Nigeria: Undermining Issues in Public Interest for Financial Gains. *International Journal of Innovative Research and Development.*

Cottle, S. (2009). *Global Crisis Reporting: Journalism in the Global Age*. United Kingdom: Open University Press.

D'Silva, M. (2000). Global media and cultural identity: Experiences from an Indian town. *Intercultural Communication Studies*, *10*(2), 55–63.

Drula, G. (2015). Forms of Media Convergence and Multimedia Content – A Romanian Perspective. *Media Education Research Journal*, *44*(20), 131–140.

Ekeanyanwu, N. (2005). *International communication: Issues, concept and researches in the 21st century. Akure*. Standard Mass Concept Company.

Ekwo, U. (1996). Commercialization of the news in Nigerian media: An Impediment to Information flow. In I. Nwosu, & U. Ekwo (Eds.), *Mass Media and Marketing Communications* (pp. 61–77). Enugu: Thought Communications Publishers.

Endong, F. P. (2014). Audience westernisation as a threat to the indigenization model of media broadcast in Nigeria. *Journal of Media and Communication Studies, 6*(8), 121-129.

Entman, R. M. (2004). *Projection of power: Framing news, public opinion and US foreign policy*. Chicago, IL: University of Chicago Press.

Examples of Americanization. (n.d.). Retrieved January 12, 2018, from https://ardeavujica.weebly.com/examples-of-americanization.html

Fadahunsi, A. (1999). *Philosophy and society: An introduction for beginners.* Ibadan: Hope Publication.

Fraser, N. (2019). How the world was won: the Americanization of everywhere review a brilliant essay. *The Guardian*. Retrieved from https://ardeavujica.weebly.com/examples-of-americanization.html

Gross, L. (2001). *Up from invisibility*. New York: Columbia University Press.

Hafez, K. (2007). *The Myth of Media Globalization*. United Kingdom: Polity Press.

Haynes, J. (2011). African cinema and Nollywood: Contradictions. *Situations: Project of radical imagination, 4*(1), 67-90.

Herkman, J. (2012). Convergence or Intermediality? Finnish Political Communication in the New Media Age. *Convergence: The International Journal of Research into New Media Technologies, 18*(4), 369–384. doi:10.1177/1354856512448727

Hjarvard, S. (n.d.). Global media cultures. In A Research Programme on the Role of Media in Cultural Globalization (pp. 71–78).

Ibagere, E. (2015). Globalization and Nollywood: Carving a niche on the global plane. *International Journal of African Society, Cultures, and Traditions, 2*(4), 1–10.

Igbinoba, A. (2014). Public perception of the cultural relevance of BBA II reality TV show: A study of covenant university staff and students. *International Journal of Social Science and Humanities Review, 2*(2), 19-30.

Impacts of Americanization. (n.d.). Retrieved January 12, 2018, from https://ardeavujica.weebly.com/impacts-of-americanization.html

Iyorza, S., & Ekwok, L. (2014). Global media and cultural hybridization in the 21st Century in Nigeria. *Journal of Social Sciences (COES&RJ-JSS), 3*, 408-416.

Jaja, J. M. (2010). *Globalization or Americanization: Implication for Sub-Saharan Africa Globalization-Today, Tomorrow*. InTech.

Kamalipour, Y. R. (2007). *Global communication* (2nd ed.). Belmont: Thomson Wadsworth.

Kleinsteuber, H. J. (n.d.). Modes and models of global communication. In *Communication Technology Policy* (pp. 1–23). Session CTP VIII Modes.

Ksiazek, T. B., & Webster, J. G. (2008). Cultural proximity and audience behavior: The role of language in patterns of polarization and multicultural fluency. *Journal of Broadcasting & Electronic Media, 52*(3), 485–503. doi:10.1080/08838150802205876

Magu, S. (2015). Reconceptualizing cultural globalization: Connecting the 'cultural global' and the 'cultural local'. *Social Sciences, 4*(1), 630–645. doi:10.3390ocsci4030630

Majidi, A. F. (2017). Globalization and economic growth: The case study of developing countries. *Asian Economic and Financial Review*, *7*(6), 589–599. doi:10.18488/journal.aefr.2017.76.589.599

McChesney, R. W. (1999). The New Global Media: It's a Small World of Big Conglomerates. *Nation (New York, N.Y.)*, (November): 2, 11–15.

Media's role in the globalization process. (2018). Retrieved January 12, 2019, from https://www.bartleby.com/essay/Medias-Role-in-the-Globalization-Process-PKAJCC8EJDMRS

MillerS. (2010). Global media.

Morales, F., & Simelio, N. (2016). Television and identities: Analysis of the consumption of 'telenovelas' by the Latin American community in Spain. *Global Studies in Audience and Power*, *23*(5), 591–609.

Nye, J. (2018). The Americanization of the world: myth or reality? Retrieved January 12, 2018, from https://baripedia.org/wiki/The_Americanization_of_the_World:_Myth_or_Reality%3F

Obeidat, M. (2010). Beyond American Borders: The Middle East and the Enigma of Anti-American Sentiments in the Aftermath of 9/11. *American Studies Today Online, 17*.

Oberiri, A. D. (2016). Journalists' Perception of News Commercialization and its implication on Media Credibility in Nigeria. *World Scientific News*, *55*, 63–76.

Oduaran, C., & Okorie, N. (2018). Community radio, family and psychological support for sexual harassment issues against women: A study of Yoruba usage. *Media Watch Journal*, *10*(1), 11–20.

Okorie, N. (2010). Media Concentration and its threat to Nigeria's Indigenous culture. In N. Ekeanyanwu (Ed.), *T & Okeke, C. Indigenous Societies and Cultural Globalization in the 21st Century: Is the Global Village truly real?* Germany: VDM Verlagon.

Okorie, N., & Bigala, P. (2016). Creating HIV/AIDS awareness through localized communication for health development in South Africa. *Journal of Health Management*, *18*(3), 439–446. doi:10.1177/0972063416651567

Okorie, N., & Bwala, N. (2017). Measuring media campaigns effectiveness for environmental health for Sustainable Development: A study of Ebola outbreak in Lagos State, Nigeria. *Journal of Health Management*, *19*(4), 1–10.

Okorie, N., & Salawu, A. (2016). Effective use of media awareness campaigns for breast cancer care among women: A comparative study. *Journal of International Women's Studies*, *17*(4), 160–173.

Okorie, N., & Salawu, A. (2017). Can my wife be virtual-adulterous? An experiential study on Facebook, emotional infidelity and self-disclosure. *Journal of International Women's Studies*, *18*(2), 166–179.

Olausson, U. (2011). *Explaining global media: a discourse approach. The Systemic Dimension of Globalization*. IntechOpen; doi:10.5772/17557

Onoja, I. (2009). The Impact of Commercialization on News Selection by Three Broadcast Station in Nigeria. *Maiduguri Journal of Arts and Social Sciences*, *7*(1), 86–99.

Owolabi, L., Ibrahim, A., Musa, B., Gwaram, B., Dutse, A., Hamza, M., ... Borodo, M. (2014). Prevalence and Burden of Human Immunodeficiency Virus and Hepatitis B Virus Co-infection in Nigeria: A Systematic Review and Meta-Analysis. *Journal of AIDS & Clinical Research*, *5*(308), 2.

Padovani, C. (2008). The extreme right and its media in Italy. *International Journal of Communication*, *2*, 18.

Roudometof, V., & Robertson, R. (1998). The space between the boundaries: Globalization and Americanization. *American Culture in Europe Interdisciplinary Perspective*, 181-195.

Tindi, S., & Ayiku, C. (2018). Local reception of global media texts: Telenovelas as sites of cultural mixture in Ghana. *Legon Journal of the Humanities*, *29*(1), 259–283. doi:10.4314/ljh.v29i1.10

Tomlinson, J. (2012). 'Watching Dallas': The imperialist text and audience research. In F. J. Lechner, & J. Boli (Eds.), *The globalisation handbook* (pp. 365–375). Sussex, UK: Wiley Blackwell.

Yanitsky, O. (2017). Current globalization: A challenge for the humanities. *Advances in Social Sciences Research Journal*, *4*(12), 131–140. doi:10.14738/assrj.412.3370

KEY TERMS AND DEFINITIONS

Americanization: In this context, it is the process whereby a person or a group of people share, imbibe and partake in American values, norms, and beliefs by assimilating into the American society.

American Values: These are American norms, ideologies, morals and standards of behaviour practised by people of American descent.

Digital Pay TV: This can also be known as premium or subscription television, which are based on people subscribing to the service periodically, through digital terrestrial, and streaming television. They provide multiple channels to customers according to a particular payment plan.

DSTV: This: is an abbreviation for Digital Satellite Television. It is a satellite service owned by Multichoice that is broadcast to about 11.9 million people.

Global Media: It is the communication through the media on a worldwide platform.

Television: This is any programme produced for transmission via a television set, through cable, or the internet.

Western Programmes: This refers to television content packaged by media professionals from the west (principally Europe or the United States) for a mass audience.

Young Africans: These: are young (typically immature and inexperienced) people that are of African descent, who grew up with African values, norms and beliefs.

Section 4
Indigenous Language Media/Communication and Education-Related Issues

Chapter 12
Health Education and Indigenous Language Media:
Issues, Trends, and Perspectives

Olujoke Funmilayo Asekere
Yaba College of Technology, Nigeria

Olunike Rachael Asaolu
Yaba College of Technology, Nigeria

ABSTRACT

Indigenous language health programmes have potentials to create knowledge, accelerate, and transform Nigeria's health burden narratives as well as create awareness on national health policies, goals, and objectives. This chapter takes the stand that not only is government disinterested in policy implementation, as suggested by the lack of practical synergy between government, policy implementation committee, and media organizations. Exploring the values of indigenous language in development media theory, this chapter sets out to demonstrate merits of media support in health policy execution via dynamics of indigenous language programmes towards achieving sustainable development goals. The chapter therefore recommends that constitutional gap in health provision should be bridged to eliminate the question of accountability at all levels and on the long run decentralize health education; and it will make it much easier for state government to embark on holistic health communication strategies that suits their geopolitical terrain.

DOI: 10.4018/978-1-7998-2091-8.ch012

INTRODUCTION

The centrality of health to proper functioning of a nation has long been established. The health burden of Nigeria, coupled with her bulging population since the 1990s has made her a flash point of reference of a failed healthcare system. With entry of new diseases around the World, Nigeria appears to be one major disease away from health collapse or outright disaster. The World Health Organization (WHO) since inception has been monitoring global health as well as providing financial and technical support to Nigeria to alleviate her health burden.

Yet, in spite international support from government and private agencies, as at 2019, challenges such as accessibility, affordability, poor quality healthcare, lack of trust and unfriendly medical personnel and many more deprive Nigerians in urban areas from obtaining medical care let alone the millions of people in rural areas. The problem posed by lack of quality healthcare was surmised aptly by Dr, Ngozi Azodoh, Head of Special Projects, Federal Ministry of Health when she attributed ten to 15 percent of all death in low and middle-income countries to poor quality of healthcare and that approximately, 8.6 million people in low- middle income countries die each year from inadequate access to quality care; out of the 8.6 million, about 3.6 million never get any heath service at all, and 5 million die because of poor quality healthcare.

It is in this context this paper examined the importance of the mass media in alleviating health burden through consciously packaged health information in indigenous language to transforming the narrative of Nigeria health system from that of apathy to a cherished one via reduction in preventable deaths. Taking advantage of media reach, massive heath education at all levels in indigenous language is believed to connect people to their roots. This study examined the implication of near non-existent health literacy at all levels of formal and informal education institutions; the implication of not actively involving the mass media at the planning and execution of health policies, the consequences of the predominant use of English language as a medium of communication in a country with high level of illiteracy in a few existing health programmes; the lackadaisical attitude of Nigerian government to unbundle the health system and ultimately, the implication of these in achieving the Sustainable Development Goals (SDGs) (3). The study suggested a way forward.

BACKGROUND TO THE STUDY

The centrality of heath and health education to sustainable development of man and his environment cannot be overemphasized. Global concern for health development and cooperation began with the 1851 first International Sanitary Conference in

Paris, Dresden and another Paris Conference in 1893 and 1894 respectively to address Cholera and the 1899 Venice Conference which dealt with preventing the spread of plague. These conventions were consolidated into a single International Sanitary Convention in 1903. With the outbreak of the Second World War, the United Nations in 1945, based on the proposal of a technical preparatory committee, drafted and adopted the Constitution of the World Health Organization (WHO) by representatives of 51

Members of the United Nations and ten (10) other nations. Since then, health issues became fundamental concern of government Worldwide (WHO, 1986). As an organ of the United Nations, WHO is charged with the responsibility of monitoring global health trends and proffering appropriate course of action as at when due is a testimony to the primary of health to continual survival of human and the universe (Mustapha, 2008).

Nigeria is signatory to several global initiatives and agenda on health and development, including the Millennium Development Goals (MDGs), now Sustainable Development Goals (SDGs). The thrust of the third goal of the SDGs is to ensure healthy lives and promote well-being for all at all ages. This also aligns with the Nigerian Vision 20:2020 goals, proposed to enhance access to quality and affordable care through the establishment of at least one general hospital in each of the 774 Local Government Areas (FMoH, 2016). According to the Constitution of the Federal Republic of Nigeria, Chapter 11 subsection 14(2b), "the security and welfare of the people shall be the primary purpose of Government" (Nigeria 1999 Constitution as Amended). Embedded in welfare is health in all ramifications.

Although, Nigeria launched several healthcare plans before it finally drafted the Health policy and strategy to Achieve Health for all Nigerians in 1988. This was subsequently revised in 2004. Then, due to necessity to develop a new national health policy to reflect new realities and trends, including the unfinished agenda of the MDGs, and new SDGs, emerging health issues (especially epidemics) and the provision of the National Health Act 2014, the new Primary Health Commitment to Universal Coverage, the 2016 National Health Policy came into existence (FMoH, 2016) with the goal: To strengthen Nigeria's health system, particularly the primary health care sub-system to deliver effective, efficient, accessible, affordable, acceptable and comprehensive health care services to all Nigerians. Yet, these policies impact in real terms is not visible in the health conditions of Nigerians. While policies are guidelines to solving practical problems, knowledge of such policies as disseminated by the media to target audience and active participation of key holders, determine, to a large extent, the success of policies. Though the media can play supportive role in health advocacy, if the language of dissemination is not suitable for specific target audience members, such advocacy will record very little success. The development media theory lays emphasis on the use of indigenous language in media text to reduce ambiguity; but colonialism robbed Nigeria of its gains by shear neglect of indigenous language for English language and political concentration at the center, which has been identified as the bane of Nigeria's development.

Several health related issues which could be nipped in the bud through deliberately packaged programmes in indigenous languages to maximize comprehension are not only few, they are mostly disseminated in Standard English. This way, most Nigerians are cut off from their roots as well as the cultural healing inherent in indigenous language. When health programmes are disseminated in indigenous language on the mass media, in community gatherings in both rural and urban centers, comprehension and retention is enhanced through grass root participation and collective action as done before the advent of colonialism. Majority of Nigerians today are ignorant of the medicinal efficacy of "Efirin and Ewuro"(Scent Leaves and Bitter Leaves) for the treatment of pile, stomach upset and blood purification; let alone the functions of "Ata Ile" and " Kanafuru" (Turmeric and Cloves) and other spices. The knowledge and application of these herbs and spices would have taken care of 60% of ailment cases attended to at primary healthcare centers thereby forestalling preventable deaths.

In addition, at the macro level, with globalization comes individuality and the use of English language alienates the people further from their ancestral root. This perhaps explains the reason Nigerian's health indicators are among the worst in the World. Nigeria shoulders 10% of the global disease burden and is making slow progress towards achieving the 2030 agenda for sustainable development (GHWA, 2014). To appreciate the extent of the slow progress, as at 2016 for instance, Nigeria still has high prevalence of communicable diseases and an increasing burden of non- communicable diseases. Communicable disease account for 66% of the total health burden of morbidity, malaria and pregnancy related deaths are other major drivers of the disease burden. Nigeria currently has a maternal mortality ratio of 576 per 100,000 and infant mortality rate of 69 per 100,000. By comparison, the maternal mortality ratio in the more developed regions is 12 per 100,000 live births. (FMOH, 2016; UN, 2017).

With a population of over two hundred thousand (200,000) people, Nigeria still grapple with essential elements of the right to health, namely: availability, accessibility, affordability, acceptability and quality (UNFPA, 2013). Other environmental challenges to health ranging from religion, political, cultural and socioeconomic factors remain key barrier in health communication. Health communication tends to be limited to health personnel in hospitals, who have little or no luxury of time to profitably engage patients, let alone communicate with community members on health-related issues. Ordinarily, mobilization of the public for health instruction is expected to cut across board of which media intervention takes precedence, particularly for national issues.

The 2016 health policy like its 1988 and 2004 predecessors are fantastic on paper and the justification for the draft is apt. However, the absence of two major stakeholders at the consultative stage in health policy formulation and implementation remain the repeated mistake of government policies. Studies have shown that undermining the active participation of the people and the media are necessary ingredient of policy failure. In fact, it is instructive to note that real development cannot be achieved with health policies that alienate the messenger and the audience at the planning stage. This perhaps explains why Mustapha (2008; P. 19) declares that "policies that have performed wonder in other countries become strategic poison when introduced into Nigeria". Since policies are meant to be executed and monitored for performance, what is the percentage success of the on-going 2016 policy, how many indigenous health programmes exist for whom, at where, in what form and to what effect in Nigeria? Can Nigeria health indicators improve significantly in real terms? Can Nigeria make significant progress in SDGs indicators? Provided Nigeria government summon the political will to partner with the Nigerian media alongside other stakeholders and do things differently.

HEALTH EDUCATION IN NIGERIA

The World Health Organization (1946) defined health as a state of complete physical, mental and social wellbeing and not merely the absence of disease or infirmity. It also defined health education as comprising of consciously constructed opportunities for learning involving some form of communication designed to improve health literacy, including improving knowledge, and developing life skills which are conducive to individual and community health. Furthermore, health education was defined by (Sharma & Gupta, 2017) as the combination of learning experiences, designed to help individuals and communities improve their health by increasing knowledge or influencing their attitudes towards health. Sharma and Gupta definition of health education encapsulates five major activities, namely: dissemination of health related information, inspiring and motivating the population for taking necessary action (behavioural change) improve health and maintaining healthy behavioral lifestyle.

Naveem (2015) notes that health is a complex concept that involves not just the soundness of a person's body but also the state of a person's mind and the quality of social environment in which people lives. Health education is a profession of educating people about health (Mckensie, Neiger and Thackeray, 2009). Areas within this profession encompass environmental, physical, social, emotional, intellectual, spiritual as well as sexual and reproductive health. The dictum "Health is Wealth" and "a healthy nation is a wealthy nation" sum the importance of health education to the fifteen (15) SDGs when perspective is properly focused on the people as the proximate determinant of change, rather than number. In essence, health is a key determinant of other achievements in life.

Health education takes place through health communication. Health communication is a multifaceted and multidisciplinary approach to reach different audiences and share health related information with the goal of influencing, engaging and supporting individuals, communities, health professionals, special groups, policy makers and the public to champion, introduce, adopt or sustain a behavioural practice or policy that will ultimately improve health outcomes (Schiavo, 2007). Health education is an integral component of learning that starts from childhood and never ends. As such, it is a complex concept that cuts across all disciplines of which media role in awareness creation is indispensable. No doubt, the mass media being an important social companion have massive potential in disseminating health information, awareness, instruction thus ultimately changing attitude of audience for healthy health choices.

However, the situation is not so due to lack of enabling incentive for both media and health promotion units at both Federal, State and Local Government levels, inadequate political commitment to healthcare. Absence of understanding of the concepts of health promotion, consumer rights and many others are few of the lacunas in Nigerian health sector. As an institution and intermediary between policy formulator and the society, the strategic and social importance of the mass media lies in their ability to disseminate information far beyond the reach of the source simultaneously. More importantly, the media report issues that demand policy formulation as much as they suggest appropriate implementation strategies. In fact with internet technology, the function of the mass media in the society is more enhanced. In health promotion, the media help health workers expand their audience reach, which is crucial, considering the fact that interpersonal channels of communication have limited reach coupled with huge human resources and reach only a small number of people in large, underserved rural areas. They are equally effective in persuasive behavioral communication as well as remind audience members of critical information that could lead to socio-economic well being of the audience. In essence, the mass media is a game changer and development accelerator due to their innate ability to educate, inform and give instructions to large number of people on issues germane to national development. Specifically, (Flora, Maibach, Maccoby, 1989) divided media promotion intervention into four levels- education, supporter, promoter and supplement. As an important ally in development agenda, the media can serve as a source of correct and credible information as well as advocate for positive health behaviour in both urban and rural areas.

Since health education is health communication, such communication must be correct, clear, concise, complete and comprehensive. The language of communication must be tailored to meet the needs of target audience. To accomplish this task, the media must understand the nitty-gritty of health issues before dissemination. Also, the language of communication must be appropriate for target audience members.

INDIGENOUS LANGUAGE HEALTH PROGRAMMES

Language of communication has been identified as one of the barriers to effective communication. . As Oyesomi, Salawu, & Olorunyomi, 2017, Oyesomi, Salawu, & Onyenankeya, 2019 and Oyesomi & Salawu, 2019 note that the language of communication is critical in conveying messages to the people. In a country like Nigeria with diverse cultural, socio-economic and religious orientation, health communication must be properly planned. The reason is that media texts are polysemic and if not properly contextualized, could result in dysfunctional output. Chibita and Salawu (2016) observed that language plays a crucial role in the media as a key public domain, to the extent that the languages people use in the media determine their chances of being heard.

According to Sobowale (1992, pp. 23-24) the basic tool of a communicator, particularly a mass communicator is language. Language is a power tool in communication. It is more than a choice or means of communication. It is a symbol of culture, origin, identity which reflects the values, morals, norms and practices of a given culture.

Paradoxically, language also may be the very hindrance to the efforts of the communicator. Indigenous language helps reduce text ambiguity and connects media audience with their cultural identity. The indigenous language of these various entities constitutes their main identity. It is the foundation of individual and collective identity and its erosion can adversely affect health and wellbeing, leading to depression, anxiety, substance abuse and even suicide (Kicmayar, Brass & Tait, 2000). In fact, (Cohen, 2001, p. 143 cited in Weigles, 2016) notes that language suppressed, particularly for indigenous people is "a form of disempowerment and oppression", that impacts on self-identity, well-being, self-esteem and empowerment, all of which are key ingredients, for individual and community healing. Meaning embedded in indigenous languages is stripped of its origin and usefulness when said in English language.

Embedded in Indigenous languages is cultural identity of the people -norms, values, folk, idioms, and morals and so on. Development is participatory, hence, after programmes, if action should be taken by audience members, it means discussions and consultation with significant other, and families and so on should be ongoing. In a situation where the meaning is not clear, further discussion for clarification becomes impossible and media efforts, in vain, particularly for rural dwellers.

McQuail (2005) certainly recognized the depth and importance of development communication as sine quo non to meaningful communication when he states: the need for the media to accomplish positive development efforts in conformity with nationally established policy. Development media theory suggests the type of relationship expected from media and government for development effort. In Nigeria like other countries of the world, the mandate of the media in their traditional responsibilities is not in doubt. The assertion of Siebert et al on the normative theories that political milieus of a nation determine its media coloration has proved positive. McQuail's foresight gave priority to national language as a sine quo non for development. Relevant to this discourse are these two assumptions: media must accept and carryout provide development tasks in line with nationally established policy, freedom of the media should be open to economic priorities and development needs of the society and media should give priority in their content to the national culture and languages.

Sadly, (Kunczick 1988 cited in Daramola 1998: p. 32) observed that McQuail failed to see the problem, of internal colonialism i.e. the smashing of local and/or regional, culture and languages. And there lies the problem of Nigeria. In the context of this discourse, efforts will be made we to explain how foreign and elitist media hegemony alongside declining indigenous health programmes in both oral media and electronic media undermine health security in Nigeria.

Unlike pioneering indigenous press set up for social reasons, the need for profit motivates media organization in programme content selection and language deployment. Largely, the Nigerian mass media is elitist in programme content and delivery; a fact which explains the few number of indigenous broadcast stations and programme contents profitable for ordinary people. In programme conceptualization, the cost burden becomes a minor issue provided there are sponsors and if such programme is targeted at elites in the society. Government activities, sponsored documentary, feature, and propaganda activities are major programme content of the day. The situation is same in print media; Umon and Oloyede (2014) laments near neglect of health issues in the Nigerian press. Their study shows that the front pages and back pages were occupied by other issues in politics, business, and crime stories not health stories and when health shows were reported 82.7% were reported in less than half a page inside The Guardian and the Punch Newspapers.

Few broadcast stations are interested in corporate social responsibility. Thus, to disseminate health programmes sponsored by stations is inimical to station viability. Since most media programmes are commercial in nature and programme content respond to audience demand, the political economy of media production takes precedence over indigenous health programmes with largely unknown audience. This is not to say that health related stories are not regular feature of broadcast content, the point is that consciously planned health educational programmes, targeted at specific audience in specific indigenous language are very few in number in a country where a state of emergency ought to have been declared on health as far back as four decades. Worst still is the fact that government owned broadcast stations lack regular schedule of health education programmes in indigenous language. This shows the lackadaisical attitude of government to health education; the point is that government expects media to support health demand generation through awareness creation without funding its own media organization. How then do Nigerians expect privately owned stations to venture into indigenous health education when public health personnel in the three tiers of health tiers can mobilize the populace even more with better outcomes? Every day, presents an opportunity for government to partner with local community, engage them to identify their health challenges, engage them for possible solutions and partner with them to get their health priorities right. The Nigerian government is not unaware of these possibilities but corruption and politicking remain our major issue in health education. The truth is that the Nigerian government may be sincere in alleviating the health burden of Nigerians; the major problem is the people. How do I mean?

Certainly, the media are not alone in this hegemonic conspiracy. Media pioneers are more knowledgeable in the importance of indigenous language communication more than media audience. This perhaps explains the indigenous language root of Nigerian Journalism with the first being Iwe Irohin and subsequent where such as Eko Akete (1903), Eleti Ofe (1933), Akede Eko (1927), Gaskoya Tafi Kwabo (1939), Iwe Irohin Osose (1925), Albashir published in Kanwi (1981), Jadadya Zaruma, Sakkawat anchi of 1951, 1948 and 1951, all published in Hausa, other modern, vernacular newspapers include Iwe Irohin Yoruba, Gbohun Gbohun, Isokan, Amana, Udoka (Ibo) and lately Alaroye (Daramola, 2006). Electronic indigenous stations include: Faji Fm, Eko Fm, Wazobia Fm and Radio Lagos 107.5 FM to mention a few. Health related programmes are least of programme priority of these stations due to programme commercialization and other related factors.

Through indigenous language, children are socialized into the larger society from their immediate families, as they progress socially and educationally, they learn to read and speak their indigenous language, know common illnesses and cures. On its part, the mass media through its programmes built on and develops latent norms and morals embedded in indigenous language as well as expand their horizon in health education. In local communities, it is expected that children should be familiar with local curative herbs and roots by the age of ten. Indigenous language, more than any other factor signpost cultural identity of people. Through indigenous language children are socialized into the larger society from their immediate families, as they progress educationally, indigenous language subjects are taught to solidify their cultural ties, as they grow older, realities of life through folklore, idioms, proverbs, songs, riddles, jokes, dance and so on becomes not only familiar but integral part of their personal psychology. In fact, Ogweezy (1999) and Akpabio (2013) believed that African communication systems through their various categorized have sustained the rural people over the years.

According to them, the rural people never experienced underdevelopment until the colonial period. This is because whatever they needed to make their lives meaningful was available to them within their environment. The adoption of English language as the official language adversely affects the esteem of indigenous language. Worst still, certain parents do not communicate in indigenous language and some are out rightly indifferent to the learning and speaking of indigenous language at homes. Thus, aliening their wards from their cultural root. Children, even take pride in saying, they do not understand their mother tongue (Ayakoroma, 2017). In school, indigenous language is termed vernacular and students are prohibited from speaking it. This mistake perpetuated for a decade was further fueled by new media, which to a large extent; undermine the collective cultural ties of Africans. The general effect of this on meaningful indigenous health programme is massive. The minister of informational cultural his Mohammed in his address at the 2017 Annual Round Table on cultural orientation expressed concerns that the country's indigenous languages are endangered and could go into extinction in no distant future if urgent steps are not taken to reverse the trend (Premium Times, 2018). Ayakoroma (2017) notes that the Nigerian society over the years have been plagued by many challenges brought about by the domineering influence of foreign cultures on our national psyche. Since the media constitute on integral part of societal dynamic, most programmes are aired in English language to the disadvantage of millions of rural and urban illiterates, whose health burden remains with them.

Nigeria operates three tiers of health-federal, state and local governments. Unfortunately, provision for the 1999 constitution did not lay emphasis on health and fails to clearly indicate the roles and responsibilities of the three tiers of government in health systems management and delivery (FMoH, 2016). While this makes coordination and effective implementation of policies difficult on the one hand, its negative impact in real term as documented by (ibid p.13) states thus

The availability of health services does not translate into the availability of quality healthcare services. Certain services are not generally available to a large percentage of the population. There is consistent disruption of Health care services, due to incessant industrial action by all cadres of health care providers in public facilities.... Many health facilities are situated far away from the people, especially in rural and hard to reach areas. The most common problem barriers to accessing health services by the population are the cost of services, distance to the health facility, and the attitude of health workers....the quality of health care is generally poor and does not instill confidence in the people....

Consequently, the health situation report shows abysmal performance in real terms and that is where the media come in as a major stakeholder. The electronic media unlike health providers do not go on strike and have the capacity not only to inform the government on areas of policy change and implementation, they also have the capacity to trigger demand creation for health services through health promotion and awareness among the populace. In sum, the media is expected to support health system via careful conceptualization; processing and transmission of timely programmes to enable individuals acquire information, knowledge attitudes and skills as well as change behaviors to facilitate the making of health choice a personal and collective priority. Certainly, the media has a mandate to promote healthy demand generation among populace in indigenous language but there internal and external issues, limiting the ability of the media to function well in this regard, namely populace and media commercialization.

Nigerian youths of today are not only ignorant of their health right, worst still, they seldom watch traditional media, not to mention health programmed aired in their own indigenous language. Consequently, Nigerians, miss out on opportunities of various curative herbs and roots around their environment, coupled with ignorance of modern cure for common illnesses, hence, the overwhelming crowd at primary health centers on daily basis

CONCLUSION

Scholars have argued that the advent of colonialism marked the starting point of underdevelopment in Nigeria, while others equally argued that we are not ready for development. The gains of maximal utilization of health educational broadcast programmes aired lies in going back to our root. Integrating language and culture within clinical setting can significantly improve health outcomes. Culture and religion significantly affect perceptions about illness, mental health. For instance, when health education takes place, the source culture and recipient culture may affect outcomes positively or otherwise. It is in the vein that suggests that for better outcome, health educators should and must identify with the culture of local people.

While it is one thing for programme planners and presenters to disseminate health educational programmes in indigenous languages, the percentage of audience members at the time of broadcast is uncertain, particularly for youths. Studies have shown that aside the use of Standard English as an official language, the advent of social media is contesting chances of children speaking and learning their indigenous language and by extension, learning healthy lifestyle is limited. Meanwhile, the early years are a special time for learning and absorbing language and culture from parents, families and communities, investment in early childhood development programmes that incorporate culture and language is key to improve health outcomes (NCEA 2016). Groups express its culture and social identity through language, because language is intimately linked to mental and ideological processes and to the perception of internal and external worlds. Language is the fundamental point of references by which an ethnic group finds its own identity. Many indigenous cultures have traditional knowledge that is transmitted only orally. It is in this vein other traditional medium of communication, in use before the advent of mass media should be deployed for health education.

RECOMMENDATION

The root of the poor health indicators in Nigeria is multifaceted and complicated. The federal government needs to unburden itself by decentralizing health administration and allow state and local government accountable for health burdens in their states. This way, the local people are actively integrated and their participation is key in alleviating health burden.

Aside the mass media, community health workers and other health personnel in various health centers should be empowered to give health talk in the predominant language or dialect of the community. In urban centers indigenous language should be used to carry non indigene along. Such health education should not be limited to straight forward talk alone; dance and drama could be utilized to mobilize the populace who would have been well informed of such event before the starting day. Such event should not be a one off edition but must be done regularly with collaboration with the local community development chairperson.

It is important to note that successful health communication should start and end with the audience desires and needs. The audience is not merely a target, but an active participant in the process and analyzing the health issues and finding culturally appropriate and cost effective solutions. State government should strive and engage identified communities in defining and implementing key strategies.

In addition, the constitutional gap in health provision should be bridged. This will eliminate the question of accountability at all levels, and on the long run decentralize health education. This way, it becomes easier for state government to decide on and embark on holistic health communication strategies that suits their geopolitical terrain in appropriate indigenous language, through the mass media alongside enter- educate approach via community health personnel and qualified doctors.

It is instructive to note that health communication source or educator must identify with the culture of host community and educate them within cultural and religious purview. Thirdly, health education should be integrated in school curriculum from basic level to higher institution.

CONFLICT OF INTEREST

The authors declare that there is no conflict of interest regarding the paper

ACKNOWLEDGEMENT

The authors recognize and appreciate authors whose works, books, and contributions have been of great assistance to this study.

REFERENCES

Alabi, S. (2003). The Development of Indigenous Language publications in Nigeria Journalism. In R. A. Akinfeleye, & I. E. Okoye (Eds), Issues in Nigeria Media History: 1900-200 AD, pp. 33-50. Lagos, Nigeria: Malthouse Press Limited.

Ayakoroma, B. (2017). Reviving the use of indigenous Languages in the Contemporary Nigerian Society: The National Institute for Cultural Orientation (NICO) Initiatives. *International Journal of Language and Linguistics, 4*(4).

Boyd, B., & Shaw, W. (2009). Unlocking Health Worker Potential: Some Creative Strategies from the field.

Chibita, M., & Salawu, A. (2016). Intoduction: Language Structure and Agency: Optimizing Media Diversity in Africa Using the Indigenous Languages. In A. Salawu, & M. B. Chibita (Eds.), *Indigenous Language Media, Language Politics and Democracy in Africa*. London, UK: Palgrave Macmillan.

Daramola, Y. (2008). Mass Media and Society in Nigeria Selected Functional Perspectives. In R. Akinfeleye (Ed.), *Mass Media and Society: A multi-perspective Approach*. Lagos: Integrity Press.

Federal Ministry of Health (2016). National Health Policy: Promoting the health of Nigerians to Accelerate Socio-Economic Development.

Mustapha, L. (2008). Mass Media and Optimization of health policy in Nigeria: The participatory Option. In R. Akinfeleye (Ed.), *Mass media and Society: A Multi Perspective Approach Lagos*. Integrity Press.

National Collaboration Centre for Aboriginal Health (NECAH). (2016). *Social Determinants of Health Culture and Language as Social Determinants of First Nations*. Inuit and Metis Health.

Oyesomi, K. O., & Salawu, A. (2019). Assessing the Uniqueness of Indigenous Language in Advertising: Analysis of Figurative Language Used in Selected Telecommunication Yoruba Advertisement in Nigeria. *Qualitative Report*, *24*(10), 2574–2591. Retrieved from https://nsuworks.nova.edu/tqr/vol24/iss10/12

Oyesomi, K. O., Salawu, A., & Onyenankeya, K. (2019, March). Newspapers' Compliance with the Code of Election Coverage of the 2015 Elections and citizens participation: Implication for Journalism Education and Professionalism. *African Renaissance*, *16*(1), 41–64. doi:10.31920/2516-5305/2019/V16n1a3

Oyetade, S (2002). Language Policies and Planning in Nigeria. Research in African Languages and Literature (6): 51-66.Oyesomi, K. O., Salawu, A., & Olorunyomi, B. (2017). Indigenous Communication: Socio- Economic Characteristics Influencing Contemporary Female Political Participation. [JIWS]. *Journal of International Women's Studies*, *18*(4), 164–181.

Premium Times. (2018). *Nigeria's Indigenous Languages endangered, may go into Extinction*. Lai Mohammed.

Sharma, S., & Gupta, Y. (2017). Mass Media for Health Education: (A Study in the state of Rajasthan). Retrieved from www.researchgate.net

Sobowale. (1992). Television for whom and at what price in Odukomaya (Ed.), Television and film Media Issues. Lagos: Unique publication (1986). Origin and Development of Health Cooperation. Retrieved from http://www.who.int/global.health./en/

Uwom, O., & Oloyede, B. (2014). Newspaper Coverage of Health Issues in Nigeria. A study of the Guardian and The Punch Newspapers January 2010 to December 2011, In International Journal of African and Asian Studies, 4.

World Health Organization. (1946). Preamble to the constitution of the WHO as adopted by the International Health Conference, New York.

World Population Review. (2019). Nigeria Population World Populationreview.com. Retrieved May 18, 2019.

KEY TERMS AND DEFINITIONS

Health Education: Learning about issues related to the physical, mental, social and economic outcomes of life. It is central to the wellbeing of individual.

Indigenous: Aboriginal attributes of culture. It represents the identity, root, norms, morals, values, beliefs and other tangible and intangible attributes of life.

Issues: Problems militating against proper functioning of a particular thing.

Language: A medium of expression peculiar to a particular group of people.

Mass Media: Mechanical means of getting messages across to a large number of heterogeneous and diversified people simultaneously.

Perspectives: Correctives opinions on how to do something better.

Trends: Current happenings regarding a particular issue.

Chapter 13
Corporate Communication, Indigenous Languages, and Community Relations:
A Discourse on Practices by Nigerian Universities

Thelma Ekanem
Covenant University, Nigeria

Rotimi Olatunji
Lagos State University, Nigeria

Lanre Amodu
Covenant University, Nigeria

Oscar Odiboh
https://orcid.org/0000-0001-5870-6223
Covenant University, Nigeria

Olusola Oyero
https://orcid.org/0000-0001-7795-5516
Covenant University, Nigeria

ABSTRACT

This conceptual work examines corporate communication as a tool for coordinating universities' internal and external messages in Nigeria. It explores universities' attempts to harness, link-up, and interact with their publics. This chapter presents effective corporate communication as the unifying principle in many institutional decisions. It emphasizes that sometimes, universities' efforts to communicate

DOI: 10.4018/978-1-7998-2091-8.ch013

effectively and profitably with their host communities end up in futility especially where indigenous language is a key environmental factor. University-neighbour relationship globally ought to be symbiotic and mutually-reinforcing. This chapter reviews scholarly commentaries on corporate communication, the relevance of indigenous language to community relations; and highlights in conclusion, the implications for universities in neglecting indigenous language during community engagements. It recommends that universities should motivate their employees to apply indigenous languages in enhancing understanding between the institutions and their host communities.

INTRODUCTION

Corporate communication is a tool for harmonizing internal and external messages by institutions all over the world. This tool is extremely important in universities' community relations where indigenous languages are inevitable means of communication. Universities' harness corporate communication activities to transact, link-up, send messages and interact with internal and external publics. In the corporate communication manual of the University of Gothenburg (2014, p. 2), proper corporate communication within universities could increase the awareness of universities' activities; create, maintain and further develop relations within and outside of universities to enhance a clear and positive representation of universities. Though complex at times, nothing is as valuable to corporate entities as their ability to relate effectively and harmoniously with their various stakeholders through communication. As such, universities need corporate communication to establish, extend, maintain and sustain mutually beneficial relationships with their stakeholders (Mamuli, Mutsotso & Namasaka, 2013).

Sometimes, universities' efforts to communicate effectively and profitably with their host communities end up in futility (Fashiku, 2016). This is because, communication for universities is becoming more complex given the fact that wherever a university is founded in Nigeria and many other places, it has to contend with the indigenous language of that environment. Language plays a vital role in all fields of human endeavour since it is a channel through which people interact. The Nigerian university structure comprises a liberal socio-educational mix of people who do not only communicate but expect to be understood. Communication in indigenous languages has been observed to enhance social attachment between all concerned (Salawu, 2006). For a harmonious existence of a university in a community, it is important for that university to be able to interact and send out messages to this external public in the appropriate language of that community.

Some communities would desire to benefit from universities around them. For universities also, fostering mutually beneficial relationships with their host communities is top priority (Onabajo, 2013). Thus, community relations becomes imperative. Community relations activities are those actions that a university undertakes to enhance itself and build a mutually beneficial relationship and of course, goodwill with its host community. In its absence, peaceful communities could become hostile; and inactive communities could become restive. Communication experts believe that indigenous language holds the key to avoiding host communities' hostilities and dampening their restiveness (Chima, 2012; Olatunji 2013; Siddiqui, 2019). However, applying appropriate language to create favourable relationships with host groups upon which an institution depends is a huge challenge for universities in Africa, especially Nigeria. The rationale for this, Popoola (2014) notes, is as a result of the colonial history and diverse ethnic composition of Nigeria. English is the official language of the country which has been adopted by institutions of learning and for this reason, indigenous languages do not appear valuable. Moreover, the local communities are also investing in their wards to acquire and speak in the English language. Also, managerial activities such as planning, coordinating, counselling and advisory in corporate communication are best tied to appropriate indigenous languages for courting neighbour publics of an institution. Conversely, these are dependent on how effective corporate communication is within that institution (Goodman, 2006; Fashiku, 2016).

As an integrator of both internal and external communication, the objective of corporate communication goes beyond building, maintaining and protecting a university's reputation to include creating and sustaining mutually beneficial relationships through communication with the university's various publics (Cutlip, Centre & Broom, 2006; Odiboh & Ekanem, 2018; Ekanem, Olatunji, Amodu, Odiboh, Yartey, Adesina & Adeyeye, 2018; Ndubueze *et al.*, 2019; Olabanjo *et al.*, 2019). Lacuna arises when a university transacts with its surrounding rural or semi urban community using non-indigenous language. The implication of this lacuna is the focus of this chapter which examines the problem of universities' abandonment of indigenous languages in engaging their host communities.

LITERATURE REVIEW

Human communities are distinguished by their language of communication. It means message, interaction, signs, symbols, processes and transfers, stimulations, intentions, questions and answers, power and control (Iordache-Platis & Josan, 2009) form the essence of communal existence. Communication is the process of transmitting information, ideas, feelings (attitudes, opinions) from a source to a receiver (Olatunji,

2013). It drives the exchange of meaning among people. Though, there are different types of communication such as verbal, non-verbal, intrapersonal, interpersonal, intergroup, internal, external, public and mass communication; Communication is a necessity for the existence of a society and the people in it. Irrespective of the type in use, communication is only effective and complete when there is *shared meaning* to facilitate necessary response. As simple as shared meaning sounds, communication could be complex and ineffective. This is because of its process which Iordache and Josan (2009) identify as an integrated communication process. Accordingly, a complete communication process must have a source, an understandable message, proper communication channels, receiver (an able interpreter); noise filters and evaluative feedback. Recipients as decoders of messages must not be bewildered by messages but appropriately pin expectations to actions.

The onus is always on universities to accomplish set goals and objectives. More often than not, Mamuli, Mutsotso and Namasaka (2013) assert, institutional goals falter when communication strategies are mere linguistic fads. Miscommunication, over-communication and under-communication have such linguistic bearings and further, transactional misunderstanding (Steyn, 2004). Nevertheless, how an institution appropriates the lingo of communication per time, especially in dealings with next door neighbour separates mutually beneficial understanding from reciprocally estranging misinterpretation. Effective corporate communication is the organizing principle behind many institutional decisions and sometimes, it could encounter hiccups. Fractures of corporate communication for Nigerian universities include but not limited to strikes, protests, riots, rumours and host community restiveness. These challenges could arise as a result of unfair treatment, miscommunication or even delayed response by university management to an issue that affects its publics (Iruonagbe, Imhonopi & Egharevba, 2015). For instance, in addition to its core mandate of teaching and research, universities, embrace the giving-back to lift their hosts into forward integrated development. Community hostility and restiveness appear where an expected benefactor is perceived as an unexpected exploiter. Whatever the situation may be, corporate communication is a significant tool to douse such tensions (Alabi, 2002; Wessels, 2017; Varsity, 2018).

Corporate Communication

Corporate communication is a core aspect of public relations in pedagogy and practice. Scholars (Cutlip, 1995; Supa & Zoch, 2009; Cornelissen, 2017) explain that though public relations is a strategic function in organizations, the practice in the 90s was inadequate because it largely consisted of communication with the press. It neglected other forms of communication within the organization leading to the emergence of corporate communication. Either in error or as a matter of fact, corporate communication is sometimes used to describe the promotion of a product, service or an organization (Johan & Noor, 2013). However, on a larger platform, it is seen as an accessory of corporate identity and institutional ownership which creates consistent and coherent corporate image for institutions (University of Nairobi, 2014, p. 2). Argenti and Forman (2002) articulate corporate communication as "the corporation's voice and the images it projects of itself on a world stage populated by its various audiences, or what we refer to as its constituencies" and as "an attitude toward communication that employees internalize." Similarly, Van Riel (1992, p. 26) sees corporate communication as an instrument of management by means of which all consciously used forms of internal and external communication are harmonized as effectively as possible, with the overall objective of creating a favourable basis for relationships with groups upon which the company is dependent. The definitions above shows not only the importance of corporate communication but that institutions engage corporate communication to lead, motivate, persuade and inform both their internal and external publics.

Odiboh (2002, p. 116) characterises corporate communication as a long-term plan for executing public and media relations, issue and crisis management programmes thereby aiding institutional growth. This mirrors corporate communication as a management function, responsible for overseeing and coordinating the actions of communication experts in a corporate setting. It also shows that corporate advancement and survival depends, to a large extent, on how much of goodwill, support and understanding an institution gets from its publics. Corporate communication in its totality, provides a potential route for competitive advantage, sustains an institution and its image both within and outside it. Saha's (2014) understanding of corporate communication is pigeonholed into crisis management which could be adopted to describe the relationship between universities and their social environments. For the purpose of this study, corporate communication is defined by the researcher as a strategic management function that offers a framework for the effective coordination of all internal and external communication with the purpose of establishing and maintaining mutually beneficial relationships, understanding and goodwill with all stakeholder groups within and outside an organisation upon whom its successes and failures depend. This definition shows that corporate communication is an essential multifaceted institutional commodity. Thus, it is important for universities to have effective strategic corporate communication within the university which could in turn flow to the external context for the sustenance of peace, harmony, understanding, countering of rumors amongst others.

Excellent corporate communication lies at the heart of institution's ability to build a superior organisational performance and culture (Cureteanu & Maxim, 2011). Its management demands a two-way strategic plan through optimal use of all its tools and functions to boost both internal and external university communications.

External communication, which is pivotal to this study, aims to obtain and transfer information between university and its host community. External communication builds network, goodwill, establishes a positive reputation for a university, ensures continued existence and growth, create and maintain mutually beneficial relationships between universities and their host communities. Other benefits include, development of trust, order, expand opportunities, social responsibility, and transparency between parties involved. The lack of effective external communication could result in problems and distortion that could lead to miscommunication (Kotler & Keller, 2009). External communication could be speaking face-to-face with community members, written message, advertising and promotion (on billboards, posters, television, and radio), etc. Proper external communication shapes positively, how a host community perceives a university in its environs. External corporate communication creates and maintains desirable public image for a university. It shapes the publics' opinion on issues that are important to the university.

Common mechanisms used to communicate with host communities are: formal and informal dialogue, town hall meetings, public relations officers, opinion leaders, workshops, signals, information days, conventional media, surveys, colours, etc. External publics are just as important as internal publics. It is through communication that institutions make contacts with their external publics especially, the host community. In sending out corporate messages to a university's host community, the use of proper language to facilitate understanding and goodwill cannot be overlooked.

The Notion of Language

Language is an integral part of human behaviour. It serves as the main channel of interaction between people in the society to share ideas and experiences (Salawu, 2006, Oyesomi, Salawu &Olorunyomi, 2017). Language is a set of symbols which embodies beyond its literal meaning, all the customs, ideas, beliefs, values, orientation and disposition of a group of people. It brings about social bonding and interactivity between parties concerned; and no language is superior to the other. It is a definite way of identifying a people besides their culture. Emeka-Nwobia (2015) affirms that the storehouse of a people's identity and way of life is their language which could be transferred to other people as well as newer generations. As such, language, whether indigenous or foreign, is an indispensable tool in life because there is no aspect of human activity that can be successful without the use of language.

Language is the mainstay of any society, institution or group of people; a lack of it renders a society incommunicado (Jibri-Daura, 2014). Its evolution can be traced as far back as between 3000-2000BC when the first symbols in form of primitive alphabets of over 600 characters came into existence (Bittner, 1989). Adzer (2012) sees language as both individual property (when it exist as knowledge) and a social property; an indispensable resource of man, necessary for his day to day transactions and activities. In actual fact, language bridges the gap between knowledge and ignorance and helps man to access and express his thoughts (Adedimeji, 2009). Since, language is innate and unique to man, it gives man the ability to express issues, concepts as well as moods, feelings and attitudes. It captures man's world of reality, fosters development, peaceful co-existence, cultural transmission, and knowledge advancement. Language is the unique property of man and all his developments, be it intellectual, ethical, political, social or economic revolves entirely on the instrumentality of language (Adedimeji, 2009).

Beyond cultural transmission, language allows people to relate with those from other communities, ethnic groups, clans, races and nations. Language is a powerful tool which must be wield judiciously. It has engendered close ties with countries of the world in terms of trade relations, political relation, educational relations, and so on. At the same time, language has also been used as a tool of cruelty and domination through the realities of slavery and colonization. For institutions and organizations, language is critical. Institutions that have employees who are skillful in language can communicate and achieve the aim of the institution. Though every living creature communicates, the ability to speak and understand a language makes it possible for individuals and groups to interact freely, communicate and share experiences amongst themselves (Oso, 2006; Popoola, 2014). Ani (2012, p.110) moves this thesis further by stating that:

The appeal of language resides precisely in its capacity to meet the needs of man for self-expression and for communication of experience in his day-to-day engagements with the world around him. Man needs language for the dissection and analysis of material reality and spiritual experience as well as for formulation of hypothetical statements, theories and belief as well as value systems. In other words, beyond facilitating communication of experience, a language must enhance man's cognitive abilities and functioning, if it is to be of permanent relevance or survive through the ages.

Accordingly, language reflects the culture of a people; in fact, it is itself, part of culture. Thus, people express themselves and their cultures better in the language of their culture which is popularly known as local or indigenous language.

Indigenous Languages

Adedeji (2014) deepens our understanding of indigenous language by presenting it as spoken, owned, shared and free among a set of people. It is central to ethnicity, homo nativity, culturality and identity of indigenous people within a geographical definition (Oyero, 2003). According to Oyesomi and Salawu (2019), Indigenous language is a language that is spoken by a group of people that resides in a locality or region It refers to tribal, vernacular, local or autochthonous language. It often originates from a distinct community of early settlers in an area for many generations (Jibir-Daura, 2014). In Nigeria, multiple indigenous languages such as Yoruba, Hausa, Igbo, Efik, Ibibio, and others shows the microcosmic nature of the social delineator. Scholars are not sure of the number of indigenous languages in Nigeria. But as a multilingual nation, Nigeria, has between 250 and 513 languages excluding the English language and French (Brann, 1990; Adegbija, 1992; Oso, 2006; Adegbite, 2010; Popoola, 2014). Both indigenous and foreign languages in Nigeria coexist.

Indigenous languages are indispensable cultural legacies without which no form of human interactions can be carried out (Solanke, 2006). . According to Oyesomi and Salawu (2019), Indigenous language is a language that is spoken by a group of people that resides in a locality or region. They are aboriginal to the people (Adeniyi & Bello, 2006). Rightly so, Olaoye (2013) recognizes indigenous language as the most effective engine of a people's culture. Olaoye (2013) further explains that indigenous languages are treasures of cultural heritage and self-identity. That is, the indicator of history and self-identification. For instance, people are sensitive about their language. People tend to tolerate, listen, understand and cooperate with those who can either understand or speak similar language with them. It portrays that those person's value and belief system are akin to theirs. In some communities, help comes easily to those who speak indigenous language. They even get to make purchases at the marketplace at lower prices instead of high prices offered to visitors. Indigenous language is part and parcel of culture. Culture is a channel through which people communicate, propagate and develop their knowledge and attitudes towards life (Siddiqui, 2019). Since, no society can function without culture, and culture is symbiotic with language; Indigenous language is a positive tool in the hands of any university that anticipate success.

Even the government recognizes the importance of indigenous language in Nigeria (National Policy on Education, 2004). Hence, every child is mandated to learn the language of the immediate environment. In schools, every child is expected to learn one of the three prominent Nigerian languages: Hausa, Yoruba, and Igbo (Omoniyi, 2012). At a special assembly of indigenous leaders held in December 2016, in Canada, Prime Minister Justin Trudeau announced the introduction of an *Indigenous Language Act*. Davis (2017) believes that Trudeau's announcement was made in the hope to preserve and revitalize the indigenous languages in Canada. In 2009, Siddiqui (2019) noted that the United Nations (UN) observed the *International Year of Indigenous Language* aimed at raising the awareness of local languages across the world and the need to preserve them. Indigenous language is a means of promoting social interaction, national cohesion and cultures globally. It is unique to people and regions. No wonder, Siddiqui (2019) sees it as the best language and a necessary tool for universities community relations activities.

Community Relations

Community relations is a sub-function of public relations, the predecessor of corporate communication that focuses on creating and maintaining mutually beneficial relationship between an organization and its host community. It is a planned corporate activity with a community to maintain an environment that benefits both the organization and the community. Robbin (2012, p.312) underscores community relations as a command function which evaluates public attitude, identifies the mission of an organization in-line with the public interest and executes a programme of action to earn public understanding and acceptance. The command function here, refers to the methods a university could use to create and manage relationship with the community in which it operates. It also describes the role of an institution to its host community. Universities are to take active interest in the well-being of their host communities. By so doing, the institution is accepting its civic responsibility and in turn, gaining long-term benefits such as community support, loyalty and goodwill from its host environment. Community relations could be outreach programmes of universities to build good relations and credibility and make life easy for them.

Universities' relationship with their neighbour publics is crucial. This neighbour supplies the organization with its workforce, raw materials, landed facility, enabling environment that could attract or fail to attract talented personnel, patronage, and can, if angered, impose restraints on that university. For instance, students, employees and visitors of a university could be harmed, kidnapped, or even killed by a hostile community; it could be instrumental to the folding up of that university. Furthermore, a comprehensive community relations activity could help universities like any other organization, to achieve visibility as a good community citizen and earn competitive advantage by having the goodwill of its host community (Hillstrom & Hillstrom, 2002; Odiboh, 2002; Amodu, Alege, Oluwatobi & Ekanem, 2017). Community relations ensures community goodwill in times of crisis management, especially in situations such as fire out-break, unethical behavior by an employee, or when journalists conduct interviews with members of a university's host community to corroborate a news story about that university. Imagine the outcome, if that university's community relations is zero!

Additionally, a university is seen in a positive light when it supports community activities that improve the quality of life of its host community. Community relations dampens the rise of rumours, bad publicity, allows party involved to mingle and interact, promotes security, increases knowledge of the institution's services, increases support, referrals and loyalty, enhances networking and opportunities, builds and enhances trust, harmony and peaceful co-existence. Community relations is a two-way communication chain involving at one end the community expectations and at the other, institution's obligations, creating a kind of symbiotic relationship (Amodu, 2013). This relationship consists of four components, namely: inform, consult, involve and collaborate. The community desires to be adequately informed, that is, get balanced and objective information about institution's plans and projects for the community and its impacts. The leaders want to be consulted. No organization should assume that they already know the needs of its host community, even if they do. Some needs are more important or pressing than others. It is, therefore, necessary that organizations consult the community to be sure that whatever project it wants to embark on is actually what the community needs and would appreciate. Also, the community wants to be involved in the decision-making process, working in collaboration as partners. This would boost the faith of the community in the institution.

Principles of Community Relations

According to Cutlip et al., (2006), the following are the underlying principles of community relations practice:

1. **Interdependence:** Here, the platform for continuing mutual relationship is dependent on the contribution of both the institution and the community to the well-being of both entities.
2. Analysis of community needs such as good roads, borehole water, healthcare, employment, and so on for efficient implementation of community relations activities.
3. **Policy:** This is the translation of institutions' good intentions about its host community into a statement of policy to guide the university's efforts towards it achievements.
4. **Participation:** Portrays institution's interest to involve members of its host community in matters concerning the university. For instance, the university could send out a special invitation to the Oba or Emir to attend the university's convocation ceremony.

Objectives of Community Relations

Hendrix (2004, p. 150) breakdowns the objectives of community relations into impact and output objectives. According to the author, impact objectives involves informing the community or modifying their attitudes and behaviours towards the university. Impact objectives as adapted from Hendrix includes the following:

1. To increase host community's knowledge of the operations of the university including its support of community well-being, projects and events.
2. To promote more favourable community opinion, attitude, interest and relationship with the university.
3. To gain greater institutional support from community leaders by inviting them to visit the university facilities, attend university functions, meet with university management, see employees at work and the students.
4. To encourage more feedback from community as a whole.

Output objectives involve efforts by the public relation's officer of the university to enhance the institution's community relations activities in the community. These are:

1. Being more responsive to community needs by ensuring that the university's contributions to the community are more pronounced.
2. To inform the community of the operations and activities of the university.
3. Correct misunderstanding, react to criticism and removal of any form of disaffection that might exist among community neighbour.
4. To create new community projects involving institutional employees and resources.
5. By being more involved in the community: The public relations expert of the university could search for community organizations (civic, professional, and religious) where the university management and employees could be members.
6. Liaise with community leaders through regular meetings.

Types of Community Relations Actions

Communities are not homogenous as the need of one differs from another's. Community relations actions are not only need-based but also aims at need-satisfaction. Thus, maintaining good relationship with a particular community entails tailored management and careful deployment of employees on behalf of the university to properly link up with each community activity. Need-based activities as noted by scholars (Hendrix, 2004; Onabajo, 2013; Olatunji, 2018) that universities could execute to uniquely cement a good relationship with host communities include:

1. An institutional open house and tour of facilities: From time to time, universities should organize a tour of the university facilities and premises for community leaders, school pupils and students of higher schools. This would encourage and educate them on what the university does. The university could also organize exhibitions and fairs; and more importantly, its employees should be allowed to participate in these events as guides and ambassadors. The participation of

employees could give them renewed pride in their workplace, especially, those from the community. It will also build their competencies and rapport.

2. Employment opportunity for community members. Educated indigenes should be employed into teaching and non-teaching positions. This would create a strong sense of belonging and investment in the higher institution. Indigenes that are not so educated or have never been to school should also be trained in different vocations and given jobs in their areas of interest.
3. Special events such as ground breaking for a new building, the completion of one, the erection of the Oba's statute at the community square, etc.
4. Sponsorship of community special events: This includes sporting events, educational programmes - scholarships, anniversary celebrations, cultural events like installation of a new Oba, chieftaincy titles and other coronation ceremonies, contribution of funds to community activities and causes.
5. Donations and charitable fundraisers: Cash and in-kind donations, pro-bono work, books, clothes, food items, etc.
6. Participation of management, employees and students in volunteer community activities: These include healthcare awareness, waste management and disposal, voluntary service for local NGOs, beautification of the community, taking part when government and other private organizations have events in the community.
7. Sensitization programmes such as workshops, trainings and seminars on empowerment, skills acquisition, etc.
8. Participation of management and employees in the political affairs of the community – serve in political office and on councils and boards.
9. Patronage: Purchase of materials and supplies from local organizations.
10. Purchase of advert space in local media which requires the use of indigenous language of the host community is also encouraged.

In all of these, indigenous language is important for the host public to fully understand and appreciate the intention behind each activity. An intention misconstrued is understanding miscarried. It is important for universities to understand that community relations is not all about donations. Sometimes, it could just be participation through same linguistic platform (Portway, 1995). The author argues that while community relations comes with benefits, institutions should not expect anything in return for its contribution to its host community nor should they boast of their deeds in the media. Rather, they should express their contributions in a language that truly depicts social responsibility. This behaviour, would enhance its public image and inevitably lead to a mutually beneficial relationship between the university and its host community. This is why Theaker (2011) counsels universities to put the philosophy of community relations into practice and make real life difference in the lives of their community members speaking the right language.

Relevance of Indigenous Language in Universities' Community Relations

The language people use could determine their chances of getting heard..To attract the attention of the locals, it should always be emphasized that indigenous language is ideal for universities to communicate in community relations activities because it gives better understanding and meaning to the members of the host community (Salawu, 2006). University should focus on facilitating dialogue rather than enabling monologue (Ekanem *et al.*, 2018). Also, the attachment people have for their native tongue, sense of pleasure and satisfaction derived from not just communicating in their indigenous language but hearing the intelligentsia do so could foster a strong bond between an institution and its host. Have you ever experienced or heard a fellow citizen of your country from a different ethnic group say something in his indigenous language and when you asked for the interpretation, he says, it will not mean the same thing in English? Or it will not sound as interesting in English? This means indigenous languages are all-encompassing, carrying with it the soul of the people.

Salawu (2006) reiterate that indigenous language is the best suitable means for universities to convey information and relate with their host communities. However, the lingo of expressing this information in writing or speech determines if the local people understand the message or if they are excommunicated (Oyero, 2007). The community has its own indigenous language in addition to the official language of a university. English language is both universal globally and local in Nigerian universities. English is the language of globalization and as such, of the media, communication, entertainment, service, workplaces, Internet, diplomacy, etc. (Adamu, 2010). It is also the language for universities' internationalization. In this web Nigerian universities tend to consciously use the same language in localization. Thus, miscommunication and misinterpretation of information are courted by the higher institutions in the drudgery of daily routine of communal transactions. On the other hand, host communities expecting communication at par with their guest universities are silently worried. Further, when expected explanations are not forthcoming, old neighbours would become disrespectful strangers in the community.

Indigenous language has value in its own right. By inculcating indigenous language into its community relations activity and other events, a university shows respect for its host community. It becomes easy for the university to win them over and co-exist harmoniously with them. Noteworthy is the fact that indigenous channels are highly credible because indigenous information dissemination is controlled locally and they are familiar to the people. If a university engages these channels to communicate with its host community, its message will not be viewed with suspicion. These channels have a wider reach because they cover those who do not know how to read or write. This means of communication is usually helpful when a university wants to organize sensitization programmes such as healthcare awareness, skills acquisition, etc. The possible consequences that universities could bear include lack of participation or low turnout since the message was not understood, inappropriate development efforts, waste of finances, resources, and time (Mundy & Lloyd-Laney, 1992).

Since communication bridges an institution with its host community, the use of appropriate language by universities for communicating, relating and transacting with host communities becomes essential. The reason is that the indigenous language of a university's environment in most cases is different from the official language of that university. To ensure that there is mutual communication between parties, it is needful for the native language of the community to be used applied conscientiously. If the university fails to do this and sticks to English language as official language, there would be dissonance and lacuna that would put university-community relationship in harm's way. For instance, Covenant University founded by Bishop David Oyedepo is hosted by the Ota community in Ogun State, Nigeria. Its indigenous neighbours speak Yoruba language while English is the official language of the university. Igbo-speaking Nsukka, Asadu, Ideke, and Alumona are host communities of English-speaking University of Nigeria, South East Nigeria. Midwest Nigeria, the official language of Ambrose Alli University is English whereas the people of Ekpoma, its host community speak Esan. These examples showcase contradictions which are antithetical to mutual understanding in a communal geo-axis. To counter this possibility, universities need to be savvy about their relationships with their stakeholders including their host communities. In other words, whenever Covenant University for instance, has to communicate with its host community, the university will have to act local and its representatives speak Yoruba. In similar circumstances, officials of University of Nigeria and Ambrose Ali University should speak Igbo and Ishan languages respectively. Appropriate language holds the key for unlocking the heart of host community as noted by Nwadike (2004).

There are many reasons why host communities desire guest universities to be language-friendly. Five reasons identified by scholars (Emeka-Nwobia, 2015; Dooga, 2012; Amery, 2017) are as follows:

1. The slow death of indigenous languages: The linguistic landscape of Nigeria is gradually eroding the demand for indigenous languages. With hundreds of indigenous languages, the country's attention is on three (Igbo, Yoruba and Hausa). Knowledge and proficiency in English language is a requirement for gaining university admission, accessing job opportunities, transacting business online, attracting friendship and attention on social media; and engaging in intertribal, interethnic and interregional marriages. Procreation through medical support and parenting are functionally based on English language.

Even the adults who attempt to speak local languages, code-mix in order to communicate. Ethnic group clashes, religious and political issues are practically being settled with English. Waning and dying languages could lead to the loss of affected peoples' heritage and culture. So, indigenous people try very hard to be attached to their language and culture even in welcoming institutions of divergent semantics. Faced with slow death of their languages indigenous people of Nigeria struggle to reverse the trend as much as possible.

2. Misinterpretations: Amery (2017) shares an experience where the Yolŋu students (north-east Arnhem Land) in Australia misinterpreted the idiomatic expression "He chucked his guts up" to mean literally "he ripped out his intestines and threw them in the air." The author explains that even simple little things that might be said, such as "let's keep an eye on it", could be baffling, because these expressions are often taken literally by the indigenous people. Thus, every human community has a language through which its members communicate and they communicate better with one another because this language is indigenous to them. Universities are not in communities to impress the indigenous people but to get and apply their lingo for mutual benefits and peaceful coexistence.
3. Different worldviews: even in a community where members seemingly speak good English, miscommunication could arise from differences in worldview. Amery again recounts an experience with a fellow health worker, about the location of a place. The colleague referred to various landmarks such as trees and rocks to describe the location. When asked about street names, the person could not come up with any. Meanwhile, they conversed with full understanding, but Amery could not follow the directions. Amery never paid attention to those landmarks and the colleague never noticed street names. This was not a linguistic issue but a matter of different worldviews. The university operates in its own world or space different from that of the community. The university must study what is more important to its host community and operate by it to succeed.

CONCLUSION AND RECOMMENDATIONS

Communication is the life blood of universities. None develops in the absence of effective corporate communication system. Corporate communication involves giving, getting, processing and highlighting information. It is essential to the delivery of data, creating awareness and ensuring public participation. The role of language in human society is indispensable. It provides means for social function, role management and mutually beneficial relationships between universities and their host communities. The relationship between universities and their host communities the world over ought to be a symbiotic one; and a mutually-reinforcing intercourse characterized by inter-dependence and solidarity. It is not expected to be otherwise, since, in addition to its core mandate of teaching and research, universities, and in particular Nigerian universities, are charged with community service and rural development.

Universities profit from having a presence in the community. Well managed community relations comes with the winning support and understanding of the community of an institution. It enhances the skills of the employees. While they are out working with the community, they often learn at an increased pace. Skills employees mostly developed through community relations activities are communication, collaboration, leadership, teamwork and creative thinking. Thus, it is recommended that when carrying out community relations activities, universities should allocate task to their employees and students to encourage creativity and personal growth. However, research shows that none of these would be possible without good communication system to enhance understanding between universities and their host communities. Also, from research, a growing number of organizations recognize the value of corporate communication and are adapting their budgets and structures accordingly (Milas *et al.*, 2014). Universities are advised to do the same for its overall benefit.

Where university public relations practitioners cannot understand indigenous languages, they could use simple English, engage interpreters, use pictures, diagrams and illustrations to encourage better interaction. Additionally, communication units in universities could look out and get an indigenous speaker as a staff of the unit to foster understanding between institutions and their host communities. Communities may not be trusting, but universities could equip or fund their vigilante group, employ their children, empower their youths, provide social amenities and so on. It is important for universities to know and understand the culture of their host communities. For instance, silence plays an important role in indigenous cultures. Indigenous people take time to open up to strangers, thus, during conversations, they often respond to questions after a prolonged pause, a concept foreign to the elite generation in universities. The pause could be to study and digest what the public relations officer is offering or proposing that the university would do for the community if they are given the privilege to be in their community.

FURTHER RESEARCH DIRECTION

The need for more discourses on the use of indigenous language for corporate communication practices in universities is pertinent, especially, for communication between universities and their host communities. Community relations activities carried out by universities in languages that are alien to their communities could result in unrests, mutual suspicion and hostilities. These problems could deny universities the steady benefits of peace, integrity and lasting goodwill. Thus, further research could look at ways in which public relations professionals in universities could study the indigenous languages and culture of their host communities; and the strategic ways they could engage the community people in the university to foster goodwill besides employment.

Studies could also be carried out on how universities could enhance their relationship and maintain smooth communication lines with their host communities using the various indigenous communication techniques and media.

REFERENCES

Adamu, A. A. (2010). The advance of the global English (language) and the future of Nigerian languages. A Journal of the Department of English, Gombe State University, Nigeria, 1, 159 – 165.

Adedimeji, M. A. (2009). Basic principles of effective writing. In V. A. Alabi, & S. T. Babatunde (Eds.), *The Use of English in Higher Education*. Ilorin, Nigeria: General Studies Division, University of Ilorin.

Adegbija, E. (1992). Survival strategies for minority languages: The case study of Oko. *ITL Review of Applied Linguistics*, *3*(104), 19–38.

Adegbite, A. B. (2010). *English language usage, uses and misuse(s) in a non-host second language context Nigeria. Inaugural lecture series 231*. OAU, Ile-Ife.

Amery, R. (2017). Recognising the communication gap in Indigenous health care. Retrieved from https://www.mja.com.au/system/files/issues/207_01/10.5694mja17.00042.pdf

Amodu, L., Alege, P., Oluwatobi, S., & Ekanem, T. (2017). The effect of human capital development on employees' attitude to work in insurance industry in Nigeria. *The Journal of Organizational Management Studies*, *2017*, 1–12. doi:10.5171/2017.494914

Amodu, L. O. (2013). *Community relations strategies and conflict resolution in Niger Delta: A study of three major oil companies*. Germany: LAP Lambert Academic Publishing.

Argenti, P., & Forman, J. (2002). *The power of corporate communication: Crafting the voice and image of your business*. New York: McGraw-Hill.

Bittner, J. R. (1989). *Mass communication: An introduction.* New Jersey: Prentice Hall.

Brann, C. M. B. (1990). The role and function of language in government language policy issues in Nigeria. *Sociolinguistics, 1*, 1–19.

Chima, A. N. E. (2012). Nigerian languages as veritable tools for conflict management. *Knowledge Review, 24*(1), 1–7.

Davis, L. (2017). Addressing indigenous language loss by unsettling the linguistic hierarchies entrenched in Canada's language policies. *Working Papers of the Linguistics Circle of the University of Victoria, 27*(1), 52-78.

Dooga, J. T. (2012). Nigeria languages: Failing health and possible healing. *An International Journal of Language, Literature, and Gender Studies. AFRREV LALIGENS, 1*(1), 76–95.

Ekanem, T., Olatunji, R., Amodu, L., Odiboh, O., Yartey, D., Adesina, E., & Adeyeye, B. (2018). A case for e-teaching and e-learning of destination public relations in Nigeria. In *Proceedings of the 31st International Business Information Management Association Conference (IBIMA)*, Milan, Italy. Academic Press.

Emeka-Nwobia, N. U. (2015). The place of indigenous Nigerian languages in national development. *Research on Humanities and Social Sciences, 5*(12), 112–117.

Goodman, M. B. (2006). Corporate communication practice and pedagogy at the dawn of the new millennium. *Corporate Communications, 1*(3), 196–213. doi:10.1108/13563280610680803

Hendrix, J. A. (2004). *Public relations cases* (6th ed.). Belmont, CA: Wadsworth/ Thomson Learning.

Iordache-Platis, M., & Josan, I. (2009). Communication efficiency within higher education institutions: The case of Romania. *European Research Studies, 12*(2), 55–70.

Johan, M. R. M., & Noor, N. A. Z. A. (2013). The role of corporate communication in building organization's corporate reputation: An exploratory analysis. *Interdisciplinary Journal of Contemporary Research in Business, 4*(12), 1230–1240.

Kotler, P., & Keller, K. L. (2009). *Marketing management* (13th ed.). London, UK: Pear Prentice-Hall.

Mundy, P., & Lloyd-Laney, M. (1992). Indigenous communication. *Appropriate Technology, 19*(2), 103–105.

Ndubueze, N., Odiboh, O., Nwosu, E., & Olabanjo, J. (2019). Awareness and perception of public relations practices in public tertiary institutions in Nigeria. In *Proceedings of the 33rd International Business Information Management Association (IBIMA)*, Granada, Spain. Academic Press.

Odiboh, O. O. (2002). Integrated marketing communication. Lagos, Nigeria: Advertising Practitioners Council of Nigeria (APCON).

Odiboh, O. O., & Ekanem, T. (2018). Teaching and learning of integrated marketing communication in three leading Nigerian universities. In *Proceedings of the 31st International Business Information Management Association Conference (IBIMA)*, 6625-6638. Milan, Italy. Academic Press.

Olabanjo, O., Odiboh, O., Nwosu, E., & Ndubueze, N. (2019). Public relations practices in local government and traditional institutions in Nigeria. In *Proceedings of the 33rd International Business Information Management Association (IBIMA)*, Granada, Spain. Academic Press.

Olatunji, R. W. (2013). Uses of semiotics in periods of hostilities, armed conflicts and peace building among the Yoruba, South-West, Nigeria. An International Journal of Arts and Humanities Bahir Dar, Ethiopia, 2(4), 8, 247-261.

Olatunji, R. W. (2018). Trends in advertising and cultures in Nigeria. *Communication Cultures in Africa*, *1*(1), 54–76. doi:10.21039/cca.5

Onabajo, O. (2013). *Elements and practice of international public relations*. Ibadan, Nigeria: College Press & Publishers Limited.

Oyero, O. S. (2003). Indigenous language radio for development purposes. In E. O. Soola (Ed.), *Communicating for Development Purposes*. Ibadan, Nigeria: Krafts Books.

Oyero, O. S. (2007). Dynamics of indigenous languages in environmental communication. In I. E. Nwosu, & O. E. Soola (Eds.), *Communication in Global, ICTs & Ecosystem Perspectives: Insights from Nigeria*. Enugu, Nigeria: Precision Publishers Ltd.

Oyesomi, K. O., & Salawu, A. (2019). Assessing the Uniqueness of Indigenous Language in Advertising: Analysis of Figurative Language Used in Selected Telecommunication Yoruba Advertisement in Nigeria. *Qualitative Report*, *24*(10), 2574–2591. Retrieved from https://nsuworks.nova.edu/tqr/vol24/iss10/12

Robbin, A. (2012). The place of the media, public relations, and consultation in community development. In O. Olufemi (Ed.), *Issues and Trends in Advertising and Public Relations Practices*. Ibadan, Nigeria: College Press & Publishers Limited.

Salawu, A. (2006). Paradox of a milieu: Communicating in African indigenous languages in the age of globalization. In A. Salawu (Ed.), Indigenous Language Media in Africa. Lagos, Nigeria: Centre for Black and African Arts and Civilization (CBAAC).

Siddiqui, M. S. (2019). *Use of indigenous language for conflict resolution.* Retrieved from https://www.researchgate.net/publication/331310662_Use_of_indigenous_language_for_conflict_resolution

KEY TERMS AND DEFINITIONS

Communication: It is the exchange of relevant information between universities and their host communities.

Community Relations: It is a specialized arm of public relations that focuses on building mutual and profitable relationships between a university and its host communities.

Corporate Communication: This refers to the deliberate and strategic creation and management of relationships between an organisation and its various publics through the use of a variety of integrated communication methods to achieve mutual understanding and realize organisational goals whilst serving that organisation's publics' interests. In this study, corporate communication refers to those activities that are carried out by information units of universities.

Indigenous: This refers to the characteristics of people inhabiting a particular region.

Indigenous Language: This refers to a tribal, vernacular, local language of a people that originated from a specified place. It is spoken, owned, shared amongst a set of people.

Mutually Beneficial Relationship: This is a polite display of friendliness, based on mutual respect, towards another person or group of people. Mutual relationship is not one that is necessarily void of unrests, mutual suspicion and hostilities, but one in which provision is made for proper settlement that is acceptable to all the parties involved.

Public Relations: This is the management function that helps to establish and maintain mutually beneficial relationships, goodwill, understanding, acceptance, agreement and cooperation between groups, organisations, and their various internal and external publics. In this study, public relations refer to those activities carried out by information units in support of universities' organisation and goals.

Chapter 14
The Language Challenge of Diabetes Information and Education in Nigeria's Multi-Lingual Setting

Chinyere Azuka Mbaka
https://orcid.org/0000-0002-1268-9904
Mountain Top University, Nigeria

ABSTRACT

Diabetes is a major health challenge in the world, but it can be effectively managed or controlled through diabetes information and education. However, none has dwelt on the language dynamics of communication interactions despite the fact that Nigeria is a multi-lingual nation. Therefore, the study investigates the language challenges faced by persons living with diabetes (PLWDs) and diabetes educators (DEs) in the course of diabetes education in the urban and semi-urban centres of Nigeria. Qualitative methods used to gather information from 120 diabetes patients selected from three health facilities in Ogun and Lagos states. The findings reveal that most diabetes educators use the English language to educate their patients. Reason being that of ease, unavailability of most diabetes education materials in the local languages and a heterogeneous audience made up of different ethnic groups. It is recommended that diabetes educators use locally prepared pamphlets and materials for inclusiveness and good understanding of their patients.

DOI: 10.4018/978-1-7998-2091-8.ch014

INTRODUCTION

The role of language in communication and hence development cannot be over emphasized. Development information given through appropriate channels using a generally acceptable and inclusive language produces the required result among the target audience. Health as a very important determinant for development is one sector where information exchange or communication between health personnel and patients should be unambiguous so as not to give room for misinformation and misconceptions which could lead to dangerous health outcomes. Language can cause divisions as well as bring unity among a people as exemplified in the Biblical story of the tower of Babel. A health message delivered in the language of the audience is more likely to be easily understood and accepted than the one in another (foreign) language. The ability of language to alienate and also disenfranchise non speakers makes it a powerful tool that should not be neglected in any development discourse, especially health care. For a development venture to be effective, all parties should be carried along from the planning stage to the implementation and evaluation stages. This participatory approach promotes just, peaceful and inclusive societies as Goal 16 of the Sustainable Development Goals (SDG 16) advocates.

BACKGROUND

Diabetes is a debilitating health condition which affects over/about 382 million cases in the world, (IDF Atlas, 2013). It occurs as a result of the inability of the body to produce enough insulin or absorb and use the already produced one. Its etiology is not fully known and is said to have no cure but can be effectively controlled or managed without leading to its many co-morbidities or even death.

According to IDF Atlas (2013), Nigeria has diabetes prevalence of 5.0% and is estimated to rise to 5.7% by 2030 because of the high rate of industrialisation and modernisation which has affected people's lifestyle negatively. The figure makes Nigeria the highest in Africa alongside Senegal and Cote d'Ivoire sharing the same figure. Efforts have been made by researchers in the health-related fields such as medicine, nursing, biochemistry and pharmacognosy at investigating the causes, signs and symptoms and the treatment and/or management options for diabetes. However, these efforts are not sufficient for the fight against diabetes without taking other social, cultural, economic and religious factors that may affect one's health into consideration. According to Parrot (2004), health determinants are not only medical or clinical as there are many other factors or variables that affect health outcome. Therefore, the application and integration of communication activities in the health sector is important to address the behavioural and other variables that affect health outcomes, which may not be addressed by the medical sciences.

Information is said to be key to diabetes prevention and management (Maina, Ndegwa, Njenga and Mucheni, 2010) as it helps PLWDs gather knowledge about the health condition and be better informed. In line with this, Diabetes Educators (DEs) are employed in diabetes clinics to educate PLWDs on the five cardinal areas of diabetes management: diet, exercise, foot care, medication adherence and blood sugar monitoring. Other media or channels (pamphlets, wall posters, and healthcare personnel-patient interaction) are also employed to disseminate information about diabetes. The knowledge acquired through these sources helps the PLWDs to assess their diabetes risk level, motivates them to seek and adhere to appropriate treatment and care and equips them with the necessary behavioural skills to be in control of their health (Moodley & Rambiritch, 2007). This holistic kind of knowledge, however, can only be gained through diabetes information and education given in a language that is mutually intelligible and culturally acceptable to the audience. In a nation such as Nigeria, with over 450 languages, this poses a big challenge. Previous diabetes health studies have focused on the communication media and strategies used by the diabetes educators and the clinical and self-management methods they advise (Mbaka, 2018) and medicinal plant research to ascertain the diabetes treatment properties of some herbs (Mbaka, G. O., Adeyemi, O. O., and Adesina, S. A. 2010). With the ongoing awareness and advocacies at different fora, such as British Council's Language and Development Conferences, about the impact of local/ indigenous languages as powerful tools for communicating culturally accessible and acceptable health messages, there is a need to investigate the language used by Diabetes Educators in some urban and semi-urban diabetes clinics in educating and informing the PLWDs about diabetes. The effectiveness or otherwise of the diabetes education needs to be measured especially in a multi-lingual nation such as Nigeria.

Nigeria's Multi-Lingual Setting

Nigeria is a country of over 190 million people in West Africa (World Population Prospects, 2019) and is easily the most populous country in Africa. The country is divided into six geopolitical zones for easy administration. Nigeria is a multi-cultural and multi-lingual nation. There are about 250 ethnic groups and over 500 indigenous languages in Nigeria. These figures portray the multi-cultural and multi-lingual dimensions of the country. The major ethnic groups in the country are Igbo, Yoruba, and Hausa and so their languages (Igbo, Yoruba and Hausa) are predominantly spoken. Other ethnicities and languages are Fulani, Ijaw, Itshekiri, Tiv, Urhobo, Kanuri, etc.

There is no unifying indigenous national language in Nigeria. The British colonized Nigeria and handed down their language, education and religion to the nation and so English became the official language of communication in the country. People felt that the language gap and mutual suspicion that exist among the various ethnic groups can be bridged by adopting a foreign language as the lingua franca. Thus English became a unifying language. A variant of the English language called 'pidgin' is also spoken by the less educated class and at informal settings.

Internal migration, which is a movement of people from one part of the country to another as a result of many factors such as economic, security, natural disasters, etc, has contributed to the influx of people, from different parts of the country, into the urban and semi-urban areas. Some of the urban and semi-urban areas include Lagos and its environs and Sagamu in Ogun state, which are the locations for the present study. The internal migrants therefore contribute to the variety of Nigerian languages spoken in the urban and semi-urban areas and also the cultures practiced. Lagos is a cosmopolitan city. It is called a mini Nigeria because almost all ethnic groups can be found in the city.

Language and Communication in Health

Health is often defined as the general condition of the mind and the body of an individual. Health is a very important aspect of life because it determines to a large extent the quality of life one lives. The maxim 'Health is wealth' aptly captures the essence. Communication has been acknowledged as a means of educating, influencing and motivating people for action. This can happen at all levels of communication through the various media. The role of communication in health care is that of information, education and motivation. The information one has about a particular health condition helps such one to assess one's risk level and seek for solutions in time in case of any danger.

Communication in health can happen at different levels – health care provider-patient level of communication, patient-patient level of communication and patient-care-giver level of communication. The most important level is health care provider-patient communication level. This is the communication between the doctor/nurse/any other health personnel and the patient. In all the levels, the channel of communication is opened through the medium of language. If there is a language gap between a doctor (for instance) and the patient, a problem has already been created. When patient and health care provider share the same language, the patient would be able to explain explicitly his/her health condition and the health personnel would be in a better position to make informed and correct diagnosis.

Scholars agree that good doctor-patient communication is necessary for effective health care delivery as it helps patients to build trust with their health care provider which in turn lead to more openness and self-disclosure, which are all important for correct diagnosis and treatment (Fernandez, Schillinger, Grumbach, Rosenthal, Stewart, Wang and Perez Stable, 2004; Jacobs, Chen, Karliner, Agger-Gupta and Mutha, 2006). It also leads to patient satisfaction which most times guarantees medication adherence and keeping of future hospital appointments. Doctor-patient communication can only be effective when it is done using the native language shared by both parties in the communicative situation.

STUDY OBJECTIVES

1. To determine the extent the local languages are used for diabetes education in Nigerian urban and semi-urban diabetes clinics.
2. To establish the knowledge level about diabetes and its management among study participants.
3. To determine the extent the local language use for diabetes education can influence improved diabetes knowledge and positive attitude to diabetes self-management practices among PLWDs.

METHODOLOGY

Qualitative study approach was adopted for the study using Focus Group Discussion (FGD), In-depth Interview (IDI) and Participant Observation (PO) as methods of collecting data. According to Marshall and Rossman (2006), qualitative research is 'pragmatic, investigative and grounded in lived experiences of people'. It is suitable for the purpose of this study as the study explores the lived experiences of PLWDs as it concerns their communications and interactions with their health care providers at the diabetes centres.

Three reputable and highly patronized diabetes clinics were purposively selected. Two of them are in Ogun state, Nigeria – Olabisi Onabanjo University Teaching Hospital (OOUTH) Sagamu and Talabi diabetes Centre (TDC) Isara, while one is in Lagos state, Nigeria – Lagos State University Teaching Hospital (LASUTH) Ikeja. The systematic sampling method was used to select 40 diabetic patients from each of the diabetes centre chosen for the study making a total of 120 participants in all. Research approval was got from the research and ethics committee of the hospitals and the informed consent of the participants obtained before the study was conducted.

Four sessions of FGD comprising 10 participants each was conducted in each centre – two in Yoruba language (the spoken native language) and two in English language (the official language). Participants were assigned to a session based on their preference and convenience. Six health professionals, two from each centre, were also interviewed. The researcher was also present at the diabetes education sessions at the centres and was able to observe the sessions firsthand. Data generated were coded and analysed using the thematic approach and explanation building for qualitative content analysis.

FINDINGS AND DISCUSSION

The findings and discussion are presented under three sub-headings, reflecting the objectives of the study. They are presented as follows:

Extent of Local Language Use for Diabetes Education

From the findings, local languages are rarely used for Diabetes Education (DE) at two of the clinics (OOUTH and LASUTH) selected for the study. The health personnel interviewed disclosed this and it was also confirmed by the researcher through participant observations of the DE sessions. A female nurse interviewed at one of the centres (LASUTH) expressed frustration at the number of ethnicities that visit the clinic. In her word:

How do you expect us to speak everyone's language? The Diabetes Educator can only speak one Nigerian language and that is Yoruba and to avoid being accused of discrimination by other non-Yoruba patients, she cannot even speak it. We speak English to everyone, it's more common.

Another female nurse in support of her colleague jokingly added, "This is Lagos now. They will understand". In order words, they assume that since Lagos is a cosmopolitan city, it is expected that all residents should be able to understand the official language of communication, which is English. Another reason adduced is lack of diabetes information, education and communication (IEC) materials in the native languages. Most of the materials are written in English.

At the OOUTH, it was observed that they make use of interpreters (nurses and other ancillary workers) who translate into English what the Diabetes Educator says in Yoruba language. Note that the location is Yoruba land and so is predominantly populated by the Yoruba speaking people of Nigeria. The problem with the interpretation method, as identified by the patients, is that most of the vital information is lost during translation. One of the patients said, "What the interpreter does is summary, not interpretation. How can you interpret a ten minutes talk in 2 minutes? So many things will be left out for sure". An elderly male patient, whose native language is not Yoruba and could barely understand English, expressed indifference at the entire scenario. He preferred to come to the clinic when the DE would have been over, see his doctor in the company of his son and go home. He said, "My daughter don't worry, I'm here to see the doctor, not all these talk talk that I don't even understand. Once I see him with my son (obviously for better communication with the doctor), I go home". The use of interpreters may not be the best option in a health care setting as studies have found that most times the interpreters omit important utterances of either the health care provider or the patient and this can affect the entire process (Sleptsova, Weber, Schopf, Nubling, Morina, Hofer and Langewitz, 2017). In another study, it was found that interpretation affects the flow of emotions and the empathy that go with the interactions between a health care provider and the patient (Krystallidou, Remael, de Boe, Hendrickx, Tsakitzidis, van de Geuchte and Pype, 2018).

TDC is the only centre where DE was done solely in the native language with no concurrent interpretation into English. The centre is the most rural of all the three centres. Most of the patients there are from Yoruba speaking part of Nigeria or speak the language.

Knowledge Level about Diabetes among Persons Living with Diabetes (PLWDs)

Discussants at the Focus Group Discussion (FGD) Sessions, who are all Persons Living with Diabetes (PLWD) showed remarkably low knowledge level in the key areas of diabetes management – diet, blood sugar monitoring, foot care and exercises. Many of them could not identify clearly the types, causes, symptoms and complications of diabetes. This corroborates the findings of Achigbu, E.O., Oputa, R.N., Achigbu, K.I. and Ahuche, I.U (2015) which found low knowledge level about causes of diabetes among their study population in south eastern part of Nigeria.

In response to the question on the causes of diabetes, one of the discussants at the FGD simply said, "Too much of anything sugary can cause diabetes". Another discussant explained further, "That is why I have stopped drinking Coke and Fanta and I don't even put sugar in my tea". The identification of sugary food and drinks as a major cause of diabetes is fast becoming a dangerous myth among the people as is also corroborated in the result of a study done in India (Rai and Kishore, 2009). This gave birth to the name 'sugar disease' used in reference to the diabetes disease among the North Indian population. This also is the case among the study population as diabetes is translated as *'ito shuga'* in Yoruba language meaning 'sugar urine'. The danger in this is that other causes of diabetes are less emphasised or totally ignored. This explains some of the misconceptions that gave birth to some of the attitudes that surround diabetes self-management behaviours among the study population. It was observed during the group discussions that most of the discussants diligently avoid taking sugary food and drinks, while still eating other forms of carbohydrates in large quantities, drinking alcohol, exercising little and missing their clinical check-ups. This, they do in the erroneous belief that taking of sugary food and drinks is the major cause of diabetes. It is somewhat ironical that some of the discussants prefer taking the so called bitter soft drinks such as 'Bitter Lemon' and 'Schwepps' in the erroneous belief that they contain less sugar as is expressed by one of the female discussants, "I take only 'Schwepps' because it is bitter. It doesn't have much sugar". When the discussants were asked to describe their daily meal plan, it was discovered that some of them did not know what constitutes a balanced meal for a diabetes patient. Carbohydrate foods dominated their daily meal plan. This simply exposed their ignorance. Carbohydrates, when broken down in the body are converted to glucose (sugar); therefore, excess of it is not good for a diabetes patient.

Many of the FGD discussants also alluded to the fact that diabetes is basically hereditary. Some of them believed that they are diabetic simply because it runs in their family, while ignoring other behaviours and habits that predispose one to developing diabetes. Findings also showed that many of the discussants could not differentiate between food types that are high in sugar content and those that are not. From the interviews conducted with the health personnel, it was gathered that the diabetes education and information given to the PLWDs covers the five cardinal areas of diabetes management which includes diet, exercise, blood sugar monitoring, medication adherence and foot care. Therefore, the issue is not the content of the education/information but in the language in which they are communicated.

From the foregoing discussion on the knowledge level of PLWDs about diabetes, it is evident from the findings that the study participants' knowledge of diabetes is coloured by misconceptions and misinformation. Some of these misconceptions are well grounded in their culture such that for them to be cleared, a culturally accessible and acceptable language and medium of communication should be adopted to reach the people and be able to change their perceptions and thus influence their attitude.

Influence of Local Language Use on Diabetes Care and Management Practices

It was observed among the PLWDs, whose clinic (TDC) conducts the DE sessions in the native language (Yoruba), a higher knowledge level about the diabetes management practices such as exercise and food types, care of the feet, identification of symptoms of high blood pressure and temporary measures to take before going to the hospital if one experiences high blood pressure. One of the FGD discussants enthusiastically narrated his surprise when he learnt that cubes of sugar can be taken by a diabetic in some situations. He said:

Before, I believed that sugar in any form is totally bad and is the cause of this condition but here, I learnt that we should keep cubes of sugar in our bags and lick them when we feel excess dizziness and head ache. This will help us temporarily until we get to the hospital to see a Doctor.

The diabetes messages were understood clearly by participants because it was explained to them in their mother tongue. Words, symbols and objects from the language were used to describe diabetes, high blood pressure, low blood pressure, diabetic sore, sugar found in carbohydrates and synthetic sugar and so the concept ceased being foreign to them.

Most of the study participants at TDC exhibited enthusiasm and willingness to come back for the next DE session. When compared with the nonchalant attitude or sheer indifference exhibited by some of their counterparts in the other centres, it was concluded that the language of DE sessions plays a major role in determining its acceptability and level of participation.

Another interesting finding is that some non-Yoruba language speakers that visit TDC complain of disenfranchisement or discrimination. They accuse the centre of being biased against other ethnic groups stating that Nigeria is a multi-cultural society and so no language should be chosen above another. They even preferred the DE sessions to be held in English. With a series of rhetorical questions showing obvious displeasure, one of the female participants (from the southern part of the country) puts it this way, "English is our official language and is understood by everybody. Why should they be speaking only in Yoruba? Is it only Yoruba people that are here? Can't they speak in English so that everyone will understand"? She ended by stating that she would only come to the clinic to get her drugs and never attend the DE session again.

The finding further reveals some of the frustrations and dilemma that health care providers face while using the native language alone for diabetes information and education. One of the diabetes educators interviewed admitted that insufficient number of trained diabetes educators in various languages of the nation and inadequate teaching aids in the various languages are some of their setbacks. Also, another female diabetes educator interviewed pointed out that for fear of being labeled 'bigots' by non-Yoruba speaking patients, they use English and then interpret in Yoruba for those who do not understand clearly. In her words, "You know this is Nigeria, before you know it, they will term it something else, weeping unnecessary sentiment and you know this is a government hospital". From the findings, it is clear that although the use of native language for diabetes education and information leads to high knowledge level of the health condition, which in turn leads to better management practices, in a multilingual society such as Nigeria, it is easier and safer to use the English language, which is the recognized official language of the nation, to avoid generating ethnic bias and sentiments among the PLWDs.

GENERAL FINDINGS

The study found that the dissemination of diabetes information and education at the diabetes clinics studied was a big challenge as a result of Nigeria's multi-lingual nature. The health care providers had a tough time selecting and sticking with a particular language for their message dissemination as any of the languages selected (native or foreign) caused some divisions and problems among the PLWDs.

It was also observed that interpreters were used in some clinics to translate from the native language to English for non-Yoruba speakers. However, some important points are sometimes left while some are misinterpreted in the interpretation process as already found by scholars both in Nigeria (Launer, 1978) and elsewhere (Sleptsova et al, 2017).

Diabetes education rendered in the native tongue of the PLWDs is more understandable, acceptable and adhered to. This is evident from the findings at the TDC, where the participants exhibited high knowledge level about diabetes and high compliance level to diabetes management practices. Majority of the diabetes educators interviewed preferred using the English language for reason of ease, availability of teaching aids and to avoid generating ethnic bias and sentiments.

CONCLUSION

Most participants preferred DE sessions in their native tongues and are more willing to accept and adopt self-management activities explained to them in their native tongue. However, the fact that many diabetics, who patronize these clinics, come from different parts of the country and so speak different languages makes the use of only one language for diabetes information and education at the centres practically unrealistic and unproductive. Hence, there is need for an alternative action which should be taken with all urgency.

RECOMMENDATIONS

There is need for IEC materials to be produced in the local languages to assist the diabetes educators. Professional Interpreters/Translators should be employed and trained in the major ethnic languages to assist diabetes educators at the sessions. There should be a profiling of the PLWDs in every diabetes centre. The native language, level of education and other preferences should be noted and arrangements made to meet the communication needs of PLWDs in the interest of inclusiveness and for better health outcomes.

REFERENCES

Achigbu, E. O., Oputa, R. N., Achigbu, K. I., & Ahuche, I. U. (2015). Knowledge and of diabetes in patients in a tertiary clinic in southeast, Nigeria. *African Journal of Diabetes Medicine*, *23*(1), 15–17.

Fernandez, A., Schillinger, D., Grumbach, K., Rosenthal, A., Stewart, A. L., Wang, F., & Pérez-Stable, E. J. (2004). Physician language ability and cultural competence. *Journal of General Internal Medicine*, *19*(2), 167–174. doi:10.1111/j.1525-1497.2004.30266.x PMID:15009796

International Diabetes Federation. (2013). IDF Diabetes Atlas, 6th Ed. Retrieved May 12, 2016, from http://www.idf.org

Jacobs, E., Chen, A., Karliner, L. S., Agger-Gupta, N., & Mutha, S. (2006). The need for more research on language barriers in health care: A proposed research agenda. *The Milbank Quarterly*, *84*(1), 111–133. doi:10.1111/j.1468-0009.2006.00440.x PMID:16529570

Krystallidou, D., Remael, A., de Boe, E., Hendrickx, K., Tsakitzidis, G., van de Geuchte, S. W., & Pype, P. (2018). Investigating empathy in interpreter-mediated consultations: an explorative study. *Patient Education Council 101*(1): 33-42. doi:. doi:10.1016/j.pec.2017.07.022

Launer, J. 1978. Taking medical histories through interpreters: practice in a Nigerian outpatient department. *British Medical Journal* 2(6142): 934-935. doi:. doi:10.1136/bmj.2.6142.934

Maina, W. K., Ndegwa, Z. M., Njenga, E. W., & Mucheni, E. W. (2010). Knowledge, and practices related to diabetes among community members in four provinces in Kenya: A cross sectional study. *The Pan African Medical Journal*, *7*, 2–5. PMID:21918691

Marshall, C., & Rossman, G. B. (2006). *Designing Qualitative Research* (4th ed.). Thousand Oaks, CA: Sage.

Mbaka, G. O., Adeyemi, O. O., & Adesina, S. A. (2010). Anti-diabetic activity of the seed extract of Sphenocentrum Jollyanum and morphological changes on pancreatic beta cells. *Journal of Medicine and Medical Sciences*, *1*(11), 550–556.

Mbaka. (2018). Influence of diabetes information and education on diabetes self-management and prevention in Ogun and Lagos states, Nigeria. Thesis, University of Ibadan.

Moodley, L. M., & Rambiritch, V. (2007). An assessment of the level of knowledge diabetes mellitus among diabetic patients in a primary health care setting. *South African Family Practice*, *49*(10), 16–18. doi:10.1080/20786204.2007.10873652

Parrot, R. (2004). Emphasizing communication in health communication. *Journal of Communication*, *54*(4), 751–787. doi:10.1111/j.1460-2466.2004.tb02653.x

Rai, M., & Kishore, J. (2009). Myths about diabetes and its treatment in North Indian population. *International Journal of Diabetes in Developing Countries*, *29*(3), 129–135. doi:10.4103/0973-3930.54290 PMID:20165650

Sleptsova, M., Weber, H., Schöpf, A. C., Nübling, M., Morina, N., Hofer, G., & Langewitz, W. (2017). Using interpreters in medical consultations: what is said and what is translated – a descriptive analysis using RIAS. *Patient Education Council, 100*(9): 1667-1671. doi:. doi:10.1016/j.pec

World Population Prospects. (2019). World Population Review. Retrieved from www.un.org.publications

KEY TERMS AND DEFINITIONS

Diabetes Education: A deliberate process through which people with, or at risk of, diabetes gain necessary knowledge and skill required to modify behaviour and successfully self-manage the disease and its related conditions.

Diabetes Information: These are basic facts and information about diabetes condition such as types, causes, symptoms, care and management which can be communicated through any medium (formal and informal) to both diabetics and non-diabetics.

Diabetes Mellitus (DM): A chronic disorder of carbohydrate, fat and protein metabolism, having hyperglycaemia (high blood sugar level) as a common feature.

Diabetes Misconceptions: These are wrong beliefs or notions about diabetes.

Health Promotion: The process of using various communication strategies to help people gain control of health determinants and achieve better health status.

Indigenous Language: This is the language that is native to a particular group of people and spoken by the indigenous people living in the locality.

Language Acceptability: The ability of a language to be termed appropriate or suitable by a group of people based on certain indices.

Language Accessibility: The ability of people to read, write and carry out other activities using a particular language.

Compilation of References

Abdulhamid, Z., Lawal, U. S., Tahir, A. A., Harande, M. M., Usman, H., & Nuhu, A. (2017). Perceptions of Hausa and Fulani Tribes on Traditional Birth Attendants in Zaria Local Government Area, Kaduna State, Nigeria. *Journal of Complementary and Alternative Medical*, *2*(2), 1–7. doi:10.9734/JOCAMR/2017/27773

Abimbola, K. (2006). *Yoruba Culture: A Philosophical Account*. Birmingham: Iroko Academic Publishers.

AbouZahr, C. (2003). Safe Motherhood: A brief history of the global movement 1947–2002. *British Medical Bulletin*, *67*(1), 13–25. doi:10.1093/bmb/ldg014 PMID:14711751

Abrahams, N., Jewkes, R., & Mvo, Z. (2002). Indigenous healing practices and self-medication amongst pregnant women in Cape Town, South Africa. [PubMed]. *African Journal of Reproductive Health*, *6*(2), 79–86. doi:10.2307/3583133 PMID:12476719

Achigbu, E. O., Oputa, R. N., Achigbu, K. I., & Ahuche, I. U. (2015). Knowledge and of diabetes in patients in a tertiary clinic in southeast, Nigeria. *African Journal of Diabetes Medicine*, *23*(1), 15–17.

Action Health. (1999). *Meeting the sexual and reproductive health needs of young people in Nigeria: A Guide for Action*. Lagos.

Adamu, A. A. (2010). The advance of the global English (language) and the future of Nigerian languages. A Journal of the Department of English, Gombe State University, Nigeria, 1, 159 – 165.

Adatara, P., Afya, A., Baku, E. A., Salia, S. M., & Asempah, A. (2018) Perspective of Traditional Birth Attendants on Their Experiences and Roles in Maternal Health Care in Rural Areas of Northern Ghana. *International Journal of Reproductive Medicine*, 2018. doi:10.1155/2018/2165627

Adedeji, O. A. (2015). Analysis of Use of English And Indigenous Languages By The Press in Selected African Countries. [OMAN Chapter]. *Arabian Journal of Business and Management Review*, *4*(8), 35–45.

Adedimeji, M. A. (2009). Globalization and the survival of the Nigerian cultural and linguistic heritage: The American paradigm. *The Sociolinguistics of English and Nigerian Languages*, 69-87.

Adedimeji, M. A. (2009). Basic principles of effective writing. In V. A. Alabi, & S. T. Babatunde (Eds.), *The Use of English in Higher Education*. Ilorin, Nigeria: General Studies Division, University of Ilorin.

Adedina, F., & Taiwo, V. (2018). Ẹkun-ìyàwo: An Aesthetical Appraisal of Nuptial Chants in Yoruba Folklore. *Journal of Communication and Media Research*, *10*(2), 161–173.

Adedokun, S., & Adedokun, A. (2016). Evaluation of the knowledge about attitude to HIV/AIDS and sexual practice among senior secondary school students in Ota Ogun State. *International Journal of Management Sciences*, *9*(1), 161–174.

Adegbija, E. (1992). Survival strategies for minority languages: The case study of Oko. *ITL Review of Applied Linguistics*, *3*(104), 19–38.

Adegbite, W. (2002) The promotion of reading habits in Yoruba and English through the media: Case study of some media. Activities in Southern Nigeria. *Literacy and Reading in Nigeria* *9*(2).

Adegbite, A. B. (2010). *English language usage, uses and misuse(s) in a non-host second language context Nigeria. Inaugural lecture series 231*. OAU, Ile-Ife.

Adegoke, S. A., & Kuteyi, E. A. (2012). Psychosocial burden of sickle cell disorder on the family, Nigeria. *African Journal of Primary Health Care & Family Medicine*, *4*(1), 1–6. doi:10.4102/phcfm.v4i1.380

Adeleke, D. A. (2003). Culture, Art and Film in an African Society: An Evaluation. *Nordic Journal of African Studies*, *12*(1), 49–56.

Adeniyi, H., & Bello, R. (2006). *Nigerian Media, Indigenous Languages and Sustainable Development. Lagos*. Nigeria: Lagos State University; http://www.lingref.com/cpp/acal/36/paper1419.pdf

Adesokan, F. O. D. (2010). *Reproductive health for all ages*: Ekiti State: Sammy prints.

Adewemimo, A. W., Msuya, S. E., Olaniyan, C. T., & Adegoke, A. A. (2014). Utilisation of skilled birth attendance in Northern Nigeria: A cross-sectional survey: Contents lists available at *Science Direct Journal* homepage: www.elsevier.com/midw

Adeyeye, B., Amodu, L., Odiboh, O., Okorie, N., Adesina, E., Yartey, D., & Ekanem, T. (2019). Data on new media use for agricultural training and research at Agricultural Services and Training Centre (ASTC). *Data in Brief*, *22*, 181–184. doi:10.1016/j.dib.2018.11.031 PMID:30581923

Adeyeye, B., Odiboh, O., Adesina, E., Yartey, D., Ekanem, T., & Ben-Enukora, C. (2018). An examination of Information Communication Technology for Agriculture-Focused Teaching, Learning and Communication Research in the 21st Century. *Proceedings of the 31st International Business Information Management Association Conference (IBIMA)*, pp. 6384- 6390. Milan, Italy.

Adhikari, S. (2018). Pillars of safe motherhood, Retrieved on September 25, 2019 from www.Publichealthnotes.com

Adia, E. A. (2014). Programme element importance: An analysis of telenovela in the Ghanaian media. *International Journal of ICT and Management*, *2*(1), 96–101.

Afolayan, A. (1995). In A. Bamgbose, A. Banjo, & A. Thomas (Eds.), *Ineffectiveness in the Presentation of English in Nigeria: Sources and Remedies. New Englishes: A West African Perspective* (pp. 113–129). Ibadan: Mosuro.

AFRRI. (2008). *Communicating with radio: what do we know? Findings from selected rural radio effectiveness evaluations, African Farm Radio Research Initiative (AFRRI)*. Ottawa, Canada: Farm Radio International.

Agyepong, A. O. (2017). "International Communication: A Narrative of Selected Indigenous Practices of the Akan Group of Ghana" in Handbook of Research on Theoretical Perspectives on Indigenous Knowledge Systems in Developing Countries.

Ahmad, W., Noor, M. A., Afzal, I., Bakhtavar, M. A., Nawaz, M. M., Sun, X., ... Zhao, M. (2016). Improvement of Sorghum Crop through Exogenous Application of Natural Growth-Promoting Substances under a Changing Climate. *Sustainability*, *8*(12), 1330. doi:10.3390u8121330

Ajzen, I. (1991). The theory of planned behaviour. *Organizational Behavior and Human Decision Processes*, *50*(2), 179–211. doi:10.1016/0749-5978(91)90020-T

Ajzen, I. (2005). *Attitude, personality, and behaviour* (2nd ed.). Maidenhead: Open University Press.

Akinleye, J. O. (1988) A comparative study of the cost effectiveness of instructional television and conventional classroom instruction in non-formal education. (Unpublished PhD thesis), University of Ibadan.

Alabi, S. (2003). The Development of Indigenous Language publications in Nigeria Journalism. In R. A. Akinfeleye, & I. E. Okoye (Eds), Issues in Nigeria Media History: 1900-200 AD, pp. 33-50. Lagos, Nigeria: Malthouse Press Limited.

Alam, M. K., & Haque, A. M. (2014). *Contribution of television channels in disseminating agricultural information for the agricultural development of Bangladesh*. Retrieved from http://digitalcommons.unl.edu/libphilprac

Al-hassan, S., Andani, A., & Abdul-Malik, A. (2011). The role of community Radio in livelihood improvement: the case of Simli Radio. *The Journal of Field Action Report*, 5. Retrieved 7th June 2019 from https://journal.openedition.org/factsreports/docannexe/image/869

Aliyu, Z., Tumblin, A., & Kato, G. (2016). Current therapy of sickle cell disease. *Haematologica*, *91*, 7–10. PMID:16434364

Allen, D. (Ed.). (1992). *Women transforming communications: Global interactions*. Thousand Oaks, CA: Sage.

Alvarez, J. L., Gil, R., Hernández, V., & Gil, A. (2009). Factors associated with maternal mortality in Sub-Saharan Africa: An ecological study. *BMC Public Health*, *9*(1), 462. doi:10.1186/1471-2458-9-462 PMID:20003411

Amery, R. (2017) Recognising the communication gap in Indigenous health care. *The Medical Journal of Australia 207*(1), pp. 13-15. doi:. doi:10.5694/mja17.00042

Amery, R. (2017). Recognising the communication gap in Indigenous health care. Retrieved from https://www.mja.com.au/system/files/issues/207_01/10.5694mja17.00042.pdf

Amodu, L. O. (2013). *Community relations strategies and conflict resolution in Niger Delta: A study of three major oil companies*. Germany: LAP Lambert Academic Publishing.

Amodu, L., Alege, P., Oluwatobi, S., & Ekanem, T. (2017). The effect of human capital development on employees' attitude to work in insurance industry in Nigeria. *The Journal of Organizational Management Studies*, *2017*, 1–12. doi:10.5171/2017.494914

Amuseghan, S. A. (2003). Prepositions in Nigerian Standard English Usage: A Study in the Domains of Science and Technology. (Doctoral Thesis), Adekunle Ajasin University, Nigeria.

Amuseghan, S. A. (2008b). *Language Policy Provisions and Curriculum Issues and Challenges in Nigeria*. A paper presented at the 53rd Annual Conference of International Linguistic Association held at Sunny College at Old Westbury, NY.

Amuseghan, S. A., Ayenigbara, G. O., & Orimogunje, T. (2010). Language and health Communication strategies towards effective public health communication programmes in Nigeria. *Journal Media and Communication Studies* 2(5), pp. 111-117, May 2010. Available at http://www.academicjournals.org/jmcs

Amuseghan, S. A. (2008a). 'Language, communication and information flow in entrepreneurship', in *African Journal of Business and Management*, *2*(10), 201–208.

Amuseghan, S., Ayenigbara, G., & Orimogunje, T. (2010, May). Language and health communication strategies towards effective public health communication programmes in Nigeria. *Journal Media and Communication Studies*, *2*(5), 111–117. https://academicjournals.org/article/article1380097791_Amuseghan%20et%20al.pdf

Amutah-Onukagha, N., Gardner, M., & Pierre, K. (2017). Progresses and challenges of utilizing traditional birth attendants in maternal and child health in Nigeria. *International Journal of MCH and AIDS*, *6*(2), 130–138. doi:10.21106/ijma.216 PMID:29367889

Anaeto, S. G., Onabajo, S. O., & Osifeso, J. B. (2008). *Models and Theories of Communication*. Maryland: African Renaissance Books Incorporated.

Anderman, S., Bamodu, G., Dine, J., Blecher, M., Brennan, F., & Freeman, M. (2006). *Human rights and capitalism: a multidisciplinary perspective on globalisation*. Edward Elgar.

Ani, A. O. (2001). *The essence of monitoring and evaluation in extension delivery*. A paper presented at a training Workshop on Extension Communication for ADPs.

Ansu-Kyeremeh, K. (1998). Perspectives on indigenous communication in Africa: Theory and applications. School of communication studies, University of Ghana, Legion.

Ansu-Kyeremeh, K. (Ed.). (2005). *Indigenous Communication in Africa: Concept, Application, and Prospects*. Accra: Ghana Universities Press.

Ansu-Kyeremeh, K., Richter, M., Villianatos, H., & Aniteye, P. (2016). Rural women's exposure to health messages and understandings of health. *Journal of Health Care Communications, 1*(3), 18.

Argenti, P., & Forman, J. (2002). *The power of corporate communication: Crafting the voice and image of your business*. New York: McGraw-Hill.

Aristotle. Poetics. (1987). Translated Stephen Hallowell. Chapel Hill, NC: University of North Carolina Press.

Aristotle.. (1987). Poetics (S. Hal, Trans.).

Attwood, F. (2007). 'Other' or 'one of us'? The porn user in public and academic discourse. *Participations, 4*, 1.

Awofata, A., & Ogundele, O. (2018). HIV epidemiology in Nigeria. *Saudi Journal of Biological Sciences, 25*(4), 697–703. doi:10.1016/j.sjbs.2016.03.006 PMID:29740232

Awoniyi, A. (1995). Determining language in education policy: The dilemma in Africa. In K. Owolabi (Ed.), *Language in Nigeria, Essays in Honour of Ayo Bamgbose*. Ibadan: Group Publishers.

Ayakoroma, B. (2017). Reviving the use of indigenous Languages in the Contemporary Nigerian Society: The National Institute for Cultural Orientation (NICO) Initiatives. *International Journal of Language and Linguistics, 4*(4).

Bagdikian, H. (2000). *The media monopoly*. New York: Beacon Press.

Baggaley, R., Sulwe, J., Burnett, A., & Ndovi, M. (1996). Forging links between the formal and traditional in Zambia. Special report: *Traditional healers*. [PubMed]. *AIDS Analysis Africa, 6*, 12–13. PMID:12290767

Ballas, S. K. (2009). The cost of health care for patients with sickle cell disease. *American Journal of Hematology, 84*(6), 320–322. doi:10.1002/ajh.21443 PMID:19415728

Bamgbose, A. (1991). *Language and the nation: The language question in sub-Saharan Africa*. Great Britain: Edinburgh University Press.

Bandura, A. (2012). Social Cognitive Theory. In P. A. M. Van Lange, A. W. Kruglanski, & E. T. Higgins (Eds.), Handbook of theories of social psychology (pp. 349-373). Thousand Oaks, CA: Sage. doi:10.4135/9781446249215.n18

Bankole, A., Sedgh, G., Okonofua, F., Imarhiagbe, C., Hussain, R., & Wulf, D. (2009). Barriers to Safe Motherhood in Nigeria, New York: Guttmacher Institute. Retrieved from https://www.guttmacher.org/sites/default/files/report_pdf/motherhoodnigeria.pdf

Barakat, P., Simon, K., Schwartz, L., & Radcliffe, J. (2016). Correlates of pain rating, Concordance for adolescents with sickle cell disease and their caregivers. *Clinical Pain Journal, 24*(5), 438–446. doi:10.1097/AJP.0b013e3181646038 PMID:18496309

Baran, S. (2014). *Introduction to Mass Communication: Media Literacy and Culture* (8th ed.). Boston, MA: McGraw-Hill.

Batista, J. (2019). *An intersectional analysis of maternal mortality in Sub-Saharan Africa: a human rights issue*. Retrieved from www.jogh.org • doi: Accessed September 25, 2019 doi:10.7189/jogh.09.01032

Bell, M., Payne, J., & Bohn, A. (2011). *ICT Options in Relation to Extension Functions*. MEAS. Available at www.meas-extension.org/resources/ict

Bello, S. (2014). Interrelationship of health communication, health literacy, therapeutic communication and other related concepts. *Journal of Communication and Media Research*, *6*(2), 175–194.

Benson, O., Victor, A., Linda, I., & Ariole, I. A. (2017). "Promoting Indigenous Language in Nigeria: Issues and Challenges for the Library and Information Professionals" Library Philosophy and Practice (e-journal). 1472. Retrieved from http://digitalcommons.unl.edu/libphilprac/1472

Berger, M. (2003). Traditional birth attendants in developing countries cannot be expected to carry out HIV/AIDS prevention and treatment activities. [PubMed]. *Reproductive Health Matters*, *11*(22), 36–40. doi:10.1016/S0968-8080(03)02286-9 PMID:14708396

Bittner, J. R. (1989). *Mass communication: An introduction*. New Jersey: Prentice Hall.

Bland, R. M., Rollins, N. C., Van den Broeck, J., & Coovadia, H. M. (2004). Child Health Group, author. The use of non-prescribed medication in the first 3 months of life in rural South Africa. [PubMed]. *Tropical Medicine & International Health*, *9*(1), 118–124. doi:10.1046/j.1365-3156.2003.01148.x PMID:14728615

Bodeker, G., Carter, G., Burford, G., & Dvorak-Little, M. (2006). HIV/AIDS: Traditional system of health care in the management of a global epidemic. [PubMed]. *Journal of Alternative and Complementary Medicine (New York, N.Y.)*, *12*(6), 563–576. doi:10.1089/acm.2006.12.563 PMID:16884348

Bolarin, O. L. (2013). Language of Communication in the Nigerian Media. *Singaporean Journal of Business Economics and Management Studies*, *1*(11).

Booth, C., Inusa, B., & Obaro, S. K. (2009). Infection in sickle cell disease: A review. *International Journal of Infectious Diseases*, *14*(1). doi:10.1016/j.ijid.2009.03.010 PMID:19497774

Borokini, T. I., & Lawal, I. O. (2014). Traditional Medicine Practices among the Yoruba People of Nigeria: A Historical Perspective. *Journal of Medicinal Plants Studies*, *2*(6), 20–33.

Boyd, B., & Shaw, W. (2009). Unlocking Health Worker Potential: Some Creative Strategies from the field.

Brann, C. M. B. (1990). The role and function of language in government language policy issues in Nigeria. *Sociolinguistics*, *1*, 1–19.

Brieger, W. (1990). Mass media and health communication in rural Nigeria. *Health Policy and Planning*, *5*(1), 77–81. doi:10.1093/heapol/5.1.77

Broughton, G., Brumfit, C., Flavell, R., Hill, P., & Pincas, A. (1978). *Teaching English as a Foreign Language*. London, UK: Routledge and Kegan Paul.

Brumfit, C. (1995). English as a Second Language and English Language Teaching: Retrospect and Prospect. In A. Bamgbose, A. Banjo, & A. Thomas (Eds.), *New Englishes: A West African Perspective* (pp. 99–112). Ibadan: Mosuro.

Bryant, M. (2015). *Conducting observational research*. Retrieved from: https://www.deakin.edu.au/__data/assets/pdf_file/0004/681025/Participant-observation.pdf

Bulterys, M., Fowler, G. M., Shaffer, N., Tih, P., Greenberg, A., Karita, E., ... De Cock, K. (2002). Role of traditional birth attendants in preventing perinatal transmission of HIV. [PMC free article] [PubMed]. *BMJ (Clinical Research Ed.)*, *324*(7331), 222–225. doi:10.1136/bmj.324.7331.222 PMID:11809647

Bunn, H. F., & Forget, B. F. (1977). *Human hematology*. Philadelphia, PA: WB Saunders.

Buor, D., & Bream, K. (2004). An analysis of the determinants of maternal mortality in sub-Saharan Africa. *Journal of Women's Health*, *13*(8), 926–938. doi:10.1089/jwh.2004.13.926 PMID:15671708

Burnett, A., Baggaley, N., Ndovi-Macmillan, M., & Sulwe, J. (1999). *Hang'Omba B*. Bennett J.

Burnett, A., Baggaley, R., Ndovi-Macmillan, M., Sulwe, J., Hang'Omba, B., & Bennett, J. (1999, August). Caring for people with HIV in Zambia: Are traditional healers and formal health workers willing to work together. [PubMed]. *AIDS Care*, *11*(4), 481–491. doi:10.1080/09540129947875 PMID:10533542

Business Dictionary. (2017) *Convenience sampling*. Retrieved from: http://www.businessdictionary.com/definition/convenience-sampling.html 3/5/2017

Cashen, M. S., Dykes, P., & Gerber, B. (2004). E-health technology and Internet Resources. Barrier for Vulnerable Population. *The Journal of Cardiovascular Nursing*, *19*(3), 209–214. doi:10.1097/00005082-200405000-00010 PMID:15191264

CDC. (2018). *Health Communication Strategies*: Available at www.npin.cdc.gov. Accessed on 25th September 2019

Chalaby, J. (2016). Television and globalization: The TV content global value chain. *Journal of Communication*, *66*(1), 1–41. doi:10.1111/jcom.12203

Champion, V., & Skinner, C. S. (2008). The Health Belief Model. In K. Glanz, B. Rimer, & K. Viswanath (Eds.), *Health behavior and health education, 4* (pp. 45–65). San Francisco, CA: Jossey-Bass.

Cheyney, A. B. (1992). *Teaching Reading Skills through the Newspaper*. Newark, DE: International Reading Association.

Chibita, M., & Salawu, A. (2016). Intoduction: Language Structure and Agency: Optimizing Media Diversity in Africa Using the Indigenous Languages. In A. Salawu, & M. B. Chibita (Eds.), *Indigenous Language Media, Language Politics and Democracy in Africa*. London, UK: Palgrave Macmillan.

Chima, A. N. E. (2012). Nigerian languages as veritable tools for conflict management. *Knowledge Review*, *24*(1), 1–7.

Chioma, P. E. (2013). News Commercialization in Nigeria: Undermining Issues in Public Interest for Financial Gains. *International Journal of Innovative Research and Development*.

Chirowa, F., Atwood, S., & Van der Putten, M. (2013). Gender inequality, health expenditure and maternal mortality in sub-Saharan Africa: A secondary data analysis. *African Journal of Primary Health Care & Family Medicine*, *5*(1), 1–5. doi:10.4102/phcfm.v5i1.471

Chiwome, E. (1996) Communicating with children on sexual Issues. In S. Mutsvairo, E. Chiwome, N. E. Mberi, A. Masasire, & M. Furusa (Eds.), Introduction to Shona Culture. pp. 51-64. Kwekwe: Juta Zimbabwe (Pvt) Limited.

Collins English Dictionary. *Language*. Retrieved from: https://www.collinsdictionary.com/dictionary/english/language

Collins, O. F., Banda, Z. M., & Albert, N. D. (2016). The impact of a Community driven Mass Media Campaign on the Utilization of maternal health care services in rural Malawi. Retrieved from https://www.ncbi.nlm.nih.gov/pmc/articles/PMC4730729/

Corcoran, N. (2010). Mass Media in Health Communication. In N. Corcoran (Ed.), *Communicating Health Strategies for Health Promotion* (pp. 73–93). London, UK: SAGE.

Cottle, S. (2009). *Global Crisis Reporting: Journalism in the Global Age*. United Kingdom: Open University Press.

CRICO. (2016) A Report of Medical Malpractice Claims from the CRICO Comparative Benchmarking System. Retrieved from https://www.vital-learning.com › blog › barriers-healthcaren communication

Crystal, D. (1987). The Cambridge Encyclopedia of Linguistics. New York: Oxford University SPress.

Crystal, D. (2000). *Language Death*. Cambridge: Cambridge University Press. doi:10.1017/CBO9781139106856

D'Silva, M. (2000). Global media and cultural identity: Experiences from an Indian town. *Intercultural Communication Studies*, *10*(2), 55–63.

Daramola, O., & Jeje, A. (1976). *Awon Asa ati Orisa Ile Yoruba*. Ibadan: Onibon Oje Press.

Daramola, Y. (2008). Mass Media and Society in Nigeria Selected Functional Perspectives. In R. Akinfeleye (Ed.), *Mass Media and Society: A multi-perspective Approach*. Lagos: Integrity Press.

Davis, L. (2017). Addressing indigenous language loss by unsettling the linguistic hierarchies entrenched in Canada's language policies. *Working Papers of the Linguistics Circle of the University of Victoria, 27*(1), 52-78.

Day, V. (2009). Promoting health literacy through storytelling. *Online Journal of Issues in Nursing, 14*(3). Retrieved from http://ojin.nursingworld.org/MainMenuCategories/ANAMarketplace/ANAPeriodicals/OJIN/TableofContents/Vol142009/No3Sept09/Health-Literacy-Through-Storytelling.html

De Jesus, M. (2013). The impact of mass media health communication on health decision-making and medical advice-seeking behaviour of U.S. Hispanic Population. *Health Communication, 28*(5), 525–529. doi:10.1080/10410236.2012.701584 PMID:22888787

Dei, G. J., Hall, B. L., & Rosenberg, D. G. (2000). Indigenous Knowledges in Global Contexts: Multiple Readings in our World (pp. 3–18). Toronto, Canada: University of Toronto Press.

Donye, A. O. (2018). Assessment of mass media performance in agricultural information dissemination to rural farmers in Girei Local Government Area of Adamawa State, Nigeria. *International Journal of Agricultural Extension and Rural Development*, *6*(5), 639–647.

Dooga, J. T. (2012). Nigeria languages: Failing health and possible healing. *An International Journal of Language, Literature, and Gender Studies. AFRREV LALIGENS, 1*(1), 76–95.

Dooley, J. A., Jones, S. C., & Desmarais, K. (2009). Strategic social marketing in Canada: Ten phases to planning and implementing cancer prevention and cancer screening campaigns. *Social Marketing Quarterly*, *15*(3), 33–48. doi:10.1080/15245000903144999

Drula, G. (2015). Forms of Media Convergence and Multimedia Content – A Romanian Perspective. *Media Education Research Journal*, *44*(20), 131–140.

Dungan-Seaver, D. (1999). Mass media initiatives and children's issues: An analysis of research and recent experiences relevant to potential philanthropic funders [Electronic version]. Paper prepared for the McKnight Foundation.

Eberhard, D. M., Simons, G. F., & Fennig, C. D. (2019) *Ethnologue: languages of the world.* Dallas, Texas: SIL International. Retrieved from http://www.ethnologue.com. Accessed on May 14, 2019.

Ebuehi, O. M., & Akintujoye, I. (2012). Perception and utilization of traditional birth attendants by pregnant women attending primary health care clinics in a rural Local Government Area in Ogun State, Nigeria. *International Journal of Women's Health*, *4*, 25–34. doi:10.2147/IJWH.S23173 PMID:22371657

Edet, I., Akpan, B., & Isaac, O. (2015). Indigenous communication media and utilization of development information in rural communities of South-South Nigeria. *International Journal of English and Literature*, *5*(1), 85–96.

Egbokhare, F. O., Oyetade, S. O., Eno-Abasi, U., & Ahmed, H. A. (2001) Language Clusters in Nigeria. CASAS Monograph Series, No. 12. Cape Town, South Africa.

Egbokhare, F. O., Oyetade, S. O., Eno-Abasi, U., & Ahmed, H. A. (2001). Language clusters in Nigeria. CASAS Monograph Series, No. 12. Cape Town, South Africa.

Egbokhare, F. O. (2004). *Breaking Barriers: ICT, Language Policy and Development. Ibadan.* Nigeria: The Postgraduate School University of Ibadan.

Ekanem, T., Olatunji, R., Amodu, L., Odiboh, O., Yartey, D., Adesina, E., & Adeyeye, B. (2018). A case for e-teaching and e-learning of destination public relations in Nigeria. In *Proceedings of the 31st International Business Information Management Association Conference (IBIMA)*, Milan, Italy. Academic Press.

Ekeanyanwu, N. (2005). *International communication: Issues, concept and researches in the 21st century. Akure.* Standard Mass Concept Company.

Ekeanyanwu, N. T. (2015). *International Communication.* Ibadan: Stirling-Horden Publishers.

Ekwo, U. (1996). Commercialization of the news in Nigerian media: An Impediment to Information flow. In I. Nwosu, & U. Ekwo (Eds.), *Mass Media and Marketing Communications* (pp. 61–77). Enugu: Thought Communications Publishers.

Elguero, E., Délicat-Loembet, L. M., Rougeron, V., Arnathau, C., Roche, B., Becquart, P., . . . Prugnolle, F. (2015). Malaria continues to select for sickle cell trait in Central Africa. *Proceedings of the National Academy of Sciences of the United States of America*, *112*(22), 1-4. 10.1073/pnas.1505665112

Elmariah, H., Garrett, M. E., De Castro, L. M., Jonassaint, J. C., Ataga, K. I., Eckman, J. R., ... Telen, M. J. (2014). Factors associated with survival in a contemporary adult sickle cell disease cohort. *American Journal of Hematology*, *89*(5), 530–535. doi:10.1002/ajh.23683 PMID:24478166

Emeka-Nwobia, N. U. (2015). The place of indigenous Nigerian languages in national development. *Research on Humanities and Social Sciences*, *5*(12), 112–117.

Emeka-Nwobia, N. U. (2015). The Place of Indigenous Nigerian Languages in National Development. *Research on Humanities and Social Sciences*, *5*(12), 112–117.

Emenyonu, P. T. (1982). Promoting the reading habit in Nigeria. In *Literacy and Reading in Nigeria*.

Encyclopaedia of Public Health. (2002). "Traditional Health Beliefs, Practices" The Gale Group Inc.

Encyclopedia Britannica. *Language*. Retrieved from: https://www.britannica.com/topic/language/Meaning-and-style-in-language

Encyclopedia of Communication and Information. (2002) *Health communication*. The Gale Group Inc. Retrieved from: https://www.encyclopedia.com/media/encyclopedias-almanacs-transcripts-and-maps/health-communication

Endong, F. P. (2014). Audience westernisation as a threat to the indigenization model of media broadcast in Nigeria. *Journal of Media and Communication Studies, 6*(8), 121-129.

English Dictionary, B. B. C. (1992). *A dictionary for the world.* London, UK: Harper-Collins Publisher.

Ensuring safe motherhood. (2019, April 22). *Vikaspedia*. Retrieved from: http://*Vikaspedia*.in/health/women-health/pregnancy-health-1/ensuring-safe-motherhood

Entman, R. M. (2004). *Projection of power: Framing news, public opinion and US foreign policy*. Chicago, IL: University of Chicago Press.

Esan, O. (2009). Nigerian Television: Fifty years of television in Africa. Retrieved 7th June 2019 from http://amvpublishingservices.com/pd-nigerian-televisionbrfifty.cfm

European Centre for Disease Prevention and Control. (2019) *What is health communication?* Retrieved from: https://ecdc.europa.eu/en/health-communication/facts

Examples of Americanization. (n.d.). Retrieved January 12, 2018, from https://ardeavujica.weebly.com/examples-of-americanization.html

Eyisi, J. (2000). Language and education: The raison d'être for political socialization. *African Journal of Research in Education, 1*(2).

Eyoh, H. N. (1986). Theatre of relevance: An interview with Ngugi Wa Thiong'o. *African Theatre Review, 1*(2), 110–114.

Fadahunsi, A. (1999). *Philosophy and society: An introduction for beginners.* Ibadan: Hope Publication.

Falle, T. Y., & Mullany, L. C. (2019) Potential Role of Traditional Birth Attendants in Neonatal Healthcare in Rural Southern Nepal. *J Health Population and Nutrition, 2009 Feb; 27*(1), 53–61.

FAO. (2006). *Framework on effective rural communication for development.* Rome, Italy: FAO.

Fathalla, M. F. (2006). Human Rights aspects of safe motherhood. *Best Practice & Research. Clinical Obstetrics & Gynaecology, 20*(3), 409–419. doi:10.1016/j.bpobgyn.2005.11.004 PMID:16469542

Federal Ministry of Health (2016). National Health Policy: Promoting the health of Nigerians to Accelerate Socio-Economic Development.

Fernandez, A., Schillinger, D., Grumbach, K., Rosenthal, A., Stewart, A. L., Wang, F., & Pérez-Stable, E. J. (2004). Physician language ability and cultural competence. *Journal of General Internal Medicine, 19*(2), 167–174. doi:10.1111/j.1525-1497.2004.30266.x PMID:15009796

FHI, & USAID. (2002). *Behaviour Change Communication (BCC) for HIV/AIDS a Strategic Framework.* Available at www.hivpolicy.org. Accessed on 25 September 2019.

Folarin, B. (2000). *Foundation of Broadcasting.* Ibadan: Atlantis Books.

Font, L. (2014). Indigenous media: From transference to appropriation. Retrieved 25th May 2019 from http://anthrovision.revues.org/668

Fossard, E. (1996). *Writing and producing radio dramas*. India: Sage.

Fraser, N. (2019). How the world was won: the Americanization of everywhere review a brilliant essay. *The Guardian*. Retrieved from https://ardeavujica.weebly.com/examples-of-americanization.html

Gaedei, B., & Versteegii, M. (2011). *The state of the right to health in rural South Africa* (p. 2011). Department of Rural Health, University of KwaZulu-Natal.

Ganle, J., Otupiri, E., Parker, M., & Fitpatrick, R. (2015). Socio-cultural barriers to accessibility and utilization of maternal and newborn healthcare services in Ghana after user-fee abolition. *International Journal of Maternal Child Health*, *3*(1), 1–14.

Gay, J., Hardee, K., Judice, N., Agarwal, K., Fleming, K., Hairston, A., ... Wood, M. (2003). *What works: A policy and program guide to the evidence on family planning, safe motherhood, and STI/HIV/AIDS interventions—Module 1 Safe Motherhood*. Washington: Policy Project; Retrieved from http://www.policyproject.com/pubs/generalreport/SM_WhatWorksps2.pdf

Geekie, R. (1995). Mali: Championing women's literacy programme' in African farmer. *The Hunger Project*, *15*, 34–50.

Gerber, A. S., Karlan, D., & Bergan, D. (2009). Does the Media Matter? A Field Experiment Measuring the Effect of Newspapers on Voting Behavior and Political Opinions. *American Economic Journal. Applied Economics*, *1*(2), 35–52. doi:10.1257/app.1.2.35

Goodman, M. B. (2006). Corporate communication practice and pedagogy at the dawn of the new millennium. *Corporate Communications*, *1*(3), 196–213. doi:10.1108/13563280610680803

Govinder, E. (2010). How effective is HIV and AIDS Communication in Africa? *African Communication Research*, *3*(2), 205–234.

Gray, A. (2018). Observations from indigenous languages in Northern Territory, Australia. *The Lancet. Global Health*, *6*(5), e496. doi:10.1016/S2214-109X(18)30075-5 PMID:29653621

Gross, L. (2001). *Up from invisibility*. New York: Columbia University Press.

Guba, E. G., & Lincoln, Y. S. (2005). Paradigmatic controversies, contradictions, and emerging confluences. In N. K. Denzin, & Y. S. Lincoln (Eds.), *The Sage handbook of qualitative research* (pp. 191–215). Thousand Oaks, CA: Sage.

Gwandure, C., & Mayekiso, T. (2012). Sexual desire and expression among girls in a traditional Shona context. *Anthropologist*, *14*(5), 415–423. doi:10.1080/09720073.2012.11891264

Hafez, K. (2007). *The Myth of Media Globalization*. United Kingdom: Polity Press.

Hanafi, A. (2013). *Indigenous Languages as Developmentals* (pp. 1–37). University of Leeds.

Haynes, J. (2011). African cinema and Nollywood: Contradictions. *Situations: Project of radical imagination, 4*(1), 67-90.

Head, S. W., Sterling, C. H., Schofield, L. S., Spann, T., & McGregor, M. (1998). *Broadcasting in America: A survey of electronic media*. Boston, MA: Houghton Mifflin.

Health communication. (2010). *Healthy People* (vol. 1). Retrieved from: https://www.healthypeople.gov/2010/document/HTML/Volume1/11HealthCom.htm

Health, P. S. U. The Public Health Bush Book Vol. 1. Strategies and Resources. Department of Health; Darwin, NT, Australia: 2007. [Google Scholar]

Healthy People. (2010). United States Department of Health and Human Services. Use Communication Strategically to Improve Health. Retrieved May 17, 2019.

Hendrix, J. A. (2004). *Public relations cases* (6th ed.). Belmont, CA: Wadsworth/Thomson Learning.

Henry, G., & Rivera, M. (1998). Public information campaigns and changing behaviours. Paper presented at the meeting of the association for Public Policy Analysis and Management, New York.

Herkman, J. (2012). Convergence or Intermediality? Finnish Political Communication in the New Media Age. *Convergence: The International Journal of Research into New Media Technologies, 18*(4), 369–384. doi:10.1177/1354856512448727

Hjarvard, S. (n.d.). Global media cultures. In A Research Programme on the Role of Media in Cultural Globalization (pp. 71–78).

Ibagere, E. (2015). Globalization and Nollywood: Carving a niche on the global plane. *International Journal of African Society, Cultures, and Traditions, 2*(4), 1–10.

Idebi, S. K. (2008). *Fundamentals of radio production*. Ibadan: Impact Motion Pictures and Media Koncept Nig.

Igbinoba, A. (2014). Public perception of the cultural relevance of BBA II reality TV show: A study of covenant university staff and students. *International Journal of Social Science and Humanities Review, 2*(2), 19-30.

Igbokwe, C., Orji, O., & Igbokwe, B. (2013). Safe motherhood practices among childbearing mothers (CBMs) in Nsukka Urban of Enugu State, Nigeria. *Journal of Applied Information Science and Technology, 6*, 27–33. Retrieved from https://www.jaistonline.org/IgbokweOrjiIgbokwe-2k13.pdf

Ikhioya, G. O. (2010). Maternal mortality and the safe motherhood programme in Nigeria: Implication for Reproductive Health. *International Journal of Education and Research, 2*(10). IPPF Factsheet 2019.

Iliyasu, Z., Aliyu, M. H., Abubakar, I. S., & Galadanci, H. S. (2012). Sexual and reproductive health related communication between mothers and their adolescent daughters in northern Nigeria. *Health Care for Women International*, *33*(2), 138–152. doi:10.1080/07399332.2011.562996 PMID:22242654

Impacts of Americanization. (n.d.). Retrieved January 12, 2018, from https://ardeavujica.weebly.com/impacts-of-americanization.html

International Diabetes Federation. (2013). IDF Diabetes Atlas, 6th Ed. Retrieved May 12, 2016, from http://www.idf.org

Interview with Chioma Obinna, assistant health editor with *Vanguard* newspaper.

Interview with Lucy Osuizogbo-Okechukwu, a Senior Correspondent with News Agency of Nigeria.

Inyang, M. P., & Anuncha, O. U. (2015). Traditional Birth Attendants and Maternal Mortality. *IOSR Journal of Dental and Medical Sciences*, *12*(2), 21–26.

Iordache-Platis, M., & Josan, I. (2009). Communication efficiency within higher education institutions: The case of Romania. *European Research Studies*, *12*(2), 55–70.

Irele, A. (1991). Culture and the Arts. In L. Thompson & ... (Eds.), *Culture and Civilisation* (pp. 52–57). Ibadan: Afrika–Link Books.

Irwin, A., Millen, J., & Fallows, D. (2003). *Global AIDS: Myths and facts tools for fighting the AIDS pandemic*. Massachusetts: Southend Press.

Itari, P. E., Beshel, C. A., & Okeme, I. (2015). Indigenous Communication Media and Utilization of Development Information in Rural Communities of South-South Nigeria. [IJEL]. *International Journal of English and Literature*, *5*(1), 85–96.

Iyorza, S., & Ekwok, L. (2014). Global media and cultural hybridization in the 21st Century in Nigeria. *Journal of Social Sciences (COES&RJ-JSS)*, *3*, 408-416.

Jacobs, E., Chen, A., Karliner, L. S., Agger-Gupta, N., & Mutha, S. (2006). The need for more research on language barriers in health care: A proposed research agenda. *The Milbank Quarterly*, *84*(1), 111–133. doi:10.1111/j.1468-0009.2006.00440.x PMID:16529570

Jaja, J. M. (2010). *Globalization or Americanization: Implication for Sub-Saharan Africa Globalization-Today, Tomorrow*. InTech.

Jepson, A. P., & MacDonald, L. D. (1988). The practice of traditional birth attendants in Zululand. [PubMed]. *Tropical Doctor*, *18*(4), 177–179. doi:10.1177/004947558801800413 PMID:3194950

Johan, M. R. M., & Noor, N. A. Z. A. (2013). The role of corporate communication in building organization's corporate reputation: An exploratory analysis. *Interdisciplinary Journal of Contemporary Research in Business*, *4*(12), 1230–1240.

John, S. (2016). The Use of Indigenous Media of Communication for Health Communication in *Olamabaro Local Government Area of Kogi State Nigeria*. Retrieved from https://www.academia.edu/33078422/The_Use_of_Indigenous_Media_of_Communication_for_Health_Commu

Jones, C. L., Jensen, J. D., Scherr, C. L., Brown, N. R., Christy, K., & Weaver, J. (2015). The Health Belief Model as an explanatory framework in communication research: Exploring parallel, serial, and moderated mediation. *Health Communication, 30*(6), 566–576. doi:10.1080/10410236.2013.873363 PMID:25010519

Kamal, S., & Islam, M. (2012) Promoting safe motherhood practices in Bangladesh: Progress and challenges. *Geneva Health Forum Archive*. Retrieved from: http://ghf.g2hp.net/2012/11/12/promoting-safe-motherhood-practices-in-bangladesh-progress-and-challenges/

Kamalipour, Y. R. (2007). *Global communication* (2nd ed.). Belmont: Thomson Wadsworth.

Kapila, M. (2006). HIV/AIDS, conflict and displacement. Retrieved June 6, 2019 from https://data.unaids.org>pub>report>2006.

Kass-Hout, T., & Alhinawi, H. (2013). Social media in public health. *British Medical Bulletin, 108*(1), 5–24. doi:10.1093/bmb/ldt028 PMID:24103335

Kaur, M., Dangi, C. B. S., & Singh, M. (2013). An overview on sickle cell disease profile. *Asian Journal of Pharmaceutical and Clinical Research, 6*(1), 25–37.

Kayombo, E. J. (2013). Impact of Training traditional birth attendants on maternal mortality and morbidity in Sub-Saharan African countries. *Tanzania Journal of Health Research, 15*(2), 1–11. doi:10.4314/thrb.v15i2.7 PMID:26591718

Khambule, N. Z. (2016). *Experiences of pregnant women from a rural community regarding antenatal care services in ethekwini district, kwazulu-natal*. Durban University of Technology.

Khan, R., Aziz, Z., & Ahmed, V. (2018). Building integrated agriculture information modelling (BIAIM): An integrated approach towards urban agriculture. *Sustainable cities and society, 37*, 594-607.

Kiptiness, E. M. (2019). Indigenous Communication Practices and Myths. Available at:https://www.slideshare.net/EvonneMwangaleKiptin/indigenous-communication-practices-and-myths

Kleinsteuber, H. J. (n.d.). Modes and models of global communication. In *Communication Technology Policy* (pp. 1–23). Session CTP VIII Modes.

Korp, P. (2006). Health in the Internet: Implication for Health Promotion. *Health Education Research, 21*(1), 78–86. doi:10.1093/her/cyh043 PMID:15994845

Kotler, P., & Keller, K. L. (2009). *Marketing management* (13th ed.). London, UK: Pear Prentice-Hall.

Krystallidou, D., Remael, A., de Boe, E., Hendrickx, K., Tsakitzidis, G., van de Geuchte, S. W., & Pype, P. (2018). Investigating empathy in interpreter-mediated consultations: an explorative study. *Patient Education Council 101*(1): 33-42. doi:. doi:10.1016/j.pec.2017.07.022

Ksiazek, T. B., & Webster, J. G. (2008). Cultural proximity and audience behavior: The role of language in patterns of polarization and multicultural fluency. *Journal of Broadcasting & Electronic Media*, *52*(3), 485–503. doi:10.1080/08838150802205876

Lagos State Ministry of Health. (2017). *Lagos State maternal and child mortality reduction (MCMR) Program.* Retrieved from: https://health.lagosstate.gov.ng/lagos-state-maternal-and-child-mortality-reduction-mcmr-program/

Lasswell, H. (1948). Mass communication, popular taste and organised social actions. In L. Bryson (Ed.), *The Communication of Ideas*. New York: Institute for Religious and Social Studies.

Lasswell, H. (1960). The structure and functions of communication in society. In W. Schramm (Ed.), *Mass Communications*. Urbana: Urbana University of Illinois Press.

Launer, J. 1978. Taking medical histories through interpreters: practice in a Nigerian outpatient department. *British Medical Journal 2*(6142): 934-935. doi:. doi:10.1136/bmj.2.6142.934

Lawal, H. O. (2015). 'Cultural Aesthetics in Nigerian Video Films: A Critical Reading of Sikiru Adesina's Ogunmola – Basorun Ibadan'. In *Repositioning Nollywood for the Promotion of Nigeria's Cultural Diplomacy & National Security*. In B. F. Ayankoroma, & A. D. Akoh (Eds.), *Book of Proceedings of the Int'l Conference of SONTA.*

Lawal, B. (1989). An analytical study of the reading habits of some secondary students in Oyo Town. In R. A. Omojuwa & ... (Eds.), *Literacy and Reading in Nigeria 4*.

Lawal, O. A. (2015). Indigenous languages as tools for effective communication of science and technology for food production in Nigeria. *Theory and Practice in Language Studies*, *5*(3), 463–468. doi:10.17507/tpls.0503.02

Lindsey, S. (2016). *Training Traditional Birth Attendants in Sub-Saharan Africa*. Liberty University.

Littlejohn, S. W., & Fuson, K. A. (2008). *Theories of Human Communication* (9th ed.). U.S.A: Thomson Wadsworth.

Mabaso, P. (2009). The compilation of a Shona children's dictionary: Challenges and solutions. *Lexikos,* 19, *Supplement* (*AFRILEX-reeks/series*), 19, 112-119.

Maguire, M., & Delahunt, B. (2017). Doing thematic analysis: A practical, step by step guide for learning and teaching scholars. *AISHE-J*, *8*(3), 3351–3369.

Magu, S. (2015). Reconceptualizing cultural globalization: Connecting the 'cultural global' and the 'cultural local'. *Social Sciences*, *4*(1), 630–645. doi:10.3390ocsci4030630

Maina, W. K., Ndegwa, Z. M., Njenga, E. W., & Mucheni, E. W. (2010). Knowledge, and practices related to diabetes among community members in four provinces in Kenya: A cross sectional study. *The Pan African Medical Journal*, *7*, 2–5. PMID:21918691

Majidi, A. F. (2017). Globalization and economic growth: The case study of developing countries. *Asian Economic and Financial Review*, *7*(6), 589–599. doi:10.18488/journal.aefr.2017.76.589.599

Makinde, T. (2004). Motherhood as a Source of Employment of Women in Yoruba Culture. *Nordic Journal of African Studies*, *13*(2), 164–174.

Makoe, L. N. (2000). *The role of traditional birth attendants in the provision of mayterrnal health in lesotho*. University Of South Africa.

Mano, W. (2004). Renegotiating tradition on Radio Zimbabwe. *Media Culture & Society*, *26*(3), 315–336. doi:10.1177/0163443704041176

Manyozo, L. (2009). Mobilizing rural and community radio in Africa. *Ecquid Novi: African Journal Studies*, *30*(1), 1–23. doi:10.1080/02560054.2009.9653389

Maputseni, C. (2006). *Using radio for advocacy and communication of issues affecting farm communities in Zimbabwe*. (Thesis), Malmo University, Sweden.

Marshall, C., & Rossman, G. B. (2006). *Designing Qualitative Research* (4th ed.). Thousand Oaks, CA: Sage.

Maune, A. (2017). Indigenous knowledge intelligence and African development, In P. Ngulube (Ed.), Handbook of research on theoretical perspectives on indigenous knowledge systems in developing countries (pp. 173-197). Hershey, PA: IGI Global. doi:10.4018/978-1-5225-0833-5.ch008

Maunganidze, L. (2016). A moral compass that slipped: Indigenous knowledge systems and rural development in Zimbabwe. *Cogent Social Sciences*, *2*(1), 1–12. doi:10.1080/23311886.2016.1266749

Mavesera, M. (2009). *Empowerment through language: exploring possibilities of using African languages and literature to promote socio-cultural and economic development in Zimbabwe* (Doctoral dissertation).

Mbaka. (2018). Influence of diabetes information and education on diabetes self-management and prevention in Ogun and Lagos states, Nigeria. Thesis, University of Ibadan.

Mbaka, G. O., Adeyemi, O. O., & Adesina, S. A. (2010). Anti-diabetic activity of the seed extract of Sphenocentrum Jollyanum and morphological changes on pancreatic beta cells. *Journal of Medicine and Medical Sciences*, *1*(11), 550–556.

Mbaya, M. (2002). Linguistic taboo in African marriage context: A study of the Oromo Laguu. *Nordic Journal of African Studies*, *11*(2), 224–235.

McChesney, R. W. (1999). The New Global Media: It's a Small World of Big Conglomerates. *Nation (New York, N.Y.)*, (November): 2, 11–15.

McKenzie, R. (2006). *Comparing media from around the world.* Boston, MA: Pearson.

McQuail, D. (2010). *McQuail's Mass Communication Theory* (6th ed.). London, UK: Sage.

Meadows, M. (2009). Walking the talk: Reflections on indigenous media audience research methods. *Journal of Audience and Reception Studies*, *6*(1).

Meadows, M., & Molnar, H. (2002). Bridging the gaps: Towards a history of Indigenous media in Australia. *Media History*, *8*(1), 9–20. doi:10.1080/13688800220134473

Media's role in the globalization process. (2018). Retrieved January 12, 2019, from https://www.bartleby.com/essay/Medias-Role-in-the-Globalization-Process-PKAJCC8EJDMRS

Meekers, D., Rossem, R., Zellner, S., & Berg, R. (2004). Using behaviour change Communications to overcome social marketing sales plateaus. Case study of Nigeria and India. Retrieved from https://www.shopsplusproject.org/sites/default/files/resource/910_file_07_Nigeria_and_India

Melaku, Y. M., Berhane, Y., Kinsman, J., & Reda, H. L. (2014). Sexual and reproductive health related communication and awareness of contraceptive methods among secondary school female students, northern Ethiopia: A cross-sectional study. *BMC Public Health*, *14*(252), 1–11. PMID:24628909

Merenu, I., Diwe, K., Uwakwe, K., Duru, C., Duru, C., Iwu, A., ... Ohale, I. (2017). To assess the utilization of safe motherhood practices among women in a rural community, in Nigeria. *Unique Research Journal of Medicine and Medical Sciences*, *5*(3), 17–24.

Meribe, N., & Oke, B. (2017). Climate change reporting in Nigeria: Challenges and implications for development. *The Nigerian Journal of Communication*, *14*(1), 133–162.

Meuter, R., Gallois, C., Segalowitz, N., Ryder, A., & Hocking, J. (2015). Overcoming language barriers in healthcare: A protocol for investigating safe and effective communication when patients or clinicians use a second language. *BMC Health Services Research*, *15*(1), 371. Retrieved from https://www.ncbi.nlm.nih.gov/pmc/articles/PMC4566365/pdf/12913_2015_Article_1024.pdf. doi:10.118612913-015-1024-8 PMID:26357948

Mfrekemfon, P. I., & Okere, U. A. (2015) Traditional Birth Attendants and Maternal Mortality: IOSR *Journal of Dental and Medical Sciences (IOSR-JDMS) 14*(2) Ver. III (Feb. 2015), pp. 21-26. Retrieved from www.iosrjournals.org

MillerS. (2010). Global media.

Miller, T., & Smith, H. (2017). Establishing Partnership With Traditional Birth Attendants For Improved Maternal And Newborn Health: A Review Of Factors Influencing Implementation. *Miller And Smith Bmc Pregnancy And Childbirth*, *17*(365), 1–10. PMID:29052533

Moemeka, A. (1980). *Mass media in a mass literacy campaign: guidelines for action in Africa.* Discussion paper. Federal ministry of education.

Momodu, M. O. (2002). Information needs and information seeking behaviour of rural dwellers in Nigeria: A case study of Ekpoma in Esan West local government area of Edo State, Nigeria. *Library Review*, *51*(8), 406–410. doi:10.1108/00242530210443145

Moodley, L. M., & Rambiritch, V. (2007). An assessment of the level of knowledge diabetes mellitus among diabetic patients in a primary health care setting. *South African Family Practice*, *49*(10), 16–18. doi:10.1080/20786204.2007.10873652

Moore, M. K. (n.d.). A literature review on behalf of and under the overall guidance of WHO'S Division of Reproductive Health. Retrieved from https://apps.who.int/iris/bitstream/handle/10665/69834/WHO_RHT_97.34_eng.pdf;jsessionid=F8AC617DE6A670C4BF5362D87EB1512E?sequence=1

Morales, F., & Simelio, N. (2016). Television and identities: Analysis of the consumption of 'telenovelas' by the Latin American community in Spain. *Global Studies in Audience and Power*, *23*(5), 591–609.

Moyo, R., & Salawu, A. (2018). A survey of communication effectiveness by agricultural extension in the Gweru district of Zimbabwe. *Journal of Rural Studies*, *60*, 32–42. doi:10.1016/j.jrurstud.2018.03.002

Mpofu, N. (2003). Cultural aspects in the Shona monolingual dictionary Duramazwi Guru reChiShona. *Lexikos,* 13, *(AFRILEX-reeks/series),* 13, 232-239.

Mpofu, P., & Salawu, A. (2019). Interrogating the autonomy of previously marginalised languages in Zimbabwe's indigenous language press. *Language Matters: Studies in the Languages of Africa*, *50*(1), 25–44. doi:10.1080/10228195.2018.1541925

Mpofu, P., & Salawu, A. (forthcoming). Sex and sexual fantasies on Zimbabwe's Ya FM and Star FM radio stations. *African Identities*.

Mtawasli, G., Pina, M., Angle, M., & Murphy, C. (1997). *The Menstrual Cycle and Its Relation to Contraceptive Methods: A Reference for Reproductive Health Trainers. United State of America: INTRAH Publication.* University of North Carolina.

Mubonderi, B., & Mpofu-Hamadziripi, N. (2018). Speaking the unspeakable: A socio-cultural analysis of tabooed language in Shona society. *The Fountain Journal of Interdisciplinary Studies*, *2*(1), 104–118.

Mufwene, S. S. (2002). Colonisation, Globalisation and the Future of Languages in the Twenty first Century. *MOST Journal on Multicultural Societies*, 19-48.

Mumvana, O. V. (2018). *Transformations and challenges of sex education in selected radio programmes*, (Honours Dissertation), Midlands State University, Zvishavane.

Mundy, P., & Lloyd-Laney, M. (1992). Indigenous communication. Appropriate Technology, 19(2), IT Publications Ltd, 103-105 Southampton Row, London, UK.

Mundy, P., & Lloyd-Laney, M. (1992). Indigenous communication. *Appropriate Technology, 19*(2), 103–105.

Musa, E., Nasidi, A., Shuaib, F., Nguku, P. M., & Vaz, R. G. (2016). Nigeria's Ebola Outbreak Response: Lessons for Future Epidemic Preparedness. *Arch Med, 8*(6). doi:10.21767/1989-5216.1000171

Museka, J., & Kaguda, D. (2013). The school and the 'second sex': A feminist response to verbal and non-verbal sexual harassment of girls by boys in Zimbabwe's secondary schools. *Journal of Emerging Trends in Educational Research and Policy Studies, 4*(2), 308–314.

Mustapha, L. (2008). Mass Media and Optimization of health policy in Nigeria: The participatory Option. In R. Akinfeleye (Ed.), *Mass media and Society: A Multi Perspective Approach Lagos*. Integrity Press.

NACA. (2017). National strategic framework on HIV and AIDS: 2017-2021. Retrieved from https://naca.gov.ng>2013-national-hiv-Nigeria National Agency for the control of AIDS (2021). National HIV/AIDS strategic plan 2010-2015. Abuja Nigeria. Retrieved April 26 2019 from http://nigeria.unfpa.org/pdf/nsp

National Collaboration Centre for Aboriginal Health (NECAH). (2016). *Social Determinants of Health Culture and Language as Social Determinants of First Nations*. Inuit and Metis Health.

National Health Service. (2017) *Your antenatal care-Your pregnancy and baby guide*. Retrieved from: https://www.nhs.uk/conditions/pregnancy-and-baby/antenatal-midwife-care-pregnant/

National Research Council. (2011). The US Health Disadvantage Relative to Other High-Income Countries Findings from a National Research Council/Institute of Medicine Report.

Ndaghu, A. A., & Taru, V. B. (2012). Role of mass media in agricultural productivity in Adamawa State, Nigeria. *Global Journal of Agricultural Sciences, 11*(2), 111–116.

Ndamba, G. T. (2008). Mother Tongue Usage in Learning: An Examination of Language Preferences in Zimbabwe. *The Journal of Pan African Studies, 2*(4).

Ndhlovu, K., & Botha, R. (2017). Euphemism vs explicitness: A corpus- based analysis of translated taboo words from English to Zimbabwean Ndebele. *South African Journal of African Languages, 37*(2), 235–243. doi:10.1080/02572117.2017.1378278

Ndlovu, S., & Hove, E. F. (2015). Old wine in new skins: Revisiting counselling in Traditional Ndebele & Shona societies. *Journal of the Humanities and Social Sciences, 20*, 101–105.

Ndubueze, N., Odiboh, O., Nwosu, E., & Olabanjo, J. (2019). Awareness and perception of public relations practices in public tertiary institutions in Nigeria. In *Proceedings of the 33rd International Business Information Management Association (IBIMA)*, Granada, Spain. Academic Press.

Ngigi, S., & Busolo, D. (2018). Behaviour Change Communication in Health Promotion: Appropriate Practices and Promising Approaches. *International Journal of Innovative Research and Development*, (7), 9.

Ngunyulu, R., & Mulaudzi, F. (2009). Indigenous practices regarding postnatal care at Sikhunyani Village in the Limpopo Province of South Africa. *Africa Journal of Nursing and Midwifery*, *11*(1), 48–64.

Ngwenya, S. (2016). Communication of reproductive health information to the rural girl child in Filabusi, Zimbabwe. *African Health Sciences*, *16*(2), 451–461. doi:10.4314/ahs.v16i2.13 PMID:27605960

Nigussie, H. (2015). Folk media and their use in HIV/AIDS prevention campaign. Retrieved May 10, 2019 from www.waccglobal.org>articles>folk-media.

Nolte, A. (1998). Traditional birth attendants in South Africa: Professional midwives' beliefs and myths. [PubMed]. *Curationis*, *21*, 59–66. PMID:11040590

Nye, J. (2018). The Americanization of the world: myth or reality? Retrieved January 12, 2018, from https://baripedia.org/wiki/The_Americanization_of_the_World:_Myth_or_Reality%3F

Obeidat, M. (2010). Beyond American Borders: The Middle East and the Enigma of Anti-American Sentiments in the Aftermath of 9/11. *American Studies Today Online, 17*.

Oberiri, A. D. (2016). Journalists' Perception of News Commercialization and its implication on Media Credibility in Nigeria. *World Scientific News*, *55*, 63–76.

Obono, K. (2011). Indigenous media preferences for reproductive health diffusion among the Yakur of Southern Nigeria. *Journal of Environment and Culture*, *8*(1), 62–77.

Obono, K. (2011). Media Strategies of HIV/AIDS Communication for behaviour change in South West Nigeria. *Africana*, *5*(2), 148–170.

Ocholla, D. N., & Onyancha, O. B. (2005). The marginalized knowledge: An informetric analysis of indigenous knowledge publications (1990-2004). *South African Journal of Library and Information Science*, *71*, 247–248.

Ochonogor, C., & Ikems, K. (2014). Attaining safe motherhood through communication campaigns in Rivers state Nigeria. *Journal of Communication and Media Research*, *6*(2), 195–210.

Odiboh, O. O. (2002). Integrated marketing communication. Lagos, Nigeria: Advertising Practitioners Council of Nigeria (APCON).

Odiboh, O. O., & Ekanem, T. (2018). Teaching and learning of integrated marketing communication in three leading Nigerian universities. In *Proceedings of the 31st International Business Information Management Association Conference (IBIMA)*, 6625-6638. Milan, Italy. Academic Press.

Odiboh, O., & Ajayi, F. (2019). Integrated Marketing Communication And Carbonated Drinks Consumers in Nigeria: A Consumerist Analysis. In *Proceedings of the 33rd International Business Information Management Association (IBIMA)*, April 10-11, 2019, Granada, Spain. Academic Press.

Odiboh, O., & Oladunjoye, A. (2019). Application of Integrated Marketing Communication Tools for Promoting Computers in Nigeria. In *Proceedings of the 33rd International Business Information Management Association (IBIMA)*, April 10-11, 2019, Granada, Spain. Academic Press.

Odiboh, O., Adeyeye, B., & Ekanem, T. (2018). Awareness of e-Transaction among Consumers of Indigenous Herbal Remedies in Ota, Nigeria: A Case for e-Herbals. In *Proceedings of the 4th IEEE International Conference on Information Management, (ICIM 2018)*, Oxford, UK, pp. 179-183. 10.1109/INFOMAN.2018.8392831

Odiboh, O., Ezenagu, A., & Okuobeya, V. (2019). Integrated Marketing Communication Tools and Facials Consumers in Nigeria: Applications and Connexions. In *Proceedings of the 33rd International Business Information Management Association (IBIMA)*, April 10-11, 2019, Granada, Spain. Academic Press.

Odiboh, O. O. (2002). *Integrated Marketing Communication*. Lagos: APCON.

Odiboh, O. O. (2011). *A Philosophy of Marketing Communication: Through Gabriel Marcel's Theory of Intersubjectivity*. Germany: VDM.

Odiboh, O., & Ekanem, T. (2019). *Mass Communication Book of Book Reviews* (Vol. 1). Germany: Academy Publishers.

Odiboh, O., Salawu, A., & Doghudje, C. (Eds.). (2019). *Introduction to Philosophy of Mass Communication for Higher Institutions*. Ibadan: Stirling Horden.

Oduaran, C., & Okorie, N. (2018). Community radio, family and psychological support for sexual harassment issues against women: A study of Yoruba usage. *Media Watch Journal*, *10*(1), 11–20.

Ofili, A. N., & Okojie, O. H. (2005, June). Assessment of the role of traditional birth attendants in maternal health care in Oredo Local Government Area, Edo State, Nigeria. *Journal of Community Medicine and Primary Health Care*, *17*(1), 55–60. doi:10.4314/jcmphc.v17i1.32428

Ogundoyin, O. (2016). Perception and attitudes of respondents in Ibadan to fear appeal-based messages on HIV/AIDS. *Journal of Communication and Media Research*, *8*(1) Sp. 1: 66-81.

Ogundoyin, O. (2016). Information and communication strategies for improving adherence to anti-retroviral drugs among patients with Human Immunodeficiency Virus infection. *International Journal of Management Sciences*, *9*(1), 1–10.

Ogundoyin, O., & Soola, E. (2014). Trends in methodological and theoretical approaches to interpersonal health communication research. *Journal of Communication and Media Research*, *6*(2), 163–174.

Ogungbemi, S. (2017). Traditional Religious Belief System. In T. Falola, & A. Akinyemi (Eds.), *Culture and Customs of Yoruba* (pp. 309–324). Austin, TX: Pan-African University Press.

Ogunyombo, O., & Azeez, O. (2018). Exploring the perspectives of selected public relations professionals on the made-in-Nigeria campaign. *Media &Communication Currents*, *2*(2), 1–20.

Ohaeri, J. U., & Shokunbi, W. A. (2001). Attitudes and beliefs of relatives of patients with sickle cell disease. *East African Medical Journal*, *78*(4), 180–186. doi:10.4314/eamj.v78i4.9058 PMID:12002066

Ojebode, A. (2004). Radio as Development Communication Medium: Types, Formats, Roles and Limitation. In E. O. Soola (Ed.), *Communicating for Development Purposes* (pp. 87–99). Ibadan: Kraft Books Limited.

Okereke, E., Aradeon, S., Akerele, A., Tanko, M., Yisa, I., & Obonyo, B. (2013). Knowledge of safe motherhood among women in rural communities in northern Nigeria: Implications for maternal mortality reduction. *Reproductive Health*, *10*(1), 57. doi:10.1186/1742-4755-10-57 PMID:24160692

Okorie, N. (2010). Media Concentration and its threat to Nigeria's Indigenous culture. In N. Ekeanyanwu (Ed.), *T & Okeke, C. Indigenous Societies and Cultural Globalization in the 21st Century: Is the Global Village truly real?* Germany: VDM Verlagon.

Okorie, N., & Bigala, P. (2016). Creating HIV/AIDS awareness through localized communication for health development in South Africa. *Journal of Health Management*, *18*(3), 439–446. doi:10.1177/0972063416651567

Okorie, N., & Bwala, N. (2017). Measuring media campaigns effectiveness for environmental health for Sustainable Development: A study of Ebola outbreak in Lagos State, Nigeria. *Journal of Health Management*, *19*(4), 1–10.

Okorie, N., & Salawu, A. (2016). Effective use of media awareness campaigns for breast cancer care among women: A comparative study. *Journal of International Women's Studies*, *17*(4), 160–173.

Okorie, N., & Salawu, A. (2017). Can my wife be virtual-adulterous? An experiential study on Facebook, emotional infidelity and self-disclosure. *Journal of International Women's Studies*, *18*(2), 166–179.

Okoro, N. (2001). Mass communication research: Issues and methodologies. Nsukka: AP Express publishers.

Okunna, C. S. (1999). *Introduction to Mass Communication* (2nd ed.). Enugu: New Generation Books.

Olabanjo, O., Odiboh, O., Nwosu, E., & Ndubueze, N. (2019). Public relations practices in local government and traditional institutions in Nigeria. In *Proceedings of the 33rd International Business Information Management Association (IBIMA)*, Granada, Spain. Academic Press.

Olabimtan, A. (1999). The Relevance of Yoruba Communication Arts to National Development in the Twenty-First Century. Lecture Delivered on May 1, 1999, Lagos State University, Ojo, Lagos.

Olajubu, O. (1978). *Ìwé Àṣà Ìbílẹ̀ Yorùbá*. Lagos: Longman Nigeria Ltd.

Olakunle, O. S., Kenneth, E., Olalekan, A. W., & Adenike, O. B. (2014). Knowledge and attitude of secondary school students in Jos, Nigeria on sickle cell disorder. *The Pan African Medical Journal*, *15*(1), 12–15.

Olaoye, A. A. (2013).The Role of Indigenous Languages in National Development: A Case Study of Nigerian Linguistic Situation. *International Journal of Applied Linguistics and English Studies, 2*(3). Available at http://www.journals.aiac.org.au/index.php/IJALEL/article/view/847 Assessed on 20/3/2019

Olatunji, R. W. (2013). Uses of semiotics in periods of hostilities, armed conflicts and peace building among the Yoruba, South-West, Nigeria. An International Journal of Arts and Humanities Bahir Dar, Ethiopia, 2(4), 8, 247-261.

Olatunji, R. W. (2013). *"Uses of Semiotics in Periods of Hostilities, Armed Conflicts and Peace Building among the Yoruba, South-West Nigeria." An International Journal of Arts and Humanities*. Ethiopia: Bahir Dar.

Olatunji, R. W. (2018). Trends in advertising and cultures in Nigeria. *Communication Cultures in Africa*, *1*(1), 54–76. doi:10.21039/cca.5

Olausson, U. (2011). *Explaining global media: a discourse approach. The Systemic Dimension of Globalization*. IntechOpen; doi:10.5772/17557

Olise, F. P. (2008). Communication for Development and Modern ICTs: Nigeria at Cross Roads. In E. M. Mojaye, O. O. Oyewo, R. M'Bayo, & I. A. Sobowale (Eds.), Health Communication, Gender Violence, and ICTs in Nigeria; Ibadan: Ibadan University Press, pp. 269-283.

Olise, P. (2007). *Primary health care for sustainable development*. Ibadan, Nigeria: Omoade Printing Press.

Olonade, O., Olawande, T. I., Alabi, O. J., & Imhonopi, D. (2019). Maternal Mortality and Maternal Health Care in Nigeria: Implications for Socio-Economic Development. *Open Access Macedonian Journal of Medical Sciences*, *7*(5), 849–855. doi:10.3889/oamjms.2019.041 PMID:30962850

Olúbòdé-Sàwè, F. O. (2010). Digital communication in indigenous languages. In R. Taiwo (Ed.), *Handbook of research on discourse behaviour and digital communication: Language structures and social interaction* (pp. 564–578). Hershey, PA: IGI Global; doi:10.4018/978-1-61520-773-2.ch036

Olukotun, A. (2006). The Indigenous Language Press and Democratic Mobilisation in Nigeria: A Historical Structural Overview. In A. Salawu (Ed.), Indigenous Language Media in Africa, Lagos: Center for Black and African Arts and Civilisation (CBAAC), pp. 126-140.

Omoloso, I. A., & Abdu rauf-Salau, A. (2014). May Indigenous Language Newspapers in Nigeria from 1914-2013: Review, A. A Paper presented at the Amalgamation National Conference of the Department of Political Science & Department of History and International Studies. Ibrahim Badamasi Babangida University. Lapai, Niger State, Nigeria. Retrieved from: https://www.academia.edu/17562000/

Omotade, O. O. (1995). Perception of sickle cell haemoglobinopathy among would be counselors. *African Journal of Medicine and Medical Sciences*, *24*(2), 315–320. PMID:8886144

Omu, F. I. A. (2008). "Ethnicity, Nationalism, and Federalism in Nigeria: An Interactive Trinity of Relationship" in F. I. A. Omu, & G. E. Oboh (Eds.), Mass Media in Nigerian Democracy. Ibadan: Stirling-Hordens Publishers (Nig) Ltd.

Onabajo, O. (2013). *Elements and practice of international public relations*. Ibadan, Nigeria: College Press & Publishers Limited.

Onabajo, S. (1999). *Essentials of Broadcast Writing and Production*. Lagos: Gabi Concept Ltd.

Onoja, I. (2009). The Impact of Commercialization on News Selection by Three Broadcast Station in Nigeria. *Maiduguri Journal of Arts and Social Sciences*, *7*(1), 86–99.

Osgood, C. E. (Ed.). (1954). *Psycholinguistics: A survey of theory and research problem. Journal of Abnormal and Social Psychology, 49 (Oct.)*. Morton Prince Memorial Supplement.

Oso, L. (2006). A Political Economy of Indigenous language press in Nigeria. In A. Salawu (Ed.), Indigenous Language Media in Africa. Lagos: Centre for Black and African Arts and Civilisation (CBAAC) pp. 175-195.

Owolabi, T. O. S. (2014). Media Coverage of SMEs in Nigeria: An Imperative for National Development, (Doctoral thesis), University of Strathclyde, Glasgow, UK.

Owolabi, L., Ibrahim, A., Musa, B., Gwaram, B., Dutse, A., Hamza, M., ... Borodo, M. (2014). Prevalence and Burden of Human Immunodeficiency Virus and Hepatitis B Virus Co-infection in Nigeria: A Systematic Review and Meta-Analysis. *Journal of AIDS & Clinical Research*, *5*(308), 2.

Owolabi, T. O. S., Ezika, E. A., Lewitt, M., & Beth, C. (2016). Communication Media and Cardiovascular Health Promotion as Factors for Sustainable Development in Nigeria, *Journal of Sustainable Development in Africa. Clarion University of Pennsylvania*, *18*(1), 156–172.

Owolabi, T. O. S., & O'Neill, E. (2014). Communication, MSMEs, and Women Empowerment for National Development in Nigeria. *Asian Journal of Research in Social Sciences and Humanity*, *4*(3), 21–34. Retrieved from https://aijsh.com/shop/articlepdf/org/socialscience/paper686.pdf

Oxford Living Dictionaries. *Language*. Retrieved from: https://en.oxforddictionaries.com/definition/language

Oye-Adeniran, B., Odeyemi, K., Gbadegesin, A., Akin-Adenekan, O., Akinsola, O., Ekanem, E., & Osilaja, O. (2019). Causes of maternal mortality in Lagos State, Nigeria. Ann Trop Med Public Health. Retrieved from http://www.atmph.org/text.asp?2014/7/3/177/149501

Oyero, O. S. (2003). Indigenous language radio for development purposes. In E. O. Soola, (Ed.), Communicating for Development Purposes. Ibadan: Krafts Books.

Oyero, O. S., Oyesomi, K. O, Abioye, T, Ajiboye E, & Kayode-Adedeji, K. T. (2018). Strategic \ communication for climate change awareness and behavioural change in Ado-Odo/Ota Local Government of Ogun State. *African Population Studies, 32*(1), (Supp.).Oyesomi, K, Okorie, N, Ahmadu, F., & Itsekor, V. (2014). Where is the African culture? Assessing the uniqueness of indigenous communication in galvanising women's political participation at the local level. *Journal of New Media and Mass Communication, 25,* USA. pp. 1-8.

Oyero, O. S., Oyesomi, K. O., Abioye, T., Ajiboye, E., & Kayode-Adedeji, K. T. (2018). Strategic communication for climate change awareness and behavioural change in Ado-Odo/Ota Local Government of Ogun State. African Population Studies, 32(1), (Supp.), 2018.

Oyero, O. (2007). Dynamics of indigenous languages in environmental communication. In I. Nwosu, & O. Soola (Eds.), *Communication in global, ICTs and ecosystem perspectives- Insights from Nigeria*. Enugu: Precisions Publishers.

Oyero, O. (2007). Dynamics of indigenous languages in environmental communication. In I. Nwosu, & O. Soola (Eds.), *Communication in global, ICTs, and ecosystem perspectives- Insights from Nigeria*. Enugu: Precisions Publishers.

Oyero, O. S. (2003). Indigenous language radio for development purposes. In E. O. Soola (Ed.), *Communicating for Development Purposes*. Ibadan, Nigeria: Krafts Books.

Oyero, O. S. (2007). Dynamics of indigenous languages in environmental communication. In I. E. Nwosu, & O. E. Soola (Eds.), *Communication in Global, ICTs & Ecosystem Perspectives: Insights from Nigeria*. Enugu, Nigeria: Precision Publishers Ltd.

Oyesomi, K. O, Salawu, A., & Olorunyomi, B. (2017). Indigenous Communication: Socio-Economic Characteristics Influencing Contemporary Female Political Participation. *Journal of International Women Studies (JIWS), 18*(4), pp. 164-181.

Oyesomi, K. O., & Salawu, A. (2019). Assessing the Uniqueness of Indigenous Language in Advertising: Analysis of Figurative Language Used in Selected Telecommunication Yoruba Advertisement in Nigeria. *Qualitative Report, 24*(10), 2574–2591. Retrieved from https://nsuworks.nova.edu/tqr/vol24/iss10/12

Oyesomi, K. O., Salawu, A., & Olorunyomi, B. (2017). Indigenous Communication: Socio-Economic Characteristics Influencing Contemporary Female Political Participation. [JIWS]. *Journal of International Women's Studies, 18*(4), 164–181.

Oyesomi, K. O., Salawu, A., & Onyenankeya, K. (2019, March). Newspapers' Compliance with the Code of Election Coverage of the 2015 Elections and citizens participation: Implication for Journalism Education and Professionalism. *African Rennaisance, 16*(1), 41–64. doi:10.31920/2516-5305/2019/V16n1a3

Oyesomi, K., Salawu, A., & Olorunyomi, B. (2017). Indigenous Communication: Socio-Economic Characteristics Influencing Contemporary Female Political Participation. *Journal of International Women's Studies, 18*(4), 164–181. Available at http://vc.bridgew.edu/jiws/vol18/iss4/12

Oyetunde, T. O., & Umolu, J. J. (1991). The current view of the reading process and its implications for English reading instruction in Nigeria: An afterword. *Literacy and Reading in Nigeria 5.*

Ozowa, V. N. (2005). Information needs of small-scale farmers' in Africa: The Nigerian example. Quarterly Bulletin of the International Association of Agricultural Information Specialists, IAALD/CABI, 40(1).

Ozowa, V. N. (1995). Information needs of small-scale farmers' in Africa: The Nigerian example. Quarterly *Bulletin of the International Association of Agricultural Information Specialists*, *40*(1).

Padovani, C. (2008). The extreme right and its media in Italy. *International Journal of Communication*, *2*, 18.

Padre, S., Sundarshana, N., & Tripp, R. (2003) Performing farm journalism: the experience of Adike Parttirike. Agricultural research and extension Network (AGREEN) Network paper No. 128, London, UK.

Palermo, T. M., Riley, C. A., & Mitchell, B. A. (2008). Daily functioning and quality of life in children with sickle cell disease pain: Relationship with family and neighborhood socioeconomic distress. *The Journal of Pain: Official Journal of the American Pain Society*, *9*(9), 833–840. doi:10.1016/j.jpain.2008.04.002 PMID:18550443

Panepinto, J. A., Pajewski, N. M., Foerster, L. M., Sabnis, S., & Hoffmann, R. G. (2009). Impact of family income and sickle cell disease on the health-related quality of life of children. *Quality of Life Research: An International Journal of Quality of Life Aspects of Treatment, Care and Rehabilitation*, *18*(1), 5–13. doi:10.100711136-008-9412-8 PMID:18989755

Panford, S., Nyaney, M., Amoah, S., & Aidoo, N. (2001). Using folk media in HIV/AIDS prevention in rural Ghana. *American Journal of Public Health*, *9*(10), 1559–1562. doi:10.2105/AJPH.91.10.1559 PMID:11574305

Parrot, R. (2004). Emphasizing communication in health communication. *Journal of Communication*, *54*(4), 751–787. doi:10.1111/j.1460-2466.2004.tb02653.x

PATH. (2010). *Improving maternal and child health in South Africa.* Johannesburg, South Africa: www.path.org

PATHS. (2005). Maternal and child health. *Journal of World Health Forum*, *7*(21), 11–21.

Paulino, N., Vázquez, M. & Bolúmar, F. (2018). *Indigenous language and inequitable maternal health care, Guatemala, Mexico, Peru, and the Plurinational State of Bolivia*. Geneva: World Health Organization 97: 59-67. doi: . doi:10.2471/BLT.18.216184

Peltzer, K., & Henda, N. (2006). Traditional birth attendants, HIV/AIDS and safe delivery in the Eastern Cape, South Africa - evaluation of a training programme. *SAJOG*, *12*(3), 140–145.

Piel, F. B., Hay, S. I., Gupta, S., Weatherall, D. J., & Williams, T. N. (2013). Global Burden of Sickle Cell Anaemia in Children under Five, 2010–2050: Modelling Based on Demographics, Excess Mortality, and Interventions. *PLoS Medicine, 10*(7). doi:10.1371/journal.pmed.1001484 PMID:23874164

Platt, O. S., Thorington, B. D., Brambilla, D. J., Milner, P. F., Rosse, W. F., Vichinsky, E., & Kinney, T. R. (1991). Pain in sickle cell disease – rates and risk factors. *The New England Journal of Medicine, 325*(1), 11–16. doi:10.1056/NEJM199107043250103 PMID:1710777

Pope, R. (2002). *The English Studies Book: An Introduction to Language, Literature and Culture* (2nd ed.). London, UK: Routledge.

Popoola, I. S. (2006). Print on the Air, an Appraisal of Koko Inu Iwe Iroyin, a Newspaper Review Programme on Metro FM, Lagos. In A. Salawu (Ed.), Indigenous Language Media in Africa. Lagos: Centre for Black and African Arts and Civilisation (CBAAC) pp. 326-346.

Porter, J. R., Xie, L., Challinor, A. J., Cochrane, K., Howden, S. M., Iqbal, M. M., ... Travasso, M. I. (2014). Food security and food production systems. Cambridge University Press. *Climatic Change, 2014*, 485–533.

Prah, K. K. (1999) *Workshop working paper on the harmonization and standardization of Nigerian languages*. Lagos.

Prah, K. K. (1999). Workshop Working Paper on the Harmonization and Standardization of Nigerian Languages. Lagos.

Prah, K. K. (2001) The idea of an African Renaissance, the languages of the Renaissance and the challenges of the 21st century. In E. Kurimoto (Ed.), *JCAS Symposium Series 14*. JCAS, Osaka, Japan.

Prah, K. K. (2001). The idea of an African Renaissance, the languages of the Renaissance and the challenges of the 21st century. In E. Kurimoto (Ed.), *JCAS Symposium Series 14*. JCAS, Osaka, Japan.

Prasad, S. (2012) Safe motherhood practice in Dalit community. *Academic Voices, 2*(1). Retrieved from: https://www.nepjol.info/index.php/AV/article/view/8291/6759

Premium Times. (2018). *Nigeria's Indigenous Languages endangered, may go into Extinction*. Lai Mohammed.

Putri, D., Malini, H., & Basmanelly, B. (2019). Living with HIV/AIDS: Stigma and social discrimination. *Journal The Messenger, 11*(1), 10–17. doi:10.26623/themessenger.v11i1.875

Quinn, C. T., Rogers, Z. R., & Buchanan, G. R. (2004). Survival of children with sickle cell disease. *Blood, 103*(11), 4023–4027. doi:10.1182/blood-2003-11-3758 PMID:14764527

Rai, M., & Kishore, J. (2009). Myths about diabetes and its treatment in North Indian population. *International Journal of Diabetes in Developing Countries, 29*(3), 129–135. doi:10.4103/0973-3930.54290 PMID:20165650

Ransome-Kuti, O. (2009). Health Care and the Mass media. In R. Akinfeleye (Ed.), *Health and Behavioural Change Communication for Development* (pp. 38–47). Ibadan: Spectrum Books Limited.

Rees, D. C., Williams, T. N., & Gladwin, M. T. (2010). Sickle-cell disease. *Lancet*, *376*(9757), 2018–2031. doi:10.1016/S0140-6736(10)61029-X PMID:21131035

Reinard, J. C. (2001). *Introduction to communication research*. McGraw-Hill Humanities, Social Sciences & World Languages.

Rice, E. S., Haynes, E., Royce, P., & Thompson, S. C. (2016). Social media and digital t echnology use among Indigenous young people in Australia: A literature review. *International Journal for Equity in Health*, *15*(81). PMID:27225519

Ritu, A. (2010). Know your folks: Traditional folk media in India. Retrieved October 13, 2019 from https;//www.youthkiawaaz.com/2010/11/know-your-folks-traditional-folk-media-in-india

Robbin, A. (2012). The place of the media, public relations, and consultation in community development. In O. Olufemi (Ed.), *Issues and Trends in Advertising and Public Relations Practices*. Ibadan, Nigeria: College Press & Publishers Limited.

Robson, C. (2011). *Real world research* (Vol. 3). Chichester: Wiley.

Rodrigues da Silva, L. B. V. (2018). Communication strategies of adolescent sexual and reproductive health programmes in Mozambique: Cultural challenges. *Open Access Journal of Public Health*, *2*(3), 1–11.

Rogers, E. M. (2003). *The diffusion of innovation* (5th ed.). New York: Free Press.

Rogers, E. M., & Antola, L. (1985). Telenovelas in Latin America: A Success Story. *Journal of Communication*, *35*(4), 24–35. doi:10.1111/j.1460-2466.1985.tb02970.x

Rommy, N. R. A. (2017). Researching Indigenous Ways of Knowing-and-Being, University of South Africa, South Africa. Doi:10.4018/978-1-5225-0833-5.ch002

Roudometof, V., & Robertson, R. (1998). The space between the boundaries: Globalization and Americanization. *American Culture in Europe Interdisciplinary Perspective*, 181-195.

Sakwa, C. P. (2012). *Gender stereotyping in radio programming: the case of Kenya Broadcasting Corporation* (Master's Thesis), University of Nairobi, Kenya.

Salawu, A. (2004). The intrinsic value of oramedia for development. *Humanities Review Journal*, 4, 18-30.

Salawu, A. (2006). Paradox of a milieu: communicating in African indigenous languages in the age of globalization. In A. Salawu (Ed.), Indigenous Language Media in Africa (pp. 1-20). Lagos, Nigeria: Centre for Black and African Arts and Civilization (CBAAC).

Salawu, A. (2006). Paradox of a milieu: Communicating in African indigenous languages in the age of globalization. In A. Salawu (Ed.), Indigenous Language Media in Africa. Lagos, Nigeria: Centre for Black and African Arts and Civilization (CBAAC).

Salawu, A. (2016). Indigenous Language Media and Democracy in Africa. In A. Salawu, & M. B. Chibita (Ed.), Indigenous Language Media, Language Politics and Democracy in Africa (pp. 13-27), Palgrave Macmillan, UK doi:10.1057/9781137547309_2

Salawu, A. S. (2001) An evaluation of development communication content of Yoruba newspapers. (Unpublished PhD thesis), University of Ibadan.

Salawu, A. S. (2004b) Social status as a factor for the readership of Yoruba newspapers in Nigeria. *Nordic Journal of African Studies 13*(2), pp. 200-215.

Salawu, A. (2004). Development Communication in Yoruba Newspapers. In E. O. Soola (Ed.), *Communicating for Development Purposes* (pp. 172–184). Ibadan: Kraft Books Limited.

Salawu, A. (2006). Indigenous language media: A veritable tool for African language learning. *Journal of Multicultural Discourses, 1*(1), 86–95. doi:10.1080/10382040608668533

Salawu, A. (2011). Breaking the culture of mute sensation: Female expression of power in Sexual contest with men in Yoruba newspapers. *Soc Sci, 27*(1), 39–51.

Salawu, A. (2015). Oramedia as a vehicle for development in Africa: The imperative for the ethical paradigm of development. *Journal of Sociology and Social Anthropology, 6*(2), 209–216. doi:10.1080/09766634.2015.11885660

Salawu, A. (2019). Alaroye, Isoleszwe and the Adoption of Digital Technologies. In A. Salawu (Ed.), *African Language Digital Media and Communication* (pp. 33–45). London, UK: Routledge Taylor and Francis Group.

Salawu, A. S. (2004a). The Yoruba and their language newspapers: Origin, nature, problems, and prospects. *Studies of Tribes and Tribals, 2*(2), 97–104. doi:10.1080/0972639X.2004.11886508

Salawu, A. S. (2004c). Contents and styles of Alaroye news publications. In O. Ndimele (Ed.), *Language and Culture in Nigeria: A Festschrift for Okon Essien. Aba: NINLAN.*

Salawu, A. S. (2004d). A readership survey of Yoruba newspapers for development messages. *Journal of Social Sciences, 8*(3), 197–202. doi:10.1080/09718923.2004.11892414

Sanyaolu, A., Okorie, C., Kumar, A., LaMoure, D., Rabadi, M., Hermandez, J., & Omoli, G. (2017). Current trends of HIV/AIDS in Asia. *South East Asia Journal of Public Health, 7*(2), 3–11. doi:10.3329eajph.v7i2.38850 PMID:28857056

Sarmento, D. R. (2014). Traditional Birth Attendance (TBA) in a health system: what are the roles, benefits and challenges: A case study of incorporated TBA in Timor Leste. *Asia Pacific Family Medicine, 13*(1), 12. doi:10.118612930-014-0012-1 PMID:25469105

Schramm, W. (Ed.). (1954). How communication works. In the Process and Effects of Mass Communication (Ch. I). Urbana: University of IIlinois Press.

Severin, W. J., & Tankard, J. W. Jr. (1992). *Communication Theories: Origins, Methods and Uses in the Mass Media*. London, UK: Longman.

Sewell, W. H. Jr. (2005). The Concept(s) of Culture. In G. M. Spiegel (Ed.), *Practicing History: New Directions in Historical Writing after the Linguistic Turn*. UK: Routledge Publishing.

Shaikh, T. B., Khan, S., Maab, A., & Amjad, S. (2014) Emerging role of traditional birth attendants in mountainous terrain: a qualitative exploratory study from Chitral District, *Pakistan. BMJ Journals, 4*(11).

Shangase, M., Pengpid, S., Peltzer, K., Henda, N., Mosala, T., Dlamini, N., & .... (n.d.). Traditional Birth Attendants and HIV/AIDS in South Africa: A Trainer's Manual. *Department of Health: Republic of South Africa.*

Sharma, S., & Gupta, Y. (2017). Mass Media for Health Education: (A Study in the state of Rajasthan). Retrieved from www.researchgate.net

Shizha, E. (2005). Reclaiming our memories: The education dilemma in postcolonial African school curricula. In A. Abdi, & A. Cleghorn (Eds.), *Issues in African education: Sociological perspectives* (pp. 65–83). New York: Palgrave Macmillan. doi:10.1057/9781403977199_4

Shizha, E. (2007). Critical analysis of problems encountered in incorporating indigenous knowledge in science teaching by primary school teachers in Zimbabwe. *The Alberta Journal of Educational Research, 53*(3), 302–319.

Sibeko, L., Dhansay, M. A., Charlton, K. E., Johns, T., & Gray-Donald, K. (2005). Beliefs, attitudes, and practices of breastfeeding mothers from a periurban community in South Africa. [PubMed]. *Journal of Human Lactation, 21*(1), 31–38. doi:10.1177/0890334404272388 PMID:15681633

Siddiqui, M. S. (2019). *Use of indigenous language for conflict resolution*. Retrieved from https://www.researchgate.net/publication/331310662_Use_of_indigenous_language_for_conflict_resolution

Siddiqui, S., Schunk, K., Batista, M., Adames, F., Ayala, P., Stix, B., ... Green, N. S. (2012). Awareness of sickle cell among of reproductive age: Dominicans and African Americans in northern Manhattan. *Journal of Urban Health, 89*(1), 53–58. doi:10.100711524-011-9618-x PMID:22009200

Singleton, K., & Krause, E. (2009). Understanding cultural and linguistic barriers to health literacy. *Online Journal of Issues in Nursing, 14*(3). Retrieved from http://ojin.nursingworld.org/MainMenuCategories/ANAMarketplace/ANAPeriodicals/OJIN/TableofContents/Vol142009/No3Sept09/Cultural-and-Linguistic-Barriers-.html

Skutnabb-Kangas, T. (2000). *Linguistic Genocide in Education or Worldwide Diversity and Human Rights?* London, UK: Erlbaum.

Sleptsova, M., Weber, H., Schöpf, A. C., Nübling, M., Morina, N., Hofer, G., & Langewitz, W. (2017). Using interpreters in medical consultations: what is said and what is translated – a descriptive analysis using RIAS. *Patient Education Council, 100*(9): 1667-1671. doi:. doi:10.1016/j.pec

Smith, J., & Abel, S. (2008). Ka Whawhai Tonu Matou: Indigenous television in Aotearoa/New Zealand. *New Zealand Journal of Media Studies, 11*(1), 1–14. doi:10.11157/medianz-vol11iss1id58

Smith, M. T. (2015). *Factors That Contribute To the Knowledge, Health Beliefs, Attitudes, and Behaviors Regarding Sickle Cell Disorder among College Students.* Heritage Press.

Sobowale. (1992). Television for whom and at what price in Odukomaya (Ed.), Television and film Media Issues. Lagos: Unique publication (1986). Origin and Development of Health Cooperation. Retrieved from http://www.who.int/global.health./en/

Sokey, P. P., Adjei, E., & Ankrah, E. (2018). Media use for health information dissemination to rural communities by the Ghana Health Service, 1. *Journal of Information Science Systems and Technology, 2*(1), 13–22.

Sonderling, S. (2009). Media, language and discourse. In P. J. Fourie (Ed.), *Media Studies: Media Content and Media Audiences* (pp. 83–115). Cape Town, South Africa: Juta & Co. Ltd.

Stefano, L. A., Hendriks, S. L., Stilwell, C., & Morris, C. (2005). *Printed information needs of small-scale organic farmers in Kwazulu-Natal.* Available at www.librijournal.org/pdf/005 1pp56-66.pdf

Svalastog, A. L., Donev, D., & Gajovic, S. (2017). Concept and Definition of Health and Health Related Values in the Knowledge Landscape of the Digital Society. *Croatian Medical Journal, 58*(6), 432–435. doi:10.3325/cmj.2017.58.431 PMID:29308835

Swallow, D. (2010). Meaning of Colours Across Cultures. Online Material. Retrieved from June 17, 2017: http://www.deborahswallow.com/2010/02/20/meaning-of-colours-across-cultures/

Taff, A., Chee, M., Hall, J., Hall, M., Martin, K., & Johnston, A. (2018) Indigenous language use impacts wellness, In K. Rehg, & L. Campbell (Eds.), The Oxford Handbook on Endangered Languages. Doi:10.1093/oxfordhb/9780190610029.013.41

Talabi, F., Ogundeji, B., & Adedowole, F. (2016). Influence of online editions on newspaper readership in south-western Nigeria. *Journal of Communication and Media Research, 8*(2), 141–162.

The Fourth Estate . (2000). No. 9., Nov./Dec. Lagos: IJC/JODER.

The University of Auckland. (2018). *About thematic analysis.* Retrieved from: https://www.psych.auckland.ac.nz/en/about/our-research/research-groups/thematic-analysis/about-thematic-analysis.html 11/6/2018.

Thomas, R. K. (2006) Introduction to Health Communication. Retrieved from eknygos.lsmuni.lt/springer/189/1- 7.pdf

Tindi, S., & Ayiku, C. (2018). Local reception of global media texts: Telenovelas as sites of cultural mixture in Ghana. *Legon Journal of the Humanities, 29*(1), 259–283. doi:10.4314/ljh.v29i1.10

Tomlinson, J. (2012). 'Watching Dallas': The imperialist text and audience research. In F. J. Lechner, & J. Boli (Eds.), *The globalisation handbook* (pp. 365–375). Sussex, UK: Wiley Blackwell.

Troskie, T. R. (1997). The importance of traditional midwives in the delivery of health care in the Republic of South Africa. [PubMed]. *Curationis, 20*, 15–20. PMID:9287548

Turner, T. (2002). Indigenous media and political imaginaries in contemporary Bolivia. Retrieved May 21, 2019 from https://bools.google.com.ng/books

Tylor, E. B. (1871). *Primitive Culture*. London, UK: John Murray.

Uche, L. U. (1989). *Mass Media, People, and Politics in Nigeria*. New Delhi, India: Concept Publishing.

Ugboaja, F. (2000). Communication for Social Change Anthology: Historical and Contemporary Readings.

Ugboaja, J. O., Oguejiofor, C. B., Oranu, E. O., & Igwegbe, A. O. (2018) Factors associated with the use of traditional birth attendants in Nigeria: A secondary analysis of 2013 Nigeria national demography and health survey. *The Nigerian Journal of General Practice, 16*(2), 45.

Ugboaja, F. (1985). *Communication: An Overview* (p. 1). International Keynotes.

Ugboajah, F. O. (1985). Oramedia in Africa. In F. O. Ugboajah (Ed.), *Mass Communication, Culture, and Society in West Africa* (pp. 165–176). New York: K. G. Saur.

UNAIDS. (1997). Report on the global HIV/AIDS epidemic. Geneva. Switzerland: UNAIDS/WHO Working Group on Global HIV/AIDS. Retrieved May 16, 2019 https://www.data.unaids.org>report>2000gren.

UNAIDS. (2017). HIV and AIDS in Nigeria. Retrieved March 8, 2019 from https://www.avert.org/professionals/hiv-around-world/sub-saharan-africa/nigeria

UNESCO. (1974). *Television traffic _ a one-way street? Reports and Papers on Mass Communication, No. 70*. Paris, France: UNESCO.

UNESCO. (2005). Convention on the Protection and Promotion of the Diversity of Cultural Expressions Quadrennial Periodic Report on Measures to Protect And Promote the Diversity of Cultural Expressions.

United States Agency International Development. (2014). Orphans and Vulnerable Children Affected by HIV and AIDS. Retrieved April 9, 2019 from https://www.usaid.gov>technical-areas.

United States Central Intelligence Agency (CIA). (2016). *World Fact Book[Online]*. Retrieved from https://www.cia.gov/library/publications/the-world-factbook/. Accessed September, 25 2019.

University of Twente. (2017). *Health Belief Model: Explaining Health Behaviors.* Available at www.utwente.nl. Accessed on September 25, 2019

Uno, S. O. (1987). Information Dissemination: How effective through local (Nigerian) languages. In S. O. Uno (Ed.), *Tropical Issues in Communication Arts. Uyo.* Modern Business Press Ltd.

Unyime, I. E., Idongesit, L. J., & Akpabio, E. A. (2016). High Patronage of Traditional Birth Homes: A Report from Akwa Ibom, Southern Nigeria. *AASCIT Journal of Health.*, *3*(1), 17–22.

Urua, E. E. (2005). Exploiting Information Technology Resources in the Human Development of Nigerian Languages. In O. M. Ndimele (Ed.), *Globalization and the Study of languages in Africa. Port-Harcourt: Grand Orbit Communications.*

Uwom, O., & Oloyede, B. (2014). Newspaper Coverage of Health Issues in Nigeria. A study of the Guardian and The Punch Newspapers January 2010 to December 2011, In International Journal of African and Asian Studies, 4.

Van Beek, S. (2016) *Intersections: Indigenous language, health and wellness: First peoples' cultural council deliverable for FNIS UBC Practicum 2016.* Retrieved from: http://www.fpcc.ca/files/PDF/Language/Intersections_Indigenous_Language_Health_and_Wellness_WebVersion.pdf

Van Biljon, J., & Kotzé, P. (2008). Cultural Factors in a Mobile Phone Adoption and Usage Model. *Journal of Universal Computer Science*, *14*(16), 2650–2679.

Van der Kooi, R. (2006). Theobald S. Traditional medicine in late pregnancy and labour: Perceptions of Kgaba remedies amongst the Tswana in South Africa. *Afr J Trad CAM.*, *3*(1), 11–22.

wa Thiong'o, N. (1986). Decolonizing the mind: The politics of language in African literature. Portsmouth: Heinemann.

Wallace, L. (1996). Media, writers, arts session summary. In G. Cantoni (Ed.), *Stabilizing Indigenous Languages.* Flagstaff: Northern Arizona University.

Wang, T., Wu, G., Chen, J., Cui, P., Chen, Z., Yan, Y., ... Chen, H. (2017). Integration of solar technology to modern greenhouse in China: Current status, challenges and prospect. *Renewable & Sustainable Energy Reviews*, *70*, 1178–1188. doi:10.1016/j.rser.2016.12.020

Waqas, M. A., Khan, I., Akhter, M. J., Noor, M. A., & Ashraf, U. (2017). Exogenous application of plant growth regulators (PGRs) induces chilling tolerance in short-duration hybrid maize. *Environmental Science and Pollution Research International*, *24*(12), 11459–11471. doi:10.100711356-017-8768-0 PMID:28316047

Webster, P. (2018). Language barriers restricting access to health care for Indigenous populations. *Canadian Medical Association Journal*, *190*(24), E754–E755. doi:10.1503/cmaj.109-5613 PMID:29914917

Weller, J., Boyd, M., & Cumin, D. (2014). Teams, tribes and patient safety: Overcoming barriers to effective teamwork in healthcare. *Postgraduate Medical Journal*, *90*(1061), 149–154. doi:10.1136/postgradmedj-2012-131168 PMID:24398594

Westley, B. H., & MacLean, M. (1957). A conceptual model for communication research. *Journalism Quarterly, 34,* 31-38.

Whalen, D., Moss, M., & Baldwin, D. (2016). Healing through language: Positive physical health effects of indigenous language use. *F1000 Research, 5,* 852. doi:10.12688/f1000research.8656.1

WHO. (2000). *Strategies for promoting safe motherhood in Nigeria by the year 2010.* Abuja: The Author World Health Organization (WHO). (2010). Trends in Maternal Mortality: 1990 to 2008[Online]. https://www.who.int/reproductivehealth/publications/monitoring/9789241500265/en/. Accessed September 25 2019

Willock, J., Deary, I. J., Edwards-Jones, G., Gibson, G. J., McGregor, M. J., Sutherland, A., ... Grieve, R. (1999). The role of attitude and objectives in farmer decision making: Business and environmentally-oriented behaviour in Scotland. *Journal of Agricultural Economics, 50*(2), 286–303. doi:10.1111/j.1477-9552.1999.tb00814.x

Wilson, P., & Stewart, M. (2008). "Introduction: Indigeneity and Indigenous Media on the Global Stage." In P. Wilson, & M. Stewart (Eds.), *Global Indigenous Media: Cultures, Poetics, and Politics.* Durham, NC: Duke University Press, 2008. Doi:10.1215/9780822388692-001

Wilson, P., Hearne, J., Córdova, A., & Thorner, S. (2017). Indigenous Media "Native Americans" Oxford Bibliographies article Doi:10.1093/OBO/9780199791286-0229

Wilson, P., & Stewart, M. (2008). *Global indigenous media. cultures, poetics and politics.* Durham, NC: Duke University Press. doi:10.1215/9780822388692

Wimmer, R. D., & Dominick, J. R. (2013). *Mass media research.* London, UK: Cengage Learning.

Wójcik, M., Jeziorska-Biel, P., & Czapiewski, K. (2019). Between words: A generational discussion about farming knowledge sources. *Journal of Rural Studies, 67,* 130–141. doi:10.1016/j.jrurstud.2019.02.024

World Health Organisation. (2009). *Track2: Health literacy and health behavior.* Retrieved from: https://www.who.int/healthpromotion/conferences/7gchp/track2/en/

World Health Organisation. (2016) *WHO Recommendations on Antenatal Care for a Positive Pregnancy Experience.* Retrieved from: https://www.ncbi.nlm.nih.gov/books/NBK409110/

World Health Organization & UNICEF. (2015). Trends in maternal mortality: 1990 to 2013: estimates by WHO, UNICEF, UNFPA, The World Bank and the United Nations Population Division. Retrieved from http://apps.who.int/iris/bitstream/.

World Health Organization Fact Sheet. (2014). *Global update on the health sector response to HIV.* Geneva.

World Health Organization. (1946). Preamble to the constitution of the WHO as adopted by the International Health Conference, New York.

World Health Organization. (1994). AIDS: Images of the epidermic, Geneva, Switzerland. Retrieved April 2, 2019 from https://apps.who.int>iris>handle

World Health Organization . (2008). "Traditional Medicine: Definitions".

World Health Organization. Fact sheets. (2012).

World Health Organization. Fact sheets. (2019).

World Health Organization. International Confederation of Midwives, & International Federation of Gynecology and Obstetrics. (2004). Making pregnancy safer: The critical role of the skilled attendant. *Bulletin of the World Health Organization.* Geneva. Retrieved from http://apps.who.int/iris/bitstream/10665/42955/1/9241591692.pdf

World Population Prospects. (2019). World Population Review. Retrieved from www.un.org.publications

World Population Review. (2019). Nigeria Population World Populationreview.com. Retrieved May 18, 2019.

Yanitsky, O. (2017). Current globalization: A challenge for the humanities. *Advances in Social Sciences Research Journal*, *4*(12), 131–140. doi:10.14738/assrj.412.3370

Ybarra, M. L., Strasburger, V. C., & Mitchell, K. J. (2014). Sexual media exposure, sexual behaviour, and sexual violence victimization in adolescence. *Clinical Paediatrics*, 1-9.

About the Contributors

Evaristus Adesina is a Researcher and a Lecturer of Mass Communication in Covenant University with high enthusiasm for identifying social problems and proffering solutions through positional and empirical research. Evaristus obtained his Bachelor of Science and Masters Degree from Bowen University and University of Lagos respectively. He recently defended his Ph.D thesis from the prestigious Covenant University, Ota, Nigeria His areas of research include among others; Health communication, Public relations, Development Communication, Mass Media and Society.

Babatunde Adeyeye is a Faculty in the Department of Mass Communication, Covenant University, Ota, Ogun State with special interest in Communication for Development, Social Media trends, Agricultural Communication and Crises Management/Communication

Tayo-Adigboluja Afolayan is a post-graduate student in the Department of Mass Communication, Covenant University, Ota, Ogun State. Her research interests are in journalism, development communication and political communication.

Lanre Olaolu Amodu (Ph.D) is a communication lecturer whose area of interest is public relations. He is currently a Senior Lecturer at Covenant University, Ota, Ogun State, in the Department of Mass Communication. He is also the immediate past Registrar of the University.

Semiu Bello is a seasoned international teacher, researcher and trainer in the field of Media and Communication. Bello bagged his PhD in Media and Communication in the Department of Media and Communication University of Canterbury, New Zealand. His areas of research interest cover health and development communication, communication theories, mass media research, media and society, media literacy, new media and media literacy. Bello has published creditably well in the field of mass communication in several international and national leaned journals. He has also presented various papers at national and international conferences across the world. He is currently with the Department of Mass Communication, Kwara State University Malete, Nigeria. Bello has acquired intensive pedagogical teaching experience in five universities both in Nigeria and abroad.

Charity Ben-Enukora is a Ph.D. student in the department of mass communication, Covenant University, Ota. Her research interests include health and development communication, media studies and gender issues. she has reviewed a good number of research articles and also has published articles to her credit.

Ayobami Busari is a Civil and Environmental Engineering faculty and researcher with PhD in Civil Engineering (Transportation Engineering Option). She has research interest in the two broad areas of transportation engineering, which are the traditional transportation engineering (transportation planning, operations, design, and safety) and pavement design and pavement materials incorporating Highway Construction and Pavement Research. She has contributed to several areas of Sustainable Pavement Engineering and Transportation planning and travel demand modelling among others with several publications. Ayobami Busari has served on numerous technical committees of various professional organizations. She is the current chairman of Association of Professional Women Engineers in Nigeria (APWEN), Ota Chapter.

Thelma Ekanem is a Doctoral candidate and an Assistant Lecturer in the Department of Mass Communication, Covenant University, Ota, Nigeria. Thelma has published research articles in numerous international and local journals of high impact. She organised many conferences on industry and university partnerships and supervised many undergraduate projects. She is a specialist in public relations and mass communication administration. She has a B.Sc. in Public Relations and Advertising and M.Sc. in Mass Communication from Covenant University.

Funmi Falobi is a Development Journalist, Gender activist, PR consultant, journalism lecturer and Media Trainer. She holds both a Bachelor and Masters Degree in Mass Communication from the University of Lagos. She has 13 years media/newsroom experience, transcending being a reporter, correspondent and editor, with work experience as State House correspondent for Daily Independent newspapers and later as Editor, Foreign Desk of the paper. She presently writes as well as serves as Editor, Social Development news (SDN) @ www.sdnonline.net including being an adjunct lecturer at the Department of Mass Communication, Yaba College of Technology, Lagos. She is also a counselor and development advocate who have over the past five years continuously advocated on issues of social development initiatives, especially to advance the cause of women and youths, as well as mentoring young media professionals. She is an Associate member, Nigeria Institute of Public Relations (NIPR), member, Nigeria Union of Journalists (NUJ) and Nigeria Association of Women Journalists (NAWOJ. Her advocacies include using the media to promote development agenda, through journalistic endeavours through print, broadcast and online platforms, as well as through speaking engagements in training programs and conferences.

Aloysius C. Ifeanyichukwu lectures in Department of Mass Communication Legacy University Okija. He is a promising communication scholar currently studying for his Doctoral Degree in Communication Art Department at University of Uyo Akwa Ibom State Nigeria. His interest areas are public relations, traditional communication systems and new media.

Chinyere Mbaka is a Media studies and Development Communication scholar presently with the Mass Communication Department of Mountain Top University, Prayer City, Nigeria. Her research interests are in health communication, children, gender and cultural studies. She is published in local and international journals and has attended and presented papers in quite a number of academic conferences both within and outside Nigeria.

Phillip Mpofu is a Postdoctoral Research Fellow in the Indigenous Language Media in Africa research entity at North West University, South Africa. He is also a senior lecturer at Midlands State University, Zimbabwe. His research combines sociolinguistics, language policy and plan- ning, language and identity politics and indigenous language media

Nahimah Ajikanle Nurudeen is a doctoral student in the School of Communication, Lagos State University, Ojo Lagos Nigeria. She is presently the Founder/Lead Strategist, TenticP Communications Nigeria Limited and the Editor of Authentic Platform News Nigeria, an online news platform based at Ikeja, Lagos. She is very prolific and has written several news articles in the media as well as contributed articles in some academic books and journals.

Odion Odiboh obtained B. A. (Philosophy); PGD, MSc (Mass Communication), and PhD (Philosophy) from the University of Lagos. He has 28 years of combined industry and teaching experience - consulting for multinational companies locally and globally. An author of 55 industry and academic publications and specialist in Integrated Marketing Communication, Philosophy of Mass Communication, Advertising and Public Relations, he has supervised 12 academic projects at both undergraduate and postgraduate levels. He has attended several academic and professional conferences locally and overseas. He pioneered annual undergraduates advertising pitch contest and organized the first ever induction of 200 undergraduates of Covenant University into Advertising and Public Relations practice in Nigeria. He is a serial winner of awards locally and internationally; and a Fellow, Officer and member of 10 professional groups in Nigeria and overseas.

Olayinka Susan Ogundoyin is a Lecturer in the Department of Mass Communication, Bowen University, Iwo, Nigeria. She is a graduate of Obafemi Awolowo University, Ile-Ife and University of Ibadan. She has teaching experience at the University level. Her area of research interests include Development Communication and Health Communication, Gender and Media Studies. She has contributed to scholarship by publishing papers in reputable journals.

Oludare Ebenezer Ogunyombo holds a PhD in Mass Communication. Ogunyombo worked as a development communication consultant with local and international organisations including the United Nations Children Emergency Fund (UNICEF) and the National Youth Service Corps (NYSC). He is a Member of the Nigerian Institute of Public Relations (NIPR); the Association of Communication Scholars and Professionals of Nigeria (ACSPN), the Advertising Practitioners Council of Nigeria (APCON) and the African Council for Communication Education (ACCE). Ogunyombo has presented scholarly papers in communication studies at several conferences. He has published over fifteen papers in journals and edited books. His areas of interest are in journalism, public relations, media influence studies and development communication.

Nelson Okorie is an active scholar and researcher, with research interests in Development Communication and Media Performance.

Oredola Opeyemi Olaoluwa is a post-graduate student in the Department of Mass Communication, Covenant University, Ota, Ogun State. His research interests are in war and crime journalism, development communication and health communication.

Rotimi Williams Olatunji is a communication specialist and currently the Dean, School of Communication, Lagos State University, Ojo, Lagos State.

Oladokun Omojola is Associate Professor at Covenant University, Ota, Nigeria. Before his career in academics, he worked as a writer for Daily Times and senior editor with The Guardian newspapers both in Lagos, Nigeria. Dr. Omojola invented the House Sign® - an advertising design system and originated the use of computer graphics for analyzing focus group transcripts. His areas of interest include ICTs, media performance and ethics, advertising, and communication research.

Toluwanimi Onakoya is a postgraduate student of Mass Communication in Covenant University. She is research driven, goal oriented and a focused individual. She is very passionate about projects relating to the media and its influence on the community around us.

Kevin Onyenankeya is a postdoctoral research fellow at the University of Fort Hare, Alice, South Africa. He has over 20 years of industry experience spanning journalism, corporate communication and university teaching. His research interests include Development Communication, Health Communication and indigenous media. He has a growing research interest in media, journalism particularly, and cultural studies (representations and cultural transmission).

Toyosi Olubenga Owolabi has practised journalism for a decade and half and was at different times a Group Political Editor and Member of Editorial Board of Concord Group of Newspapers and Editor of Credit Market Magazine in Nigeria before he veered into lecturing. He had taught Mass Communication at Igbinedion and Benson Idahosa Universities in Edo State, Nigeria before moving to Lagos State University where he currently teaches journalism and development communication. He has co-authored two books, contributed chapters in books and published articles in many academic journals locally and internationally. Owolabi has a PhD in Journalism and Development from the University of Strathclyde, Glasgow, United Kingdom, M.A (Linguistics) and M.A (Communication and Language Arts) from the University of Ibadan, PGD (Journalism) from the Nigeria Institute of Journalism Lagos, and a B.A (Hons) Language and Linguistics of the University of Ilorin Nigeria. His research interests are in media and development communication.

Olusola Oyero obtained his B.A. and M.A. degrees from the University of Ibadan and Ph.D. from Covenant University, Ota, Ogun State, Nigeria. He was also a Post-doctoral Fellow at North-West University, South Africa. With well over a decade experience in academics, he is currently an Associate Professor and Head of Department, Mass Communication, Covenant University.

Ada Peter is an Assistant Professor, Media, and International Security, Covenant University, Ota, Nigeria. She produces comprehensive, policy-focused, nontechnical cybersecurity documents that emphasize and teach senior principal state officials how to best make informed decisions on cyber policy, strategy, and planning. She also explores the processes of terrorism and uses algorithms to analyze online big data, which she thinks may help predict acts of terror and armed conflicts. The most recent honor of her research is from the U.S Department of State, recognizing Dr. Peter as SUSI Scholar on U.S National Security and Policymaking.

Victor Tunji Taiwo did teach Media, Communication, Film and Nigeria People and Culture courses in the departments of Mass Communication and General Studies, Southwestern University, Okun-Owa, Ijebu, Ogun State and currently in the Dept. of Theatre Arts, AOCOED, Ijanikin, Lagos, (Part-Time Lecturer) where he teaches Communication, Media and Film courses. He obtained his degrees in Yoruba Language and Communication Arts and Communication Studies. He is currently a PhD research student (Awaiting Final Defence) in Media and Communication Studies at Lagos State University. His areas of interest include Indigenous Communication, Non-Verbal Communication, Theatre and Film studies, Political/Development Communication, Theories, Media Management and Indigenous PR/Advertising.

Index

S

T

U

W

Y

www.ingramcontent.com/pod-product-compliance
Lightning Source LLC
LaVergne TN
LVHW061549290926
849162LV00004B/951